Differential Diagnosis in Otolaryngology–Head and Neck Surgery

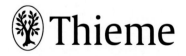

Differential Diagnosis in Otolaryngology–Head and Neck Surgery

Michael G. Stewart, MD, MPH
Professor and Chairman
Department of Otorhinolaryngology
Senior Associate Dean for Clinical Affairs
Weill Cornell Medical College
New York, New York

Samuel H. Selesnick, MD, FACS
Professor and Vice Chairman
Department of Otorhinolaryngology
Weill Cornell Medical College
New York, New York

Max M. April, MD, FAAP, FACS
Professor of Clinical Otorhinolaryngology
Professor of Clinical Otorhinolaryngology
  in Pediatrics
Department of Otorhinolaryngology
Weill Cornell Medical College
New York, New York

Patrick J. Byrne, MD, FACS
Director
Division of Facial Plastic and Reconstructive
  Surgery
Associate Professor
Department of Otolaryngology–Head and Neck
  Surgery
Johns Hopkins University School of Medicine
Co-medical Director
Greater Baltimore Cleft Lip and Palate Team
Baltimore, Maryland

Lawrence R. Lustig, MD
Professor
Department of Otolaryngology–Head and Neck
  Surgery
University of California–San Francisco
San Francisco, California

Bradley F. Marple, MD
Professor and Vice Chairman
Department of Otolaryngology–Head and Neck
  Surgery
University of Texas Southwestern Medical Center
Dallas, Texas

Jason G. Newman, MD, FACS
Assistant Professor
Department of Otorhinolaryngology–Head and
  Neck Surgery
Center for Cranial Base Surgery
University of Pennsylvania School of Medicine
Philadelphia, Pennsylvania

Thomas A. Tami, MD
Director
Cincinnati Sinus Institute
Medical Director
Cincinnati Group Health Associates
Cincinnati, Ohio

Robert F. Ward, MD, FACS
Professor of Otorhinolaryngology
Professor of Otorhinolaryngology in Pediatrics
Department of Otorhinolaryngology
Weill Cornell Medical College
New York, New York

Thieme
New York • Stuttgart

Thieme Medical Publishers, Inc.
333 Seventh Ave.
New York, NY 10001

Executive Editor: Timothy Y. Hiscock
Managing Editor: J. Owen Zurhellen IV
Editorial Director: Michael Wachinger
Production Editor: Kenneth L. Chumbley, Publication Services
International Production Director: Andreas Schabert
Vice President, International Marketing and Sales: Cornelia Schulze
Chief Financial Officer: James W. Mitos
President: Brian D. Scanlan
Compositor: Macmillan Publishing Solutions
Printer: Leo Paper Group

Library of Congress Cataloging-in-Publication Data

Differential diagnosis in otolaryngology–head and neck surgery / [edited by] Michael G. Stewart ... [et al.].
  p. ; cm.
  Includes bibliographical references.
  Summary: "Designed as a practical resource for rapid and accurate diagnosis in otolaryngology—head and neck surgery and facial plastic surgery, this comprehensive manual uses an innovative format that simulates what physicians experience in daily practice. Each symptom-based chapter opens with the patients presentation followed by an easily accessible list of potential diagnoses and supplementary data on the features of the different diseases to help the user correctly identify the problem. Features: - Chapters labeled by signs and symptoms — not by disease — enable quick clinical reference - In-depth coverage of the diagnostic evaluation, including PET/CT of the head and neck, allergy and immunologic evaluation, key information on how to assess a variety of complaints, and much more - Numerous cross-references throughout the text clearly link different symptoms and diseases to provide a solid understanding of each diagnosis - 82 high-quality illustrations and clinical photographs, including 52 in full-color, demonstrate lesions and diseases - Well-organized tables of rare diseases and syndromes aid rapid review Differential Diagnosis in Otolaryngology is a must-have reference and refresher for clinicians in otolaryngology who need to update their knowledge of their own and other subspecialties in the field of otolaryngology-head and neck surgery. It is also a valuable tool for otolaryngology residents and fellows as they prepare for daily practice or study for exams"—Provided by publisher.
  ISBN 978-1-60406-051-5 (alk. paper)
  1. Otolaryngology—Diagnosis. 2. Diagnosis, Differential. I. Stewart, Michael G., 1962-
  [DNLM: 1. Otorhinolaryngologic Diseases—diagnosis. 2. Diagnosis, Differential. WV 150 D5686 2011]
  RF48.D535 2011
  617.5'10754—dc22   2010022115

Important note: Medical knowledge is ever-changing. As new research and clinical experience broaden our knowledge, changes in treatment and drug therapy may be required. The authors and editors of the material herein have consulted sources believed to be reliable in their efforts to provide information that is complete and in accord with the standards accepted at the time of publication. However, in view of the possibility of human error by the authors, editors, or publisher of the work herein or changes in medical knowledge, neither the authors, editors, nor publisher, nor any other party who has been involved in the preparation of this work, warrants that the information contained herein is in every respect accurate or complete, and they are not responsible for any errors or omissions or for the results obtained from use of such information. Readers are encouraged to confirm the information contained herein with other sources. For example, readers are advised to check the product information sheet included in the package of each drug they plan to administer to be certain that the information contained in this publication is accurate and that changes have not been made in the recommended dose or in the contraindications for administration. This recommendation is of particular importance in connection with new or infrequently used drugs.

Some of the product names, patents, and registered designs referred to in this book are in fact registered trademarks or proprietary names even though specific reference to this fact is not always made in the text. Therefore, the appearance of a name without designation as proprietary is not to be construed as a representation by the publisher that it is in the public domain.

Printed in China

5 4 3 2 1

ISBN 978-1-60406-051-5

This book is dedicated to my teachers, who instilled curiosity in me, and to my trainees, who continue to challenge and inspire me.

Michael G. Stewart

I dedicate this book to my wife, Alex, and to my three sons, Joshua, Benjamin, and Jordan. My family is the source of greatest joy in my life.

Samuel H. Selesnick

Contents

V Differential Diagnosis in Pediatric Rhinology and Sinus Disease ... 171
Section Editors: Max M. April and Robert F. Ward

VI Differential Diagnosis in the Oral Cavity (Adult and Pediatric) 179
Section Editor: Jason G. Newman

VII Differential Diagnosis in the Larynx, Pharynx, Trachea, and Esophagus (Adult and Pediatric) 217
Section Editor: Jason G. Newman

Foreword

Prior to the twentieth century, the great weight of medical thought concerned the process of distinguishing one disease from another in order to establish a prognosis. In our era of advanced technology, the emphasis in medicine, especially a surgical subspecialty such as otolaryngology, focuses excessively upon determining what intervention offers a patient the best chance of cure and too little upon the art and science of diagnosis. According to the American poet Edward Hodnett (1841–1920): "If you do not ask the right questions, you do not get the right answers. A question asked in the right way often points to its own answer. Asking questions is the A-B-C of diagnosis. Only the inquiring mind solves problems."

This text, edited by Professors Stewart and Selesnick, seeks to guide the otolaryngologist to pose the right questions by refocusing attention upon the fundamentals of diagnosis (history, physical examination, laboratory data, and imaging), in order to reach thoughtful and accurate answers by which to guide application of modern therapies.

It is a widely quoted myth in medicine that differential diagnosis is primarily the domain of *cognitive* specialties such as internal medicine and neurology. Some would have you believe that surgeons "think only from the elbow down" and tend to derive pleasure from acting quickly and decisively rather than cogitating over complex medical differentials. To the contrary, the spectrum of diseases encountered by the otolaryngologist is as intricate and variable as those in any medical field—except that they occur in a highly compact region of byzantine anatomical complexity.

In most specialties, the clinician needs to master a single organ system. In otolaryngology, as a regional specialty of the head and neck, the clinician needs to be concerned with disorders of four special senses (hearing, balance, smell, taste), as well as functionalities as diverse as voice, swallowing, breathing, facial expression, etc. This wide spectrum of disease presentations—from minor malady to critical illness, from young to old, involving men or women, etc.—makes the study of differential diagnosis especially relevant to the otolaryngologist.

This new text is a tour de force of 82 chapters that comprehensively cover the entire field of otolaryngology from alopecia to vertigo. The organization of the chapter by symptom, rather than by disease process, facilitates practical application of the knowledge to aid diagnosis in both the clinic and at the bedside. This volume should be of value not only for students and residents seeking to learn otolaryngology for the first time, but also to seasoned practitioners seeking to enhance their diagnostic acumen. The eminent diagnostician Sir William Osler once said: "The value of experience is not in seeing much, but in seeing wisely." The quest for sophistication in differential diagnosis leads the wise physician down the path of better serving his or her patients.

Robert K. Jackler, MD
Sewall Professor and Chair
Department of Otolaryngology–Head and Neck Surgery
Associate Dean
Postgraduate Medical Education
Stanford University School of Medicine
Stanford, California

Preface

Although otolaryngologists–head and neck surgeons are drawn to medicine for many reasons, we all share a singular and profound sense of responsibility for our patients. Yet it is indeed a challenge to keep abreast of advances in diagnosis and therapeutics and to meet the expectations to which we hold ourselves and to which we are held by the public. The breadth and depth of otolaryngology-head and neck surgery continue to expand. As otolaryngologists, we now require a knowledge base that includes not just the established core of our field, but also sleep medicine, esophageal disorders, allergies, and skull base surgery, to name a few areas unfamiliar to our predecessors. The knowledge base in all areas of our field is increasingly voluminous as new studies add to the literature. Furthermore, time can separate patients with rare disorders; accordingly, our memories may fade regarding what differential diagnoses to consider.

It seems, at times, that therapeutic advances overshadow the fundamentals of diagnostic skills in otolaryngology and other medical specialties. Evolving technologies are exciting and innovative but are useless to a patient with no diagnosis. In the office, at the bedside, and in the emergency department, patients present to us with symptoms and signs, which are the clues that trigger our thoughts and ultimately our recommendations.

This book is intended to offer the clinician a practical resource for the formulation of a differential diagnosis. Although other texts on this topic exist, one distinguishing feature of *Differential Diagnosis in Otolaryngology–Head and Neck Surgery* is its innovative design. The text is organized around symptoms, the most fundamental information that our patients give us. Within the text the reader will find a hierarchical organization of potential diagnoses that are symptom based. In addition, the reader will find clear links to other areas of the text that should be considered for a given complaint.

We are proud to have the contributions of some of the brightest minds in our field in *Differential Diagnosis in Otolaryngology–Head and Neck Surgery*. It has been our pleasure to work with these contributors.

The editors and contributors hope that this book will be a useful addition to the tools each of us has available in the evaluation of patients with otolaryngologic complaints, and that ultimately, the use of this resource will translate into the best possible outcome for each patient who entrusts us with his or her care.

Michael G. Stewart, MD, MPH
Samuel H. Selesnick, MD, FACS

Acknowledgments

The editors would like to recognize the diligent work of the contributors to this project. Their research and writing have added much to the literature. The staff of Thieme Publishers has been responsive and professional throughout the process of crafting this book, and we truly appreciate their efforts. Special thanks go to Julie Fernandes here at the Weill Cornell Department of Otorhinolaryngology. Her organizational skills and enthusiasm for the project were remarkable. Finally, we recognize the efforts of the faculty of the Weill Cornell Department of Otorhinolaryngology. This team effort is one that we all value.

Contributors

Ronda E. Alexander, MD
Assistant Professor
Department of Otorhinolaryngology–Head and
  Neck Surgery
University of Texas Medical School at Houston
Houston, Texas

Jill M. Anderson, AuD, CCC-A
PhD Candidate
Department of Communication Sciences and
  Disorders
University of Cincinnati
Cincinnati, Ohio

Max M. April, MD, FAAP, FACS
Professor of Clinical Otorhinolaryngology
Professor of Clinical Otorhinolaryngology in
  Pediatrics
Department of Otorhinolaryngology
Weill Cornell Medical College
New York, New York

Devraj Basu, MD, PhD
Assistant Professor
Department of Otorhinolaryngology–Head and
  Neck Surgery
University of Pennsylvania School of Medicine
Philadelphia, Pennsylvania

Ray Gervacio F. Blanco, MD, FACS
Departments of Otolaryngology and General
  Surgery
Johns Hopkins University Hospital
Greater Baltimore Medical Center
Baltimore Maryland

Andrew Blitzer, MD, DDS
Professor of Clinical Otolaryngology
Columbia University College of Physicians and
  Surgeons
Director
New York Center for Voice and Swallowing
  Disorders
New York, New York

Joel H. Blumin, MD, FACS
Associate Professor and Chief
Department of Otolaryngology and
  Communication Sciences
Medical College of Wisconsin
Milwaukee, Wisconsin

Brian B. Burkey, MD
Section Head
Department of Head and Neck Surgery and
  Oncology
Head and Neck Institute
Cleveland Clinic
Cleveland, Ohio
Adjunct Professor
Department of Otolaryngology
Vanderbilt University
Nashville, Tennessee

J. Kenneth Byrd, MD
Resident
Department of Otolaryngology–Head and Neck
  Surgery
Medical University of South Carolina
Charleston, South Carolina

Patrick J. Byrne, MD, FACS
Director
Division of Facial Plastic and Reconstructive
  Surgery
Associate Professor
Department of Otolaryngology–Head and Neck
  Surgery and Dermatology
Johns Hopkins University School of Medicine
Co-medical Director
Greater Baltimore Cleft Lip and Palate Team
Baltimore, Maryland

Ara A. Chalian, MD
Associate Professor
Department of Otorhinolaryngology
Director, Facial Plastic Reconstruction
Patient Safety Officer
Director, Microvascular Lab
Hospital of the University of Pennsylvania
Philadelphia, Pennsylvania

Eugene A. Chu, MD
Department of Head and Neck Surgery
Kaiser Permanente
Facial Plastic and Reconstructive Surgery
Downey, California
Clinical Assistant Professor
Department of Otolaryngology–Head and Neck
Surgery
University of California–Irvine School of
Medicine
Irvine, California

David M. Cognetti, MD
Assistant Professor
Department of Otolaryngology–Head and Neck
Surgery
Thomas Jefferson University
Philadelphia, Pennsylvania

Marc A. Cohen, MD
Resident
Department of Otorhinolaryngology–Head and
Neck Surgery
Hospital of the University of Pennsylvania
Philadelphia, Pennsylvania

Samuel D. Cohen, MD
Eastern Carolina ENT–Head and Neck Surgery
Wilson, North Carolina

Terry A. Day, MD, FACS
Director
Head and Neck Tumor Center
Professor
Department of Otolaryngology–Head and Neck
Surgery
Medical University of South Carolina
Charleston, South Carolina

Paul J. Del Casino, CRNP
Critical Care Department
St. Luke's Hospital and Health Network
Allentown, Pennsylvania

Bryan C. Ego-Osuala, MD
Chief Resident
Department of Otorhinolaryngology
University of Maryland School of Medicine
Baltimore, Maryland

Adele K. Evans, MD
Assistant Professor
Department of Otolaryngology–Head and Neck
Surgery
Wake Forest University School of Medicine
Winston-Salem, North Carolina

Robert L. Ferris, MD, PhD
Professor and Vice-chair for Clinical Operations
Chief
Departments of Otolaryngology, Radiation
Oncology, and Immunology
Co-leader, Cancer Immunology Program
University of Pittsburgh Cancer Institute
Pittsburgh, Pennsylvania

Kristin B. Gendron, MD
Midwest ENT Specialists
St. Paul, Minnesota

David Goldenberg, MD, FACS
Associate Professor of Surgery and Oncology
Director of Head and Neck Surgery
Division of Otolaryngology–Head and Neck
Surgery
The Pennsylvania State University
The Milton S. Hershey Medical Center
Hershey, Pennsylvania

Stephen A. Goldstein, MD
Main Line Gastroenterology
Paoli, Pennsylvania

Suman Golla, MD
Associate Professor
Department of Otolaryngology
University of Pittsburgh Medical Center St.
Margaret's
Pittsburgh, Pennyslvania

Christine G. Gourin, MD, FACS
Associate Professor
Director
Clinical Research Program in Head and Neck
Cancer
Department of Otolaryngology–Head and Neck
Surgery
Johns Hopkins University School of Medicine
Baltimore, Maryland

Nazaneen Grant, MD
Assistant Professor
Department of Otolaryngology–Head and Neck
Surgery
Georgetown University Hospital
Washington, DC

John H. Greinwald Jr., MD, FAAP
Associate Professor
Department of Otolaryngology and Pediatrics
University of Cincinnati College of Medicine
Director
Auditory Genetics Laboratory
Cincinnati Children's Hospital Medical Center
Cincinnati, Ohio

Chia Haddad, MD
Resident Physician
Department of Otolaryngology
Hospital of the University of Pennsylvania
Philadelphia, Pennsylvania

Mary J. Hawkshaw, RN, BSN, CORLN
Research Associate Professor
Department of Otolaryngology
Drexel University College of Medicine
Philadelphia, Pennsylvania

Timothy E. Hullar, MD, FACS
Assistant Professor
Department of Otolaryngology–Head and Neck
   Surgery
Program in Audiology and Communication
   Sciences
Washington University School of Medicine
St. Louis, Missouri

Lisa Ishii, MD, MHS
Assistant Professor
Department of Otolaryngology–Head and Neck
   Surgery
Johns Hopkins University School of Medicine
Baltimore, Maryland

Stephanie A. Joe, MD
Director
The Sinus and Nasal Allergy Center
Co-director
Skull Base Surgery
Associate Professor
Department of Otolaryngology–Head and Neck
   Surgery
University of Illinois–Chicago
Chicago, Illinois

Carl E. Johnson, MD
Assistant Professor of Clinical Radiology
Department of Radiology
New York Presbyterian Hospital
Weill Cornell Medical College
New York, New York

Sasan Karimi, MD
Professor
Department of Radiology
Memorial Sloan-Kettering Cancer Center
Weill Cornell Medical College
New York, New York

James J. Kearney, MD, FACS
Associate Professor of Clinical
   Otorhinolaryngology
Department of Otorhinolaryngology
University of Pennsylvania School of Medicine
Philadelphia, Pennyslvania

Margaret A. Kenna, MD, MPH
Director of Clinical Research
Department of Otolaryngology and
   Communication Enhancement
Children's Hospital
Boston, Massachusetts

Joslyn S. Kirby, MD
Assistant Professor
Department of Dermatology
The Pennsylvania State University
The Milton S. Hershey Medical Center
Hershey, Pennsylvania

Niels Kokot, MD
Assistant Professor
Department of Otolaryngology–Head and Neck
   Surgery
University of Southern California Keck School
   of Medicine
Los Angeles, California

Stephen Y. Lai, MD, PhD, FACS
Assistant Professor
Department of Head and Neck Surgery
Assistant Professor
Department of Molecular and Cellular
   Oncology Center
The University of Texas M. D. Anderson Cancer
   Center
Houston, Texas

Miriam N. Lango, MD
Assistant Professor
Department of Surgery
Fox Chase Cancer Center
Philadelphia, Pennsylvania

Jason M. Leibowitz, MD
Resident
Department of Otorhinolaryngology–Head and
   Neck Surgery
Hospital of the University of Pennsylvania
Philadelphia, Pennsylvania

Nanette Liégeois, MD, PhD
Department of Dermatology
Johns Hopkins University School of Medicine
Baltimore, Maryland

Lindsay Lipinski, MD
Resident
Department of Neurosurgery
University at Buffalo
Buffalo, New York

Lawrence R. Lustig, MD
Professor
Department of Otolaryngology–Head and Neck
Surgery
University of California–San Francisco
San Francisco, California

Bradley F. Marple, MD
Professor and Vice Chairman
Department of Otolaryngology–Head and Neck
Surgery
University of Texas Southwestern Medical
Center
Dallas, Texas

K. Christopher McMains, MD
Clinical Assistant Professor
Department of Otolaryngology–Head and Neck
Surgery
University of Texas Health Science Center at
San Antonio
San Antonio, Texas

Michael V. Medina, MD
Assistant Professor
Department of Head and Neck Surgery
University of Florida
Gainesville, Florida

Noah E. Meltzer, MD
Clinical Fellow
Facial Plastic and Reconstructive Surgery
Department of Otolaryngology–Head and Neck
Surgery
Cleveland Clinic
Cleveland, Ohio

Thuy-Anh Melvin, MD
Resident
Department of Otolaryngology–Head and Neck
Surgery
Johns Hopkins University School of Medicine
Baltimore, Maryland

Christopher J. Miller, MD
Director of Dermatologic Surgery
Assistant Professor of Dermatology
University of Pennsylvania
Perelman Center for Advanced Medicine
Philadelphia, Pennsylvania

Jeffrey L. Miller, MB, BCh
Professor of Medicine and Clinical Director
Division of Endocrinology
Thomas Jefferson University
Philadelphia, Pennsylvania

Matthew C. Miller, MD
Assistant Professor
Department of Otolaryngology
University of Rochester Medical Center
School of Medicine and Dentistry
Rochester, New York

James W. Mims, MD
Assistant Professor
Department of Otolaryngology
Wake Forest University School of Medicine
Winston-Salem, North Carolina

Natasha Mirza, MD, FACS
Professor
Department of Otolaryngology–Head and Neck
Surgery
University of Pittsburgh
Director
Penn Voice and Swallowing Center
Chief
Department of Otolaryngology
Philadelphia Veterans Affairs Medical Center
Philadelphia, Pennsylvania

Nadia Mohyuddin, MD
Assistant Professor
Bobby R. Alford Department of
Otolaryngology–Head and Neck Surgery
Baylor College of Medicine
Houston, Texas

Zayna Nahas, MD
Resident
Department of Otolaryngology
Johns Hopkins University Hospital
Baltimore, Maryland

Melonie A. Nance, MD
Assistant Professor
Department of Otolaryngology
Indiana University School of Medicine
Indianapolis, Indiana

Jason G. Newman, MD, FACS
Assistant Professor
Department of Otorhinolaryngology–Head and
Neck Surgery
Center for Cranial Base Surgery
University of Pennsylvania School of Medicine
Philadelphia, Pennsylvania

Christopher L. Oliver, MD
Head and Neck Surgical Specialists
Englewood, Colorado

Seth M. Pransky, MD
Clinical Professor of Surgery
Division of Otolaryngology
University of California–San Diego
Director
Department of Pediatric Otolaryngology
Rady Children's Specialist Medical Foundation
San Diego, California

Edmund Pribitkin, MD
Professor
Academic Vice Chairman
Department of Otolaryngology–Head and Neck
  Surgery
Thomas Jefferson University
Philadelphia, Pennsylvania

Murugappan Ramanathan Jr., MD
Assistant Professor
Department of Otolaryngology–Head and Neck
  Surgery
Johns Hopkins University School of Medicine
Baltimore, Maryland

Jeremy D. Richmon, MD
Assistant Professor
Department of Otolaryngology–Head and Neck
  Surgery
Johns Hopkins University School of Medicine
Baltimore, Maryland

James W. Rocco, MD, PhD
Assistant Professor
Department of Otology and Laryngology
Harvard Medical School
Director
Head and Neck Oncology Research
Massachusetts Eye and Ear Infirmary
Boston, Massachusetts

David Rosen, MD
Associate Professor
Department of Otolaryngology–Head and Neck
  Surgery
Thomas Jefferson University
Philadelphia, Pennsylvania

Ravi N. Samy, MD, FACS
Program Director
Neurotology Fellowship
Department of Otolaryngology
University of Cincinnati College of Medicine
Cincinnati Children's Hospital Medical Center
Cincinnati, Ohio

Pina C. Sanelli, MD, MPH
Associate Professor of Radiology and Public
  Health
Department of Radiology
New York Presbyterian Hospital
Weill Cornell Medical College
New York, New York

Robert T. Sataloff, MD, DMA, FACS
Professor and Chairman
Department of Otolaryngology–Head and Neck
  Surgery
Senior Associate Dean for Clinical Academic
  Specialties
Drexel University College of Medicine
Philadelphia, Pennsylvania

Keith G. Saxon, MD, FACS
Assistant Professor
Department of Otology and Laryngology
Harvard Medical School
Boston, Massachusetts

Samuel H. Selesnick, MD, FACS
Professor and Vice Chairman
Department of Otorhinolaryngology
Weill Cornell Medical College
New York, New York

Duane Sewell, MD
Assistant Professor
Department of Otolaryngology–Head and Neck
  Surgery
University of Maryland School of Medicine
Baltimore, Maryland

Jo Shapiro, MD
Associate Professor
Department of Otology and Laryngology
Harvard Medical School
Chief
Division of Otolaryngology
Brigham and Women's Hospital
Boston, Massachusetts

Jeffrey M. Shaari, MD
Private Practice in Otolaryngology
West New York, New Jersey

Eric L. Slattery, MD
Resident
Department of Otolaryngology–Head and Neck
  Surgery
Washington University School of Medicine
St. Louis, Missouri

Anthony Sparano, MD
Fellow
Department of Otolaryngology–Head and Neck
    Surgery
University of Michigan
Ann Arbor, Michigan

Jacob D. Steiger, MD
Steiger Facial Plastic Surgery
Boca Raton, Florida

Michael G. Stewart, MD, MPH
Professor and Chairman
Department of Otorhinolaryngology
Senior Associate Dean for Clinical Affairs
Weill Cornell Medical College
New York, New York

Babar Sultan, MD
Resident
Department of Otolaryngology–Head and Neck
    Surgery
Johns Hopkins University Hospital
Baltimore, Maryland

Thomas G. Takoudes, MD
Clinical Instructor
Department of Surgery
Division of Otolaryngology
Yale University School of Medicine
New Haven, Connecticut

Thomas A. Tami, MD
Director
Cincinnati Sinus Institute
Medical Director
Cincinnati Group Health Associates
Cincinnati, Ohio

Bruce K. Tan, MD
Fellow
The Sinus and Allergy Center
Northwestern University
Chicago, Illinois

Mark H. Terris, MD
Service Chief
Department of Otolaryngology–Head and Neck
    Surgery
Kaiser Permanente, Mid-Atlantic States
Rockville, Maryland

Erica R. Thaler, MD
Professor
Director
Department of Otolaryngology–Head and Neck
    Surgery
University of Pennsylvania School of Medicine
Philadelphia, Pennsylvania

Dale Amanda Tylor, MDCM
Assistant Professor
Department of Otolaryngology
Vanderbilt University
Nashville, Tennessee

Robert F. Ward, MD, FACS
Professor of Otorhinolaryngology
Professor of Otorhinolaryngology in Pediatrics
Department of Otorhinolaryngology
Weill Cornell Medical College
New York, New York

Randal S. Weber, MD, FACS
Professor and Chairman
Department of Head and Neck Surgery
The University of Texas M. D. Anderson Cancer
    Center
Houston, Texas

Richard O. Wein, MD, FACS
Assistant Professor
Department of Otolaryngology–Head and Neck
    Surgery
Tufts Medical Center
Boston, Massachusetts

Mark A. Zacharek, MD, FAAOA
Associate Professor
Deparment of Otolaryngology–Head and Neck
    Surgery
University of Michigan
Ann Arbor, Michigan

Craig H. Zalvan, MD, FACS
Associate Professor of Otolaryngology
New York Medical College
Valhalla, New York
Medical Director
The Institute for Voice and Swallowing
    Disorders
Phelps Memorial Hospital Center
Sleepy Hollow, New York

Fawen Zhang, MD, PhD
Assistant Professor
Department of Communication Sciences and
    Disorders
College of Allied Health
University of Cincinnati
Cincinnati, Ohio

Lee A. Zimmer, MD, PhD, FACS
Assistant Professor
Department of Otolaryngology
University of Cincinnati College of Medicine
Cincinnati, Ohio

I Diagnostic Evaluation

Section Editors: *Michael G. Stewart and Samuel H. Selesnick*

1 Evaluation in Otology and Neurotology

Eric L. Slattery, Timothy E. Hullar, and Lawrence R. Lustig

Clinical complaints in otology and neurotology represent a diverse spectrum of disorders with many overlapping symptoms. For this reason, otolaryngologists must carefully and appropriately evaluate patients with otologic complaints to achieve timely diagnosis of potentially treatable and reversible pathologic processes.

The history is an essential component of the evaluation of patients with otologic disorders and includes defining the onset and timing of hearing loss, tinnitus, vertigo, otalgia, or otorrhea. Associated symptoms, particularly those related to the central nervous system (CNS) or cranial nerve dysfunction, should be sought. Prior history of noise exposure, potential ototoxic medication exposure, head trauma, family history of ear disease, or meningitis should be elicited. The presence of any associated medical conditions such as autoimmune disorders or diabetes is critical in the assessment.

The foundation of diagnosis in otology and neurotology rests with the clinical examination. The examination begins with a general otolaryngologic assessment, consisting of an examination of the overall facial and skull features to identify potential congenital or acquired asymmetry, integument, or pigment abnormalities. The otologic examination consists of initial visual inspection of the auricle and mastoid process. Microscopic examination of the external auditory meatus and canal is followed by subsequent inspection of the tympanic membrane. Pneumatic otoscopy with a Siegel pneumatic speculum allows visualization of tympanic membrane mobility under the microscope. Standard rhinologic, oral, and neck examination should follow. Particular attention should be given to the cranial nerve examination, as many otologic and neurotologic processes can affect cranial nerve function.

Tuning fork examination, most commonly using a 512 and 1024 Hz tuning fork, provides a rough but simple method of determining auditory function within the clinic. The two tests commonly performed are the Weber test and the Rinne test of air conduction determination. Together these tests can rapidly differentiate a conductive from a sensorineural loss and can determine which ear is likely affected.

Evaluation of hearing should be performed using objective testing. Hearing loss can occur at any stage of the auditory pathway, from the ear canal to the auditory cortex. Although simple otoscopy can identify obvious pathology in the external and middle ear, the ability to determine the cause and nature of hearing loss, particularly the evaluation of the cochlea, may not be possible by physical examination alone. The standard objective measure of hearing is audiometry. Pure tone threshold audiometry, the most fundamental of all diagnostic hearing tests, is a behaviorally based measure of hearing that is used to distinguish between sensorineural (cochlear and central auditory pathways) and conductive (external and middle ear) types of hearing loss. The primary goal of pure tone testing is to obtain a representation of the quietest sound intensities one can hear across the frequency spectrum. These data can then be compared with well-established normative population-based standards to determine the nature and degree of the hearing loss. Both air- and bone-conduction thresholds are typically identified, allowing an accurate determination of the level (mild to profound) and nature (conductive, sensorineural, or mixed) of the hearing loss. Additional testing parameters include speech audiometry, which includes both the speech reception threshold (SRT), defined as the quietest level at which a patient can repeat a word, and the speech discrimination score (SDS), calculated as the percentage of words a patient can hear and repeat at a comfortable listening level.

Acoustic immittance testing is also commonly performed during the audiogram and includes tympanometry and the acoustic reflex. Tympanometry measures the changes that occur to the tympanic membrane and ossicles as a result of a change in air pressure in the ear canal; it is important for evaluating such conditions as otitis media and eustachian tube dysfunction. The stapedius muscle reflex, or acoustic reflex, is another important component of immittance testing and represents contraction of the stapedius muscle in response to a loud auditory signal. This test is important in helping to identify otosclerosis, retrocochlear lesions, or abnormalities, such as superior semicircular canal dehiscence.

Auditory brain response (ABR) testing, also referred to as brainstem auditory evoked response (BAER) and brainstem auditory evoked potential (BAEP), is an important objective electrical test to measure cochlear and retrocochlear function. The ABR is an averaged surface recording of the sound-activated auditory pathway beginning in the cochlea. The objective nature of this test, independent of a patient's ability to respond, has made it an integral component of auditory testing in newborns, infants, and toddlers, as well any patient who might not be able to respond accurately to pure tone testing, including patients undergoing general anesthesia.

High-resolution computed tomography (CT) and magnetic resonance imaging (MRI) give the otolaryngologist an extraordinary ability to localize pathology within the inner ear and auditory pathway. Together they provide important and complementary data necessary for otologic diagnosis. The strengths of the CT scan include its superior bone detail and ability to detect bony erosive processes (eg, cholesteatoma and tumor), spongiotic changes in the otic capsule (otosclerosis), and congenital abnormalities (eg, aural atresia and congenital ossicular fixation). MRI is one of the most important modalities clinicians have to evaluate otologic and retrocochlear pathology. MRI with contrast dye, gadolinium–DTPA (diethylenetriamine penta-acetic acid), is the imaging modality of choice for identifying inflammatory processes (eg, labyrinthitis) or neoplasms (eg, vestibular schwannoma) within the temporal bone or along the central auditory pathways.

Laboratory testing, such as serum assessment for syphilis, Lyme disease, and autoimmune disease, can further elucidate diagnoses.

◆ Vestibular Evaluation

One of the challenges an otolaryngologist faces when evaluating the patient with dizziness is determining if the dizziness is due to an otologic or nonotologic pathology. Fortunately, a thorough history can often make that determination with a relatively high degree of precision. The first step in this process involves determining if the patient has true vertigo, defined as an illusory sense of motion that can be rotatory, linear, or vertical. Symptoms can be episodic or continuous; most vestibulopathies cause fluctuating or episodic symptoms, although there may be a constant sense of disequilibrium in addition. The patient's symptoms may reflect a disorder of information processing from the semicircular canals or from the otolith organs. Rotary nystagmus may be more common with semicircular dysfunction, and abnormal sensations of tilt or sudden drop attacks can be seen with otolith dysfunction. In addition, underlying medical problems could cause or exacerbate the patient's symptoms. Thyroid disease, diabetes mellitus, anemia, autoimmune diseases, hypoperfusion of the brain from postural hypotension, and cardiac arrhythmias can lead to dizziness and/or vertigo. A variety of medications can also produce symptoms that mimic vestibular disorders (**Table 1.1**). Triggers for dizziness are also important to elicit, such as changes in position (eg, benign positional vertigo), certain foods (eg, Meniere disease or vestibular migraine), and loud noises (eg, superior semicircular canal dehiscence). Lastly, dizziness may be accompanied by, for example, aural fullness and tinnitus (eg, Meniere disease), dysarthria, diplopia, and paresthesias (eg, vertebrobasilar insufficiency), or headaches and photophobia (eg, vestibular migraine).

Following a thorough history, the differential diagnosis should be relatively short. This should then be corroborated with findings on physical examination. Besides a thorough otologic examination, additional tests focus on examining ocular responses to head motion to evaluate for central and peripheral abnormalities in the vestibular pathways (**Table 1.2**). These tests include ocular smooth pursuits and saccadic motion (abnormal in central lesions) and the head-thrust sign (to evaluate for vestibular hypofunction). Frenzel goggles will facilitate examination of the eyes by preventing fixation-suppression of nystagmus. Evaluation under Frenzel goggles can include the head-shake test and Valsalva-, hyperventilation-, or sound-induced nystagmus. A Dix-Hallpike examination will test for benign positional vertigo. Additional tests might include a cerebellar examination and dynamic visual acuity, looking for degradation of vision while reading a Snellen eye chart with and without head shaking, a sensitive test for bilateral vestibular hypofunction.

Objective testing for vestibular dysfunction includes audiometry as described above, in addition to other tests depending on clinical suspicion. The most

Table 1.1 Commonly Used Medications That May Be Associated with Dizziness

Drug	Type of Dizziness	Mechanism
Aminoglycosides	Vertigo, disequilibrium	Damage to vestibular hair cells
Platinum compounds (cisplatin)	Vertigo, disequilibrium	Damage to vestibular hair cells
Antiepileptics Carbamazepine Phenytoin Primidone	Disequilibrium	Cerebellar toxicity
Tranquilizers Barbiturates Antihistamines Tricyclic amines	Intoxication	CNS depression
Antihypertensives, diuretics	Near-faint	Postural hypotension, reduced cerebral blood flow
Amiodarone (Cordarone)	Disequilibrium	Unknown
Alcohol	Intoxication, disequilibrium, positional vertigo	CNS depression, cerebellar toxicity, change in cupula-specific gravity
Methotrexate (Rheumatrex)	Disequilibrium	Brainstem and cerebellar toxicity
Anticoagulants	Vertigo	Hemorrhage into inner ear or CNS

Abbreviation: CNS, central nervous system.

commonly employed battery of tests is electronystagmography (ENG) or video ENG (VNG). The ENG records ocular movement at rest and in response to various perturbations, including positional nystagmus, saccade testing, smooth pursuit testing, optokinetic testing, and caloric testing. When combined with a thorough history, the ENG battery can be quite useful in determining the etiology of balance dysfunction. Additional tests to consider include rotatory chair testing (useful for diagnosing bilateral vestibular hypofunction), vestibular evoked myogenic potentials (for diagnosing semicircular canal dehiscence), and platform posturography (useful for monitoring response to vestibular therapy and rehabilitation, as well as identifying malingerers).

Table 1.2 Functional Classes of Eye Movements

Class of Eye Movement	Main Function
Visual fixation	Holds the image of a stationary object on the fovea
Vestibular	Holds images of the visual world steady on the retina during brief head rotations
Optokinetic	Holds images of the visual world steady on the retina during sustained head rotations
Smooth pursuit	Holds the image of a moving target on the fovea
Nystagmus (quick phase)	Resets the eyes during prolonged rotation and direct gaze toward the oncoming visual scene
Saccades	Brings images of objects of interest onto the fovea
Vergence	Moves the eyes in opposite directions so that images of a single object are placed simultaneously on both foveae

Suggested Reading

Chan Y. Differential diagnosis of dizziness. Curr Opin Otolaryngol Head Neck Surg 2009;17(3):200–203

Offiah CE, Ramsden RT, Gillespie JE. Imaging appearances of unusual conditions of the middle and inner ear. Br J Radiol 2008;81(966):504–514

Seemungal BM, Bronstein AM. A practical approach to acute vertigo. Pract Neurol 2008;8(4):211–221

Shah LM, Wiggins RH III. Imaging of hearing loss. Neuroimaging Clin N Am 2009;19(3): 287–306

Worden BF, Blevins NH. Pediatric vestibulopathy and pseudovestibulopathy: differential diagnosis and management. Curr Opin Otolaryngol Head Neck Surg 2007;15(5):304–309

Zapala DA, Shaughnessy K, Buckingham J, Hawkins DB. The importance of audiologic red flags in patient management decisions. J Am Acad Audiol 2008;19(7):564–570

2 Evaluation in Rhinology

Bradley F. Marple

The signs and symptoms of nasal disease can present a unique challenge to a practitioner. Indeed, many symptoms attributed to the nose and paranasal sinuses may simply reflect the normal physiologic function of the nose. As an example, rhinorrhea, congestion, and even subtle changes in olfaction may be normal under many circumstances, and as a result, are easily overlooked as insignificant. At times, however, these complaints may provide hints to a variety of significant, and potentially harmful, underlying pathologic conditions.

Unlike many anatomical regions, the nose and paranasal sinuses present a unique diagnostic challenge. As a result of this, it is not uncommon to find that neoplasms in this region are identified only after progressing to an advanced stage of development. Complete evaluation often requires numerous complementary modalities. The patient's history and physical examination frequently provide "signals" of underlying disease, leading to a more extensive and focused evaluation. Fortunately, the skills and tools necessary to evaluate complaints related to the nose are readily available within the scope of otolaryngologic care. Radiography, immunologic testing, serology, and endoscopy are among a few of the tools available to the otolaryngologist. Although these tools are necessary to gather information required for appropriate diagnosis and management, it is the ability to synthesize the resultant information from these modalities that yields accurate diagnoses.

Each of the chapters focuses not only on a structured overview of the differential diagnosis that should be considered when a complaint is offered by a patient, but also on an initial review of the history, physical examination, laboratory, and procedural tools that are best suited to the assessment of each particular complaint. The high points of the history, physical examination, and additional testing, however, are intended to supplement the information that is gathered in the course of a thorough overall assessment.

◆ Assessment of the Rhinologic Complaint

History

It goes without saying that the evaluation of each patient starts with a thorough assessment of the patient's individual history. For the purposes of this section, those historical features that are unique to each specific symptom will be addressed within its specific chapter.

Physical Examination

A complete exam of the head and neck is essential to fully evaluate any rhinologic complaint and should serve as the starting point for any initial evaluation.

- General examination: provides for an overall assessment of the general state of the patient. Frequently, information may be gathered that will help to direct further assessment of the patient and serve to identify areas that will require focus. An example of this may be an auricular abnormality that would suggest a destructive cartilaginous process, such as relapsing polychondritis.
- Cranial nerve examination/neurologic examination: a thorough examination of the sensory and motor function of the pertinent cranial nerves is crucial, as it may yield evidence of extension of disease beyond the confines of the nose/paranasal sinuses.
- Otoscopy: middle ear effusion may indicate pathology in the nose and/or paranasal sinuses:
  - Cerebrospinal fluid (CSF) otorrhea
  - Eustachian tube dysfunction
  - Nasopharyngeal mass or nasal mass with extension into the region of the fossa of Rosenmüller
  - Extension of an infiltrative process that results in obstruction or extrinsic compression of the eustachian tube
- Nasal examination: Many techniques are available to assess nasal obstruction:
  - Examination of the external nose provides important information and should not be overlooked. Special attention should be directed to areas of erythema, edema, peau d'orange, and soft tissue disruption/ulceration.
  - Anterior rhinoscopy can be performed using a speculum and appropriate light source. This provides access to the anterior nasal vestibule. The anterior aspect of the inferior turbinate can be easily inspected, as well as the architecture of the anterior nasal septum. Access to the midportion or posterior nasal cavity can be challenging.
- Nasopharyngeal examination: can be performed with indirect techniques. Although a nasopharyngeal mirror can be used, it provides a limited view of the structures within this area. More commonly used tools are a 0- or 30-degree rigid endoscope and a flexible laryngoscope.
- Cervical examination

Additional Assessment

Endoscopic Evaluation

- Nasal endoscopy can provide a detailed and complete examination of the more posterior reaches of the nasal cavity. Many times the information from this examination can supplement that of anterior rhinoscopy.

- ○ Evaluation of the inferior, middle, and superior turbinates and meatus should be performed. Drainage and/or polyps may be seen in any of these areas.
- ○ Posterior drainage from the middle meatus can be seen laterally to the eustachian tube orifice. Drainage from the superior meatus is often noted over the eustachian tube orifice.

- Nasopharyngoscopy can be performed using an endoscope. This procedure usually requires topical anesthetic and decongestant use (especially if there is some degree of baseline obstruction or hypertrophy). The nasopharynx should be examined for any cicatricial scars, which may indicate an extremely rare diagnosis of nasopharyngeal stenosis. The surface mucosa, the eustachian tube orifice, and the fossa of Rosenmüller should be analyzed to include or exclude physiologic and anatomical obstructions, both of which could be of benign or malignant origin.

  - ○ Rigid endoscopy: provides clear visual resolution of the nasopharynx and can be easily incorporated during nasal endoscopy. In the event of tortuous anatomy, access to the nasopharynx may be limited.
  - ○ Flexible endoscope: usually performed as an additional procedure along with rigid nasal endoscopy. The flexible scope is maneuverable and allows further evaluation of the oropharynx, hypopharynx, and supraglottic larynx.

Assessment of Nasal Patency

- Cottle maneuver: simply retracting facial soft tissue just lateral to the nasal alae in the direction of the ipsilateral ear while asking the patient to nasally inspire provides an assessment of the dynamic patency in the region of the nasal valve. A perceived improvement in nasal obstruction signals dynamic collapse in the region of the nasal valve.
- Acoustic rhinometry: involves an assessment of the patency of the nasal cavity based on reflections of an acoustic signal directed into that cavity. The changes in the reflected sound represent changes within the cross-sectional area along the nasal cavity. After these acoustic signals are registered and processed via computer, an estimate of the cross-sectional area of the nose can be determined as a distance from the nostril. This technique, which has been validated in several studies, but also criticized for being burdensome, provides an estimate of the cross-sectional areas of the nose as a function of the distance from the nostril. Thus, the site (anterior, middle, or posterior) and degree of nasal obstruction can be identified. Also, analysis can be done before and after topical decongestants are applied, allowing discrimination of mucocutaneous versus structural blockage. Standards for age, race, ethnicity, and gender exist.
- Rhinostereometry: measures the horizontal range of the anterior portion of the inferior turbinate. This is done by attaching a binocular microscope head to a nasal speculum. The view of the inferior turbinate is carefully recorded with quadrant measurements. This technique has been correlated

with acoustic rhinomanometry and has been used to evaluate the nasal cycle objectively.

Assessment for Cerebrospinal Fluid Fistula

- Provocation: placing the patient's head in a dependent position can lead to evidence of a leak of clear, watery fluid. Such a finding is suggestive of a CSF fistula from the nose or temporal bone.
- Collection of fluid sample for β_2-transferrin: β_2-transferrin is a protein found in CSF and the aqueous and vitreous humor of the eye. Nasal fluid is collected and sent for laboratory examination. Electrophoresis is performed to separate proteins and detect β_2-transferrin. When present, a CSF leak is confirmed; however, a negative test result does not exclude a diagnosis of CSF leak.
- Radionuclide study: a highly sensitive test to detect a CSF leak. It involves the intrathecal injection of a radioactive tracer, indium 111 DTPA (pentetate). Intranasal pledgets are placed and left for several hours. These are then removed and placed in a radioactive counter to detect the tracer. The patient's serum levels are drawn for comparison counts.
- Intrathecal fluorescein may be introduced via a lumbar puncture or spinal drain for better identification of a CSF fistula. Recommended doses of fluorescein (0.2–0.5 mL of 5% fluorescein diluted in 10 mL of spinal fluid and reintroduced slowly into the intrathecal space) are quite small, yet are sufficient to allow easy identification of CSF that escapes from the subarachnoid space. Identification of fluorescein can be aided by the use of a Wood lamp or a blue endoscopic filter, but these techniques are frequently not necessary.

  - Complications with fluorescein are infrequent. Although it is not approved by the U.S. Food and Drug Administration for intrathecal use, no permanent neurologic deficits have been reported with low dosing.
  - Complications, including seizures and extremity numbness, have been associated with the use of high dosages.

Radiology

- Computed tomography (CT) is the radiologic imaging mode of choice to evaluate the nasal cavity, paranasal sinuses, nasopharynx, and skull base. Visualization of all of these areas is critical in the evaluation of a nasal obstruction. The standard protocol for a sinus CT scan includes axial and coronal slices. Sagittal images may occasionally be provided. CT scans typically obtained for visualizing the paranasal sinus should include coronal and axial (3 mm) cross sections. Soft tissue and bony windows facilitate evaluation of disease processes and the bony architecture. The use of intravenous contrast material just prior to scanning can help define soft tissue lesions and delineate vascularized structures, such as vascular tumors. Contrast-enhanced CT is particularly useful in evaluating neoplastic, chronic, and inflammatory processes. For most patients with sinusitis, however, non-contrast CT of the paranasal sinuses generally suffices. For patients who may not tolerate the prone position required for coronal cuts, computer-generated reconstructed coronal views can be generated from thin axial sections. If sufficiently thin (1–2 mm) axial sections are available, sagittal reconstructions can also be helpful for teaching purposes and further delineating anatomical structures.

- Magnetic resonance imaging (MRI) scans are often ordered to further define or delineate soft tissue anatomy. In addition to viewing neural enhancement and neuronal pathways, it may help to strengthen or weaken suspicion for benign or malignant tumors or fungal disease.
- Angiography can be useful when an assessment of vascular anatomy is required. It may also be combined with embolization when needed for the control of arterial bleeding.

Suggested Reading

Bailey BJ, Johnson JT, Newlands SD, eds. Head and Neck Surgery–Otolaryngology. Vol. 1. 4th ed. Philadelphia: Lippincott Williams & Wilkins; 2006

Cummings CW, Flint PW, Harker LA, et al, eds. Otolaryngology Head and Neck Surgery. Vol. 2. 4th ed. Philadelphia: Elsevier Mosby; 2005

Snow JB Jr, Wackym PA, eds. Ballenger's Otorhinolaryngology: Head and Neck Surgery. 17th ed. Lewiston, NY: People's Medical Publishing House; 2009

3 Evaluation of the Upper Aerodigestive Tract

Marc Cohen and Jason G. Newman

A multifaceted approach is necessary for the critical evaluation of the upper aerodigestive tract. This chapter identifies the necessary elements of a comprehensive evaluation of this vital anatomical region.

◆ Patient History

A thorough history is important because it may serve as the principal or only means of diagnosis. Accordingly, once a chief complaint has been identified, the physician should proceed with a thorough medical history tailored to the patient's primary pathology.

Of primary importance in an evaluation of the upper aerodigestive tract is whether the patient has experienced any discomfort or pain, as well as the nature, location, intensity, and any alleviating factors of this discomfort. Additionally, the physician should identify symptoms of odynophagia and dysphagia, and all associated factors should be addressed. Key points relative to dysphagia are whether the dysphagia is to solids, liquids, or both, and the time patterns associated with the symptoms. The physician should inquire about other gastrointestinal complaints, including globus, heartburn, throat clearing, regurgitation, gurgling in the neck, halitosis, and a prior history of caustic ingestion.

The physician should assess symptoms present in the upper airway, including stridor. Specifically, the physician should inquire about the nature of stridor, whether breath sounds are inspiratory or expiratory, as well as the presence of alleviating factors. Voice changes, shortness of breath, wheezing, and coughing may also indicate pathology in the upper airway and should be addressed. Any history of recurrent aspiration pneumonia, intubation, or abnormal lesions is significant and should be considered by the practitioner.

Other otolaryngologic symptoms are critical to an evaluation of the upper aerodigestive tract. An inquiry should be made into otologic symptoms, including hearing loss, aural fullness, and otalgia. Likewise, nasal symptoms such as obstruction, epistaxis, congestion, discharge, and changes in olfaction should be considered. Neurologic symptoms with clinical relevance include vision changes, changes in sensation, and any symptoms related to cranial neuropathy.

The physician should consider a history of constitutional symptoms, such as fever, sweats, and weight loss. Additionally, factors such as prior radiation to the head and neck area and any history of alcohol or tobacco use should be evaluated. Of crucial importance is an inquiry into the patient's past medical history. Although the physician should consider all organ systems, any history of oncologic processes, hemangiomas, and any cardiovascular and pulmonary pathology are most pertinent. Finally, each patient should be asked about his or her medications and allergy history.

◆ Physical Examination

Subsequent to a thorough patient history, a physical examination is performed as appropriate. General characteristics of the patient should be assessed, including the patient's comfort level and ability to speak coherently, cachexia, and the presence of secretions. The presence of stridor and its nature (inspiratory or expiratory) should be noted. Additionally, vital signs, including pulse oximetry, may be crucial to a proper diagnosis.

Following the initial assessment, the physician should conduct a thorough examination of the head, face, and neck. The examination should include an inspection and palpation of all surface structures; this includes an assessment for mass lesions, disruption of the facial skeleton, abnormal lymph nodes, or any other abnormalities. Thyroid and cricoid cartilage should be palpated. The presence of a scar on the face or neck indicating prior surgery should be noted. At this time, crepitus or any other anomaly should be ruled out.

In furtherance of a thorough evaluation of the upper aerodigestive tract, an examination of the ear, nose, and throat should occur. An otoscopic exam should be performed to rule out trauma, mass lesions, or serous otitis media, which may indicate an obstructed eustachian tube. Anterior rhinoscopy should be performed with a headlight and nasal speculum to assess the nature of the inferior turbinate, mucosa, and nasal septum. An intraoral examination using a headlight and tongue depressors should be performed. Specifically, inspection of the structures of the oral cavity, including the anterior tongue, hard palate, floor of the mouth, retromolar trigone, and buccal mucosa, should be conducted. Also to be examined are the oropharynx, including the posterior one third of the tongue, posterior and lateral pharyngeal walls, tonsillar pillars, soft palate, and uvula. The practitioner should inspect and express Wharton and Stensen ducts. Finally, an evaluation of the upper aerodigestive tract includes mirror laryngoscopy. This allows proper assessment of a patient's nasopharynx, as well as the supraglottis and glottis.

◆ Further Evaluation

Following the history and physical examination, the practitioner should use office endoscopy as appropriate. This is covered in greater depth in sections VI and VII, but rigid and flexible endoscopies are critical in the evaluation of the upper aerodigestive tract. Flexible nasopharyngolaryngoscopy can be more comprehensive and is vital for assessing the nasal cavity, inferior and middle turbinates, maxillary os, skull base, sphenoethmoidal recess, nasopharynx, eustachian tubes, base of the tongue, vallecula, epiglottis, arytenoids, pyriform sinuses, and false and true cords. Vocal cord mobility and airway patency above the level of the true cords also can be assessed.

A complete radiologic assessment of the upper aerodigestive tract may involve multiple modalities and may assist the physician in the proper diagnosis. This may include plain films, computed tomography, magnetic resonance imaging, and positron emission tomography, as well as fusion techniques. A thorough discussion of these modalities is provided in sections VI and VII.

Unsurprisingly, the most definitive evaluation of the upper aerodigestive tract occurs in the operating room. Direct laryngoscopy allows systematic inspection and palpation of the oral cavity, oropharynx, hypopharynx, supraglottis, and glottis. Microlaryngoscopy can be performed with a telescope lens or microscope for more precise evaluation of these structures. Flexible or rigid bronchoscopy may be performed to assess the subglottis, trachea, and mainstem bronchi. Finally, flexible or rigid esophagoscopy can be used to diagnose and treat certain pathologies present in the esophagus.

Suggested Reading

Couch ME, Blaugrund J, Kunar D. History, physical examination, and the preoperative evaluation. In: Cummings CW, Flint PW, Haughey BH, et al, eds. Otolaryngology: Head and Neck Surgery. 4th ed. Philadelphia: Elsevier; 2005

Postma GN, Belafsky PC, Amin MR, et al. Endoscopic evaluation of the upper aerodigestive tracy. In: Bailey BJ, Johnson JT, Newlands SD, eds. Head and Neck Surgery: Otolaryngology. 4th ed. Philadelphia: Lippincott Williams; 2006

4 Evaluation of the Voice

Joel H. Blumin

Patients often present to the otolaryngologist with the chief complaint of a hoarse voice. The differential diagnosis is wide, varying from relatively benign conditions, such as chronic and acute laryngitis, to problems of greater concern, such as vocal cord paralysis and head and neck cancer. A hoarse voice can occur from an isolated laryngeal problem or be symptomatic of regional or systemic pathology. Hoarseness can be considered both a symptom and a sign. As a symptom, patients will often lump together all aberrancies of voice and language into the complaint of hoarseness. As a sign, physicians often categorize hoarseness as dysphonia and use it to describe the perceptual deviation of the patient's voice from normalcy. This is specifically different than the description of other problems of communication, such as dysarthria (problem with articulation), aphasia and apraxia (problems with language symbolization or execution), and dementia (problem with ideation).

◆ History

History taking of the dysphonic patient begins as it does with most medical conditions: answering the questions how, when, what, and where. The physician starts with generalized open-ended questions, then hones the conversation toward pointed questions that relate to the different laryngeal functions, including voice. Specific voice-related complaints include problems of hoarseness, volume, stamina, and fluency. The physician should have the patient separately describe each type of problem and how it affects his or her voice. Different patients with similar problems may perceive the impact to their voice differently. What a patient does with his or her voice not only plays an important role in the patient's own perception of the degree of dysphonia, but also can have an impact on management decisions. For instance, an operatic soprano will have different vocal demands and expectations than, perhaps, an office worker. Additionally, it is important not only to ask about the patient's profession, but also to get a sense of his or her non-work-related vocal demands. A dysphonic singer who spends his evenings working in a smoky bar will need different treatment than one who is more aware of the best laryngeal hygiene.

The larynx is a complex organ with three main functions: act as a conduit for respiration, protect the airway during swallowing, and produce voice. The physician should ask about issues that relate to these three domains of laryngeal function. Does the patient have any breathing problems? Has the patient noticed any restriction in respiration? Where is that restriction? Is it in the neck or in the chest? Does the patient make noise during respiration? Is this inspiratory, expiratory, or both? Are there any problems with swallowing? Is this to solids, liquids, or both? Has the patient had to alter his or her diet? Has there been any unintentional (or intentional) weight loss? Is there a cough, and is it associated with swallowing? Does the patient notice aspiration? Is there a history of pneumonia?

Several instruments for voice-related outcomes are used in clinical practice. The Voice Handicap Index (VHI), the Voice Outcomes Survey (VOS), and the Voice-Related Quality of Life (VRQOL) test are examples of such instruments. These are generated at the time of the patient's initial intake as well as repeat visits and help to understand the impact of the patient's voice on his or her overall health-related quality of life. Another commonly used instrument, the Reflux Symptom Index (RSI), surveys symptomatology related to laryngopharyngeal reflux, a common source of chronic laryngitis; it can be used to help gauge the impact of common inflammatory symptoms.

◆ Physical Examination

The physical examination of the dysphonic patient begins with the first moment of patient contact with the physician. Sometimes, the patient's initial utterance can be a significant clue to the underlying pathology. The astute clinician listens carefully to the voice while taking the history. This conversation provides an opportunity for the clinician to perceptually evaluate the quality of the patient's dysphonia during connected speech under a variety of conditions—spontaneous when the physician walks into the exam room, recitative when the patient explains why he or she is there, and responsive when the patient answers directed questions. Further voice-specific evaluations can be helpful when the patient reads and recites specific phrases and utterances weighted toward specific voice-related tasks. Standardized evaluation using scoring techniques such as the GRBAS (Grade, Roughness, Breathiness, Asthenia, Strain) and CAPE-V (Consensus Auditory Perceptual Evaluation–Voice) scales can be used to ascertain the degree of dysphonia and to follow the patient longitudinally or compare with other groups of patients.

A complete head and neck physical examination is performed. This includes examination of the head and neck, as well as the entire body. Many laryngeal disorders have a systemic or neurologic basis, and these problems can affect other bodily functions, as well as those of the larynx. A cranial nerve examination is always performed. The neck is carefully palpated and evaluated for masses, adenopathy, or thyromegaly. The laryngeal skeleton is palpated for structural abnormalities, asymmetries, or step-offs, especially when a history of trauma is considered. The mucosa of the head and neck is carefully examined using standard techniques of visualization and palpation. The indirect mirror examination of the larynx is appropriate but inadequate for the evaluation of most voice disorders. A detailed laryngeal examination with endoscopic instrumentation is far superior and supersedes the mirror examination.

In the patient with laryngologic symptomatology, a careful office-based endoscopic evaluation of the larynx and pharynx should always be performed. A variety of tools exist, and provider preference may dictate the chosen technique. In general, endoscopy is performed with both rigid transoral and flexible transnasal endoscopes. Compared with flexible fiberoptic endoscopes, rigid transoral instrumentation with Hopkins rod optics gives a superior detailed view of the anatomy at the expense of connected speech due to anatomical distortions imposed by the examination itself. Recent advances with chip-on-the-tip digital technology have evened the field in flexible instrumentation, and we can now get a highly detailed view of the larynx with minimal anatomical distortion from performance of the examination.

Endoscopic examination should be performed under standard continuous source halogen lighting, as well as videostroboscopic technique. Videostroboscopy refers to visualization of the larynx during phonation with a rapidly on-off flickering xenon light source. This light source is synchronized to and then flashed slightly off the fundamental frequency of the voice. The images are typically captured onto analog or digital media, giving the opportunity to review examinations in slow or stop motion, as well as providing a means for data archiving. The stroboscopic process allows for close visualization of the glottic cycle and fine evaluation of the opening and closure of the vocal fold edges, as well as propagation of the mucosal wave. In reality, the visualized glottic cycle is a bit artificial, as it is a montage of many glottic cycles and is dependent on periodic voicing. In patients with aperiodic laryngeal motion, the stroboscopic examination is less effective. Aperiodic motion can be evaluated with newer high-speed digital imaging. This technique uses a digital capture device capable of near-real-time capture of vocal fold motion. Regrettably, at the time of this writing, this device has limited use in the usual clinical evaluation because of associated high costs and nonstandardization of data evaluation.

◆ Additional Testing

Laryngeal electromyography (LEMG) is used to evaluate the neuromuscular activity of the larynx. Movement disorders of the larynx are common, and they relate to a wide range of laryngeal problems. Unfortunately, LEMG is not an absolute objective test; having the test performed by a clinician trained and experienced in this technique can diminish some of the variability related to subjectivity. This study is performed with the patient awake. After percutaneous electrodes are placed into the laryngeal musculature, the patient is asked to perform a variety of gestures (including phonation, breathing/sniffing, and chin push) that are used to excite the different muscles. Evidence of normal and abnormal innervation is inferred and used to design a specific treatment for the patient. Currently, there are no accepted methods of directly evaluating laryngeal nerve physiology in the ambulatory patient with nerve conduction studies, including conduction velocities, compound motor action potentials, and sensory nerve action potentials. The quality of laryngeal sensation can be evaluated roughly by gag or laryngeal spasm response to palpation by the flexible laryngoscope tip. More specific testing of sensation can be evaluated with specialized air-puff laryngeal adductory response equipment.

Acoustic and aerodynamic voice analyses are typically performed by the speech-language pathologist as part of a multidisciplinary voice evaluation. Standardized methods of evaluation using commercially available devices are most commonly performed. During an acoustic study, the patient voices standardized phonemes and phrases within a standardized environment. After digital capture, portions of these are used for the evaluation of perturbations of the acoustic signal. Vocal tract aerodynamics are evaluated similarly: the patient phonates into a standardized mask, and airflow and intraoral pressure are measured. Airflow resistance and subglottic pressure are calculated, and perturbations are quantified. These techniques are rarely diagnostic by themselves, but they can be helpful as part of the larger diagnostic evaluation. They also may be useful in following an individual longitudinally or comparing the individual to a larger population of patients with similar voice complaints.

Radiologic testing is used infrequently in the primary evaluation of voice disorders. Imaging studies are typically indicated when one questions the structural integrity of the larynx, such as following trauma, or in the evaluation of the laryngeal innervation when denervation is suspected, such as in a patient who presents with findings consistent with a vocal fold paralysis. Both computed tomography (CT) and magnetic resonance imaging (MRI) can be used. In general, MRI is preferred when central disorders are considered, and CT is preferred for the evaluation of peripheral (cervical) pathology, with the latter performed with much greater frequency. Ultrasound may be indicated when thyroid pathology is considered. Laboratory evaluation of the voice patient is performed infrequently.

Suggested Reading

Belafsky PC, Postma GN, Koufman JA. The validity and reliability of the reflux finding score (RFS). Laryngoscope 2001;111(8):1313–1317

Belafsky PC, Postma GN, Koufman JA. Validity and reliability of the reflux symptom index (RSI). J Voice 2002;16(2):274–277

Berke GS, Gerratt BR. Laryngeal biomechanics: an overview of mucosal wave mechanics. J Voice 1993;7(2):123–128

Karnell MP, Melton SD, Childes JM, Coleman TC, Dailey SA, Hoffman HT. Reliability of clinician-based (GRBAS and CAPE-V) and patient-based (V-RQOL and IPVI) documentation of voice disorders. J Voice 2007;21(5):576–590

Merati AL, Bielamowicz SA, eds. Diagnostic procedures in laryngology. In: Textbook of Laryngology. San Diego, CA: Plural Publishing; 2007:73–146

Merati AL, Halum SL, Smith TL. Diagnostic testing for vocal fold paralysis: survey of practice and evidence-based medicine review. Laryngoscope 2006;116(9):1539–1552

Munin MC, Rosen CA, Zullo T. Utility of laryngeal electromyography in predicting recovery after vocal fold paralysis. Arch Phys Med Rehabil 2003;84(8):1150–1153

Portone CR, Hapner ER, McGregor L, Otto K, Johns MM III. Correlation of the voice handicap index (VHI) and the voice-related quality of life measure (V-RQOL). J Voice 2007;21(6):723–727

Sulica L. Voice: anatomy, physiology, and clinical evaluation. In: Bailey BJ, Johnson JT, Newlands SD, eds. Head and Neck Surgery–Otolaryngology. 4th ed. Philadelphia: Lippincott Williams & Wilkins; 2006:817–827

5 Allergy and Immunologic Evaluation

Bradley F. Marple

Allergy testing is indicated when there is a strong suspicion of allergy despite a lack of improvement with conventional medical treatment. It is also indicated in the patient who may benefit from immunotherapy. Allergy tests are used to determine the specific antigens that trigger the allergic response in the patient: this allows treatment or allergen avoidance to be antigen specific. Allergy testing can be divided into two broad categories: in vivo and in vitro testing.

- In vivo (skin) testing is a method of determining IgE (immunoglobulin E)–mediated sensitivity to a specific antigen or set of antigens. The antigen that is to be tested is introduced into the dermis or epidermis via an intradermal injection or skin prick technique, respectively. Less frequently, a patch technique, which relies on absorption of the test antigen, may be used. A positive test is determined when the skin area to which the antigen has been applied develops a wheal-and-flare response, indicating antigen-specific degranulation of cutaneous mast cells. Both quantitative (degree of sensitivity) and qualitative (presence of sensitivity) measurement can be determined using this technique. A negative response represents either an anergic state or the absence of IgE-mediated sensitivity to the specific test antigen. Skin testing carries a small but potentially serious risk of allergic reaction, or anaphylaxis.
- In vitro testing measures the level of either total IgE or IgE specific to a particular antigen present in a patient's serum by way of an enzyme-linked immunoabsorbent assay (ELISA). Elevated IgE levels denote the IgE-mediated sensitivity to the test antigen. Given the fact that in vitro testing is performed in a laboratory setting on the patient's serum, the risk of this testing technique is limited to that of venipuncture. For this reason, in vitro testing is frequently the test of choice for patients who are at high risk for anaphylaxis or severe systemic reactions.
  - Total IgE: The simplest form of in vitro testing is a measurement of the total IgE antibody level in a patient's serum. Total IgE is a nonspecific test that nonetheless has utility in certain situations. A normal total IgE screen does not rule out an elevated IgE to a specific antigen; therefore, a normal result warrants further testing. However, measurement of total IgE may prove useful if elevated, as this may prompt more thorough allergen testing if the initial allergy screen is negative.
  - Antigen-specific IgE: Alternatively, and arguably more useful, antigen-specific IgE can be obtained. The results obtained by many in vitro methodologies can provide both quantitative and qualitative measurement of patient sensitivity to a specific antigen. This form of assessment provides analogous information to that of in vivo testing.

- Immunologic evaluation: occasionally, immunodeficiency will give rise to recurrent rhinitis and rhinosinusitis. If suspected, an appropriate immunologic evaluation should be undertaken.
  - Total immunoglobulin levels:
    - IgG
      - IgG1
      - IgG2
      - IgG3
      - IgG4
    - IgM
    - IgA
  - Qualitative response to vaccination demonstrates a patient's ability to mount an appropriate humoral immune response to an immune challenge. This can be measured by obtaining specific IgG titers to a vaccination prior to its administration and comparing those results to the postconvalescent titers 1 month later. A normal response should result in at least a doubling of specific IgG titers. Vaccines that are commonly used to perform this test include:
    - Pneumovax: titers are obtained for each of the serotypes of streptococcal pneumonia included in the vaccine.
    - *Haemophilus influenzae* type B
    - Tetanus toxoid
- Serology and other laboratory tests: there are several disease states that can lead to nasal symptomatology. Some can be identified by the following tests:
  - Wegener granulomatosis: C-ANCA (antineutrophil cytoplasmic autoantibody)/P-ANCA, urinalysis
  - Churg-Strauss syndrome: eosinophil level
  - Hypothyroidism: thyroid-stimulating hormone
  - Sarcoidosis: angiotensin-converting enzyme, calcium
  - Syphilis: fluorescent treponemal antibody, tissue plasminogen activator
  - Cystic fibrosis: sweat chloride test
  - Ciliary function: at times, either congenital or developmental disruption of mucociliary function can give rise to sinonasal disease.
- Assessment of mucus
  - Cystic fibrosis: sweat test
- Assessment of ciliary structure and function
  - Saccharine test: gross assessment of ciliary function. Saccharine is placed on the medial surface of the inferior turbinate. Gustatory identification of a sweet sensation within 10 to 15 minutes denotes the presence of ciliary function. The results of this test vary widely.
  - Transmission electron microscopy of the cilia ultrastructure can be used to identify ciliary abnormalities.

● Biopsy: tissue samples from the nose are relatively simple to obtain and should be considered when a suspicious lesion is identified on physical examination. If the lesion in question arises from the region of the skull base, it is wise to obtain a preprocedure computed tomography scan to eliminate inadvertent biopsy of masses associated with skull base dehiscence.

Suggested Reading

Adkinson NF Jr, ed. Middleton's Allergy: Principles and Practice. Expert Consult: Online and Print. 7th ed. Elsevier; 2008

King H, Mabry RL, Mabry C, Gordon B, Marple BF. Allergy in ENT Practice: The Basic Guide. New York and Stuttgart: Thieme Medical Publishers; 2004

6 Evaluation in Facial Plastic and Reconstructive Surgery

Patrick J. Byrne

A careful history is performed after discussing with the patient his or her motivations for seeking the evaluation. This includes a detailed medical history (as with any initial patient encounter), in part to determine if the patient is a candidate for any intervention. This general history and exam will not be reviewed here. The evaluation of the patient presenting to the facial plastic surgery clinic is then focused as determined by the patient's concerns.

◆ History

This first section will list some specific points in the history that are important to elicit, depending on the chief complaint. In all cases of elective cosmetic surgery in particular, one must assess the psychological health of the patient. This is typically done through the review of the patient's history and by discussing with the patient his or her motivations. In some cases, a formal referral to a psychiatrist may be warranted.

It is very important to take preoperative photographs of each and every patient. This is part of the medical record for patients undergoing facial plastic surgery, both cosmetic and reconstructive.

Aging Face

The patient who desires to look younger may have a very specific aim, such as reducing the jowls or improving the appearance of the eyes. In other cases, he or she may not have a specific goal, just a sense that he or she wants to look more attractive. It is important to include the following in the patient's history.

- Previous surgery or treatments: multiple previous operations, injectable treatments, and resurfacing are common in this population.
- History of previous Accutane use: resurfacing is best avoided if this has occurred in the recent past.
- History of dry eye: periocular surgery (eg, blepharoplasty and browlift) can impair the ability to lubricate the eye effectively, and some patients are predisposed to subsequent desiccation. Consider clearance by ophthalmology in such cases.
- Alopecia: some procedures, such as a browlift, can worsen this condition.
- Smoking: The risk of hematoma and skin necrosis as a surgical complication is increased.

Rhinoplasty

- Previous surgery of the nose: revision cases are riskier and more difficult.
- Nasal obstruction: clarify if it is bilateral or unilateral, fluctuating or constant, related to allergic rhinitis, and so on.
- Previous trauma
- Chronic or recurrent sinusitis or allergic rhinitis
- Cocaine or topical decongestant use: this may increase the risk of septal perforation.

◆ Physical Exam

The exam is generally focused, depending on the chief complaint. Some important points of inquiry to include are listed here.

Aging Face

- Hairline and hairstyle: these frequently affect the choice of technique for both browlift and facelift. A receding hairline in a patient who does not always have bangs covering the forehead, for example, will warrant a discussion regarding whether or not to perform a browlift, and if so, which technique. The position of the temporal hairline will influence the placement of facelift incisions.
- Lower lid laxity: the snap-back, inferior distraction, and lateral distraction tests should be documented. The tone and support of the lower lid have profound implications for choices of blepharoplasty, midface lift, and other cosmetic procedures.
- Skin quality: fine wrinkling and irregular pigmentation and vascularity are not addressed with lifting procedures, and alternatives should be discussed with the patient.
- Bony anatomy: the relationship of mandibular projection and hyoid position should be documented and discussed with the patient.

Rhinoplasty

- A detailed nasal and facial exam is important, including each of the analyses of the nasal proportions. This is beyond the scope of this text.
- Bony anatomy, including the length of the nasal bones: shorter bones provide less support to the midvault and thus imply potentially greater surgical risk.
- Skin and soft tissue envelope thickness: patients must be educated about the unique characteristics of their nose. The technical strategies used intraoperatively with patients at either extreme (very thin vs thick skin) are profoundly different.
- Size, orientation, and rigidity of lower lateral cartilages
- Chin projection

Facial Reanimation

- Corneal exam: this is critically important. Patients with diminished sensation are at increased risk of corneal desiccation.
- Previous history of dry eye
- Bell phenomenon: this is protective.
- Contralateral smile pattern: this is important to document, as the goals will be to modify both sides of the face as necessary to improve symmetry.
- Synkinetic pattern, if present

Facial Trauma

- Document a thorough cranial nerve exam.
- Eye exam should include extraocular movements; consider an ophthalmology referral.
- Dental occlusion
- Check for septal hematoma.
- Midface stability
- Neck crepitus
- Hemotympanum

Imaging studies are not often necessary in facial plastic and reconstructive surgery. Exceptions include computed tomography scans for facial fractures, electromyograms for some cases of facial paralysis, and magnetic resonance angiograms for fibula free flaps.

Suggested Reading

Papel ID. Facial Plastic and Reconstructive Surgery. 3rd ed. New York and Stuttgart: Thieme Medical Publishers; 2009

7 The State of the Art in Head and Neck Imaging

Pina C. Sanelli, Carl E. Johnson, and Sasan Karimi

This chapter will provide the clinician with an understanding of the basic principles and clinical applications of head and neck imaging. The discussion focuses on computed tomography (CT), magnetic resonance imaging (MRI), and positron emission tomography (PET), which are commonly used in the evaluation of otolaryngologic diseases.

◆ Computed Tomography

CT scanning has had a major impact on the diagnosis and management of otolaryngologic diseases. The use of computers to reconstruct radiograph attenuation data into an image allows the clinician to evaluate the anatomy and pathology from many different angles without overlying anatomical structures and to adjust the image contrast for better visualization of soft tissue and osseous pathology. There are continued advances in computer software allowing three-dimensional visualization of anatomical details and pathologic processes.

Basic Principles

CT provides high-resolution imaging using ionizing radiation. The x-ray tube delivers photons in a collimated beam to the patient, which represents the slice thickness of the image. The tube is linked to multiple detectors that collect these photons at a different rate of intensity, depending on the degree of absorption through the patient. It is rotated at many different angles to obtain different absorption patterns across various rays through a single slab of the patient. Current CT scanners have circumferential detectors moving in a 360-degree arc with continuous data acquisition and gantry rotation. Images are created through a mathematical reconstruction algorithm called filtered backprojection that adjusts the visibility of quantum mottle in images, known as "image noise." The filtered backprojection algorithms can be customized to adjust the image noise and resolution for optimal evaluation of soft tissue or bone.

Image interpretation and analysis are based on the qualitative observation of the different absorption values for various organs and their pathology. Quantitative absorption values can be obtained for each region of interest within a slice, referred to as Hounsfield units (HU). The scale for CT absorption generally ranges from +1000 to –1000 HU. The calculation of HU measurements are relative to water (designated as a zero value). Dense cortical bone measures approximately +1000 HU, and air measures –1000 HU. Generally, acute blood ranges from 56 to 76 HU, calcification is 140 to 200 HU, and fat is –30 to –100 HU. Metallic objects are at the highest HU range. Structures containing high protein concentrations will also have higher HU measurements in the range of clotted blood, such as tenacious sinus secretions, proteinaceous cysts, and the lens of the eye. CT absorption values that measure < 0 are mostly limited to air in the sinuses and fat in the neck and orbits.

Intravenous administration of contrast is used in otolaryngologic imaging for improved detection and further evaluation of pathologic processes. Contrast enhancement improves detection of normal-enhancing structures, such as blood vessels in the neck, to determine their location and pathologic involvement. Pathologic processes, such as infection, inflammation, and neoplasms, will demonstrate variable uptake of contrast depending on the vascularity and permeability of these vessels. The delivery of contrast to the intravascular compartment will also affect the degree of contrast enhancement for both normal and pathologic processes.

Advantages

CT remains the preferred modality for clinical use in otolaryngologic imaging because of its many advantages. CT has widespread availability throughout academic, community, and private practices, with prompt accessibility 24 hours a day without prolonged scheduling delays, allowing for immediate imaging in the emergency setting. Critically ill and claustrophobic patients are able to tolerate CT imaging because of its rapid image acquisition time and patient accessibility. Patients who are not able to undergo MRI due to incompatibility from indwelling devices, such as pacemakers, inferior vena cava filters, and mechanical pumps, are candidates for CT scanning. There are few patient contraindications for CT scanning. In comparison to MRI, CT has the ability to limit image distortion artifact from surgical clips or implantable devices by changing the angle or level of scanning.

There are software programs available for quick and easy postprocessing of the acquired images to aid in the visualization and interpretation of otolaryngologic diseases. Helical scanning allows for the volume of tissue scanned to be further reconstructed into thinner sections or imaging planes, known as multiple planar reformats. Reconstructions can be performed in any imaging plane with varying degrees of obliquity to obtain specific information. An example is the Poschl view of the petrous temporal bone used to visualize the bony covering of the superior semicircular canal. There are different reconstruction algorithms that also can be applied to highlight a particular tissue or organ. Bone disease is best visualized with a bone, edge, or detail algorithm to accentuate the interface between the bone and soft tissue. This can be particularly important in providing detailed bony anatomy needed for temporal bone, skull base, and sinus imaging. Any algorithm or reconstruction can be applied to the acquired CT data, which may be saved temporarily or permanently, depending on available storage space, for future use.

Viewing images may be performed with different window widths and levels to accentuate the differences in the CT absorption values between normal structures and their pathologic processes. Window width refers to the HU range selected for gray scale display, and the widow level refers to the center point at which the range is displayed. To visualize tissues with wide variations in CT attenuation, as in bone versus air, a larger width of 2000 to 3000 HU and a level of 300 to 600 HU are used. To visualize subtle differences in soft tissues, a smaller width of 80 to 400 HU and a level of 20 to 80 HU are recommended. The window width and level settings can be adjusted manually for each image to obtain optimal visualization.

Disadvantages

There are recognized disadvantages to CT scanning, mainly due to its use of ionizing radiation and iodinated contrast administration. In the past decade, tremendous advances in CT technology and applications have increased its clinical utilization, creating concerns about individual and population doses of ionizing radiation. The most radiosensitive organs in the head are the lens of the eye and skin, with the greatest concern for early cataract formation and permanent skin damage, respectively. With assistance from the American College of Radiology, Radiologists and Diagnostic Imaging Physicists, scanning protocols are continually adjusted according to the ALARA (as low as reasonably achievable) principle to minimize patient radiation exposure while maintaining optimal image quality. Mechanisms used for dose reduction include adjusting x-ray beam filtration and collimation, x-ray tube current modulation and adaptation for a patient's body habitus, peak kilovoltage optimization, improved detection system efficiency, and noise reduction algorithms. To further limit radiation exposure to the lens, CT scanning protocols should avoid including the orbits in the scanning field of view when appropriate. Other measures to limit total radiation exposure to patients have been employed in otolaryngologic imaging by using high-resolution helical scanning only in the axial plane, then performing reformations to avoid the additional radiation dose from direct coronal or sagittal imaging. This has been applicable particularly for imaging the petrous temporal bone, sinuses, and orbits.

The additional patient risks from exposure to iodinated contrast are considered low. Overall, intravenous administration of iodinated contrast is considered safe, with severe or life-threatening reactions rare. Immediate adverse reactions are classified as idiosyncratic or nonidiosyncratic. Idiosyncratic reactions resemble allergic or hypersensitivity reactions that are unpredictable and independent of dose, categorized as mild, moderate, or severe. Severe reactions are potentially life-threatening, with development of hypotension, cardiac arrhythmias, bronchospasm, laryngeal edema, pulmonary edema, and respiratory arrest. Nonidiosyncratic reactions reflect the physiologic effects of contrast media and direct organ toxicity. These are predictable, dose-dependent reactions, including sensations of warmth, a metallic taste in the mouth, bradycardia, vasovagal reactions, and neuropathy. Known risk factors include previous reaction to iodinated contrast, multiple allergies, and asthma. Precautionary measures are recommended in patients identified at risk of contrast reactions with premedication using corticosteroids and antihistamines to reduce the risk of anaphylaxis.

Delayed adverse reactions from iodinated contrast include contrast-induced nephropathy, estimated to occur in 2 to 7% of all patients receiving a CT scan with contrast. Generally, contrast-induced nephropathy manifests as an elevation in serum creatinine concentration within the first 24 hours that reaches a peak by 3 to 7 days, then returns to baseline within 1 to 2 weeks. In rare cases, patients require temporary or permanent dialysis. Patients with normal renal function are at very low risk for contrast-induced nephropathy. Known risk factors include preexisting renal insufficiency, diabetes mellitus, dehydration, concurrent use of nephrotoxic drugs, a high contrast dose, age > 70 years, and cardiovascular disease. Recommended precautions include adequate hydration, which is the most important method for preventing contrast-induced nephropathy. Administration of acetylcysteine (Mucomyst) and use of iso-osmolar contrast agents may also be done as precautionary measures.

In summary, an overall risk–benefit assessment should be considered for patients prior to CT scanning. This is particularly recommended for the pediatric population, patients with identified risk factors, and patients requiring multiple or repeated CT examinations.

Clinical Applications

Overall, CT scanning is the primary modality used in otolaryngologic imaging. It is preferred for imaging of the petrous temporal bone, sinuses, and orbit, given its superior spatial resolution for anatomical details and improved diagnostic imaging of bone structures compared with other modalities, such as MRI and plain films. Presently, CT scanning has replaced plain films for the detection of fractures of the orbit, petrous temporal bone, maxilla, face, and skull.

CT imaging has a leading role in the evaluation of temporal bone disease for the external, middle, and inner ear. The high resolution of anatomical details, coupled with the ability to reformat the imaging plane into any obliquity, allows for optimal imaging of the temporal bone. For example, oblique planes can be reconstructed to obtain Poschl and Stenvers views to assess details of small structures, such as the superior semicircular canal and facial nerve canal, respectively. Another strength is the visualization and interpretation of temporal bone imaging in the challenging postoperative setting. Otologic procedures may extensively alter the appearance of the temporal bone with surgical removal of small middle ear structures or implantation of various prosthetic devices. The role of imaging with CT has been expanding in this area for accurately assessing the type and extent of the surgical changes and recognizing potential complications.

Evaluation of the sinonasal cavity and the sinus drainage patterns is better with CT scanning techniques. The components of the ostiomeatal complex—the maxillary antrum, infundibulum, hiatus semilunaris, uncinate process, middle turbinate, and meatus—are well seen in the coronal plane. The sphenoethmoidal recesses are best evaluated on axial imaging. Processes that affect the nasal cavity and its turbinates are commonly viewed in both the axial and coronal planes. However, sagittal reformats provide improved visualization of the lateral nasal wall.

CT and MRI have a complementary role in the evaluation of cranial nerve pathology and together offer a full picture of bone and soft tissue changes. CT can provide a road map of the skull base and facial bone anatomy preoperatively by depicting the neurovascular skull base foramina and canals. The effect of a lesion on the adjacent bone is useful in differentiating aggressive, rapidly growing processes from benign and indolent lesions. Malignant or aggressive processes may have a permeative or erosive appearance to the adjacent bone, whereas benign lesions may expand or remodel bone.

Evaluation of the soft tissue neck is commonly performed by both CT and MRI modalities. CT provides improved detection of retained foreign bodies that are radiopaque and contain metallic elements. However, wood and glass fragments with lower lead levels may be difficult to visualize. Additional clinical indications for CT scanning are superior detection of a salivary gland calculus and calcifications on noncontrast imaging. Generally, CT and MRI are fairly comparable in the infrahyoid neck regarding the information they can provide. The fat content in the neck allows for increased conspicuity and delineation of pathology on CT. However, the ability of MRI to differentiate tumor–muscle interfaces, skull base and intracranial invasion, and perineural spread makes it a highly desirable imaging modality for otolaryngologic diseases.

◆ Magnetic Resonance Imaging

MRI is able to provide excellent anatomical detail in the evaluation of the neck without the use of ionizing radiation. The use of MRI in the evaluation of the neck has grown because of technological advances that allow for more rapid acquisitions and the ability of MRI to provide information on tissue characterization and pathologic information not available with other imaging modalities.

Basic Principles

MR image formation depends on the interaction of an applied magnetic field, radiofrequency (RF) waves, and the electromagnetic activity of atomic nuclei containing an odd number of protons and neutrons, both of which have spins. MR-active nuclei have a net spin, which induces a magnetic field as the nucleus spins around its axis. Hydrogen nuclei, or protons, are most commonly used in clinical MRI because of their abundance. An externally applied magnetic field causes the nuclei to spin at a given frequency, referred to as precessing. Also, the nuclei align parallel or antiparallel to the external magnetic field, creating a net magnetization vector. When an RF pulse is applied, the net magnetization vector is flipped to a certain angle, usually 90 degrees or less, producing two magnetization vector components, longitudinal (T1) and transverse (T2) magnetization. The transverse magnetization precessing around a receiver coil induces a current, which is the MR signal. When the RF pulse is turned off, the protons realign with the external magnetic field through the process of T1 relaxation, in which longitudinal magnetization recovers. In MR pulse sequences, there are two key parameters, the repetition time (TR) between the application of the RF excitation pulses and the echo time (TE) between the application of the RF pulse and the peak of the signal detected (spin echo).

Image interpretation is based on the variations in T1, T2, and proton density differences in tissue contrast. MR pulse sequences can be altered to accentuate the T1 and T2 signal. Substances with high (hyperintense) signal intensity are "bright" or whiter on the MR images, whereas those with low (hypointense) signal intensity are "dark" or blacker on the MR images. Some expected T1 and T2 signal intensities for various tissues are given below.

T1-Weighted Images

- Dark: air, calcified tissue (stones, cartilage, bone), fast-flowing blood
- Low: collagenous tissue (scar, tendons, ligaments), high water content tissues (simple cysts or fluid collections, edema)
- Intermediate: proteinaceous tissue (abscesses, complex cysts)
- Bright: fat, some hemorrhage (methemoglobin), fatty bone marrow, contrast agents, slow-flowing blood

T2-Weighted Images

- Dark: air, calcified tissues (stones, cortical bone), fast-flowing blood
- Low to intermediate: collagenous tissue (scar, tendons, ligaments), muscle, cartilage
- Intermediate to bright: fat, fatty bone marrow
- Bright: high free water tissue (simple cysts, cerebrospinal fluid, some hemorrhages, extracellular methemoglobin)

The MR pulse sequences commonly used in clinical imaging of the neck include T1-weighted spin echo to emphasize the T1 tissue signal and T2-weighted multiple echo train spin echo (fast spin echo, turbo spin echo) to accentuate T2 signal characteristics of the tissue. In neck imaging, it is often desirable to suppress the high signal from fat in the neck. Suppression of signal from fat can be achieved through various techniques on both T1- and T2-weighted sequences. These include spin echo chemical shift fat suppression, which relies on the precessional frequency differences between fat and water, and inversion recovery techniques (STIR, or short T1 inversion recovery), in which the signal from fat is nulled by application of an inverting (180-degree) pulse. Fat suppression is routinely used following paramagnetic contrast administration to accentuate tissue enhancement. The high signal intensity (bright) fat found in the head and neck may mask enhancement, particularly in high fat-containing regions such as the parapharyngeal space. Other sequences that can have a role in MRI of the neck include diffusion-weighted imaging, in which movement of water protons is highlighted, and MR spectroscopy, in which tissue chemical composition can be investigated.

MR images of the neck are typically acquired at 5 mm slice thickness. Thinner images (1–3 mm) are obtained when imaging smaller structures, such as the internal auditory canals, or focused imaging of the larynx. Unlike CT, where multiplanar imaging is usually achieved through image reformatting, direct multiplanar imaging is the rule with MRI. Direct axial and coronal scans are routinely acquired, although sagittal or oblique planes may be obtained as needed. Scans are often obtained after injection of paramagnetic contrast agents (gadolinium chelates) following unenhanced T1- and T2-weighted imaging. Contrast is often useful in the evaluation of neoplastic, infectious, and inflammatory diseases.

Advantages

Some advantages of MRI are better soft tissue definition and characterization, better evaluation of bone marrow spaces, and ability to obtain spectroscopic data. CT is often the preferred imaging modality because of its greater ease of acquisition, as well as the fact that less effort is often required for confident interpretation of neck CT as compared with MRI. However, MRI is often superior in providing soft tissue definition compared with CT, particularly in regions absent of motion or other artifacts, such as the tongue and oral cavity. As a general rule, the closer the pathology is to the skull base, the more often MRI will delineate the disease to better advantage than CT. Consequently, MRI can be considered as a first imaging choice to evaluate the suprahyoid neck. In addition to the tongue, the parapharyngeal space, masticator space, nasopharynx, and salivary glands are perhaps better imaged initially with MRI.

Disadvantages

Limitations of MRI include its long imaging time with associated greater difficulty with patient compliance, its marked sensitivity to motion artifact and imaging artifact, and its incompatibility associated with metallic implants. Contraindications to MRI include cardiac pacemakers and implantable cardiac defibrillators. Most, though not all, implants are safe for MRI. Some metallic implants may be MRI incompatible or have relative contraindications, having specific hardware and imaging constraints. Consequently, metallic implants should be assessed on an individual basis. MRI is also not advisable with patients suffering from claustrophobia and seriously ill or multitrauma patients who require advanced monitoring or assisted ventilation.

Gadolinium contrast agents are generally very well tolerated, although rare allergic reactions do occur. Also, contrast should be used with caution in patients with renal impairment, particularly those with a glomerular filtration rate of < 30, because of the potential for developing nephrogenic systemic fibrosis.

Clinical Applications

Although there is controversy as to when to use MRI or CT of the neck, overall, MRI can be considered equivalent to CT in the evaluation of the head and neck. MRI is the preferred imaging modality for the assessment of nasopharyngeal carcinoma. It can better show skull base bone marrow tumor invasion and intracranial tumor spread. Associated perineural tumor spread is also best evaluated using MRI. Perineural tumor extension is more commonly associated with cutaneous head and neck malignancies, although it can be found with other tumors, especially adenoid cystic carcinoma.

MRI has an important role in the evaluation of the larynx, providing information complementary to CT. High T1 signal paraglottic fat provides excellent contrast for separating the false cords in the supraglottic larynx from the true cords. MRI is also sensitive for cartilage tumor invasion, although it is not as specific as CT. False-positive findings will be more common with MRI because reactive and inflammatory changes are associated with increased T2 signal and enhancement, similar to tumor invasion.

Evaluation for lymphadenopathy throughout the neck is more easily accomplished with CT, although MRI may provide important information on pathologic nodes that cannot be determined by CT because of its better contrast resolution. Diffusion-weighted MRI sequences are also useful for differentiating benign from malignant nodes and in discriminating malignant nodes of various pathologies.

MRI can provide important information concerning the resectability of neoplasms, particularly in deciding if a tumor can be classified as stage T4a or T4b. Overall, MRI has a higher sensitivity but lower specificity than CT. It can also provide useful information in differentiating recurrent tumor from posttreatment changes. MRI findings suggesting tumor include an enlarging enhancing infiltrating mass that is intermediate to high signal intensity on T2-weighted images. Abnormal soft tissue that has decreased T2 signal intensity suggests posttreatment scarring. Diffusion-weighted imaging may also be useful in differentiating recurrent or residual tumor from posttreatment changes, with tumor showing decreased water diffusion as compared with treatment changes. In both resectability issues and evaluation of the posttreatment neck, PET-CT is assuming an ever greater role.

MRI is of primary importance in the evaluation of the temporal bone, especially in patients with sensorineural hearing loss and facial nerve dysfunction. It is superior to CT in the evaluation of cerebellopontine angle masses and lesions in the internal auditory canals. High-resolution, thin-section T2-weighted sequences can demonstrate the anatomy of seventh and eighth nerves in the internal auditory canal and the anatomy of the membranous labyrinth. Enhanced images readily show inflammatory and neoplastic lesions in the internal auditory canal and membranous labyrinth. MRI is superior to CT for imaging hearing loss associated with an enlarged vestibular aqueduct or cochlear nerve abnormality. It is also the preferred modality for detecting labyrinth inflammatory disease and has an important role in imaging inner ear dysplasia. Inflammatory middle ear disease is also evaluated with MRI. Increased T2-weighted signal intensity related to retained fluid or mucosal disease and enhancement of granulation tissue are readily demonstrated using MRI, although CT provides osseous anatomy detail unavailable with MRI. Associated intracranial complications with inflammatory disease or tumor including venous sinus thrombosis can be better shown using MRI as compared with noncontrast CT. Diffusion-weighted sequences can differentiate recurrent cholesteatoma from granulation tissue. Petrous apex cholesterol granulomas are easily diagnosed on MRI with hyperintensity on T1- and T2-weighted sequences because of chronic blood products.

MRI and CT are complementary for the evaluation of paranasal sinus neoplasms, and a combination of these is often necessary to fully evaluate the tumor and its extent of spread. CT better demonstrates osseous anatomy and associated tumor osseous destruction or erosion associated with sinonasal neoplasms, whereas MRI has greater soft tissue resolution and contrast. Multiplanar images are usually obtained with thin-section (3 mm) T1- and high-resolution T2-weighted images, which should include the orbits and skull base to assess tumor extent. Specific identification of histologic tumor type is not possible on MRI, but squamous cell carcinomas and adenocarcinomas are commonly intermediate to hypointense compared with cerebral gray matter on T2-weighted images. Adenoid cystic carcinomas have variable signal intensity, perhaps related to their cellularity, cystic changes, and necrosis. Melanomas may be hyperintense on T1-weighted images with variable T2-weighted signal intensity. Tumors characteristically enhance following intravenous administration of contrast. MRI can better differentiate tumor from sinonasal retained secretions and mucosal disease. Tumor is most commonly relatively hypointense on T2-weighted images and enhance more uniformly relative to secretions and hyperplastic mucosa. Sinonasal secretions may have variable signal intensity because of variations in protein content, requiring both T1- and T2-weighted images for a complete evaluation. Although CT shows bone destruction to better advantage, MRI is more sensitive for showing skull base bone marrow infiltration, intracranial and dural tumor invasion, and perineural metastatic disease. MRI is also useful for investigating orbital tumor invasion, although CT has overall greater accuracy.

◆ Positron Emission Tomography

PET has become a valuable tool for the diagnosis of new and recurrent neoplasms in the head and neck. It is a functional imaging method using a radioactive agent for the detection of abnormal metabolism in pathologic processes. The combination of PET and CT imaging modalities allows for improved diagnostic accuracy of neoplastic diseases by providing correlation of the functional information with the anatomical imaging.

Basic Principles

PET scanners detect coincidence photons that are produced when a positron emitted by a radioactive element undergoes annihilation. These photons are detected by the PET scanner to form an image. The most common positron emitter used in PET imaging is fluorine 18 (^{18}F). The radioactive element is incorporated into a glucose analogue, 2-fluoro-2-deoxy-D-glucose (FDG). ^{18}F-FDG is taken up by metabolically active cells by glucose transporters in the cell membrane. Once ^{18}F-FDG undergoes phosphorylation to form ^{18}F-FDG-6-phosphate, it does not undergo further metabolism but instead accumulates in the cytoplasm, allowing for its detection on imaging.

PET imaging requires specific patient preparation. Because FDG is a glucose analogue, elevated serum glucose levels and the use of insulin have influence on the FDG uptake that can adversely affect the images. The patient's activity and speech need to be restricted prior to FDG administration to prevent unwanted muscular uptake that interferes with image interpretation.

Qualitative interpretation and semiquantitative assessment of the radiotracer uptake are obtained from the acquired PET data. The Standardized Uptake Value (SUV) is a measurement of the radiotracer uptake from a static (single point in time) PET image. The SUV is calculated from the amount of tracer activity in the tissue/injected radiotracer dose/patient weight. In general, malignant tumors have SUVs > 2.5 to 3.0, and normal tissues have SUVs in the range of 0.5 to 2.5. It should be noted that the range of SUVs designated for malignant and benign conditions overlap. Therefore, some benign lesions, such as infection and inflammatory conditions, may have markedly elevated SUV measurements mimicking malignancy.

Advantages

Given its limited availability, expense, and need for lengthy patient preparation, PET imaging is not the primary modality used for the evaluation and diagnosis of otolaryngologic diseases. However, PET imaging has many advantages compared with anatomical imaging modalities, such as CT, MRI, and ultrasound. PET is able to provide whole-body coverage in a single examination using only one dose of reactive agent. Artifacts on the images due to metallic hardware and issues of intravenous contrast administration are not a concern. One of the most important advantages of PET imaging is its superior diagnostic accuracy for the detection of neoplastic processes. In the detection of metastatic adenopathy, the sensitivity and specificity of CT are estimated at 57 to 82% and 47 to 90%, respectively; those for MRI are 80 to 88% and 41 to 79%, respectively. Although there is variable diagnostic accuracy of FDG-PET, the reported sensitivity is 90%, and specificity is 94%.

The combined approach of PET and CT imaging has led to the advantage of correlating the functional information with the anatomical imaging for more accurate localization and diagnosis of pathologic processes. The PET-CT scanner is basically a unit consisting of a PET and a CT that allows for imaging the patient at the same setting without needing to move the patient. The PET and CT images obtained from this type of scanner can be fused to provide superior anatomical localization compared with other types of image fusion protocols. Imaging with PET-CT also has the advantage of shorter imaging times, as CT data can be used to correct for attenuation of the PET images. Schöder et al (2004) showed that PET-CT is more accurate in depicting cancer and that it can alter patient care.

Disadvantages

Disadvantages of PET imaging include its high cost and limited availability in the community because it requires a cyclotron to produce the radioactive elements. Patient preparation and manufacturing of the FDG agent add to its inappropriateness as an imaging modality in emergent situations. Radiation exposure is also a factor to consider in these patients. Another shortfall of PET is the lack of adequate spatial resolution resulting in poor anatomical localization of smaller neoplasms. PET images can be fused with cross-sectional imaging performed at different times and settings to better localize hypermetabolic lesions. However, image fusion protocols suffer from several technical limitations and can be misleading at times. The advent of PET-CT has ameliorated anatomical localization of FGD avid lesions.

There are multiple limitations and pitfalls that one must be aware of to prevent false interpretation of the images. Normal physiologic uptake as with the salivary glands and normal lymphoid tissue, as well as muscular activity, can lead to false interpretation of the results. Increased FGD uptake can also occur with infection and inflammation, particularly in the irradiated and operative bed. Artifacts due to technical factors related to imaging and image processing can also be misleading. Brown fat, which is most commonly present in the neck of infants, children, and women, is metabolically active as well. Warthin tumor and pleomorphic adenomas even though benign are FDG avid. False-negative results may be seen with tumors that are slow growing and not very metabolically active, such as adenoid cystic carcinoma and low-grade lymphoma, particularly mucosa-associated lymphoid tissue (MALT) lymphoma. It is important to keep in mind that PET can be insensitive to small volumes of tumor, such as melanoma recurrence at the primary site.

Clinical Applications

Squamous cell carcinoma accounts for the overwhelming majority of malignant tumors of the head and neck, and ~60% of patients have advanced disease. The presence of nodal disease in patients with head and neck cancer has significant prognostic implications in addition to its impact on patient management. This is illustrated by a decrease in the overall 5-year survival rate of 65% for patients with N0 stage cancer to 29% for those with evidence of nodal disease. Therefore, an accurate assessment for nodal disease is critical for proper TNM (tumor-nodes-metastasis) staging.

An important utility of PET imaging has been shown in the evaluation of patients with cervical metastatic adenopathy from an unknown primary malignancy. The reported rates in detecting the unknown primary malignancy are variable in different studies and should be considered with caution because these results are highly dependent on clinical skills and the evaluation methodologies used. PET has been reported to be more accurate in detecting residual disease at the primary malignancy site. This is important, as early detection allows for change in treatment or salvage surgery for some neoplasms. PET is also more specific than CT or MRI in detecting residual lymph node metastases. PET can also aid in detecting distant metastases, because as many as 10% of patients with head and neck squamous cell carcinoma (HNSCCA) can have distant metastases at the time of initial diagnosis. This is also true for second primary malignancies, as patients with HNSCCA have an ~5% annual rate of developing a secondary primary in the upper aerodigestive tract.

The posttreatment follow-up evaluation of patients with head and neck malignancies can often be challenging with cross-sectional imaging (CT and MRI). Patients often have architectural distortion and scarring from surgery or edema and fibrosis following radiotherapy, which can significantly limit follow-up evaluation. Unlike CT and MRI, which rely on morphological and structural changes, FDG-PET provides the means for metabolic assessment. The rationale for PET imaging is that neoplasms are more metabolically active than normal tissue.

Increased soft tissue and muscular uptake following surgery and/or radiation treatment can lead to false-positive and -negative PET results. Therefore, it is crucial not to rely on PET imaging alone performed immediately following treatment. Recently, it has been suggested that early follow-up PET imaging (6–8 weeks) after completion of chemoradiation in patients with advanced HNSCCA can be accurate and identify those who might need additional treatment.

In patients with thyroid cancer with tumors that do not accumulate iodine 131, PET imaging can be used for staging and posttreatment follow-up. It also can be used and is approved by the Centers for Medicare and Medicaid Services for diagnosis, initial diagnosis, and restaging of most head and neck cancers. It has been shown to be useful for the evaluation of response to therapy.

Suggested Reading

Abdel Razek AA, Kandeel AY, Soliman N, et al. Role of diffusion-weighted echo-planar MR imaging in differentiation of residual or recurrent head and neck tumors and posttreatment changes. AJNR Am J Neuroradiol 2007;28(6):1146–1152

Adams S, Baum RP, Stuckensen T, Bitter K, Hör G. Prospective comparison of 18F-FDG PET with conventional imaging modalities (CT, MRI, US) in lymph node staging of head and neck cancer. Eur J Nucl Med 1998;25(9):1255–1260

Ak I, Stokkel MP, Pauwels EK. Positron emission tomography with 2-[18F]fluoro-2-deoxy-D-glucose in oncology: 2. The clinical value in detecting and staging primary tumours. J Cancer Res Clin Oncol 2000;126(10):560–574

Anzai Y, Carroll WR, Quint DJ, et al. Recurrence of head and neck cancer after surgery or irradiation: prospective comparison of 2-deoxy-2-[F-18]fluoro-D-glucose PET and MR imaging diagnoses. Radiology 1996;200(1):135–141

Becker M, Zbären P, Laeng H, Stoupis C, Porcellini B, Vock P. Neoplastic invasion of the laryngeal cartilage: comparison of MR imaging and CT with histopathologic correlation. Radiology 1995;194(3):661–669

Borges A, Casselman J. Imaging the cranial nerves: 1. Methodology, infectious and inflammatory, traumatic and congenital lesions. Eur Radiol 2007;17(8):2112–2125

Brooks SL. Computed tomography. Dent Clin North Am 1993;37(4):575–590

Bui KL, Horner JD, Herts BR, Einstein DM. Intravenous iodinated contrast agents: risks and problematic situations. Cleve Clin J Med 2007;74(5):361–364, 367

Chong VF, Khoo JB, Fan YF. Imaging of the nasopharynx and skull base. Neuroimaging Clin N Am 2004;14(4):695–719

Dailiana T, Chakeres D, Schmalbrock P, Williams P, Aletras A. High-resolution MR of the intraparotid facial nerve and parotid duct. AJNR Am J Neuroradiol 1997;18(1):165–172

Davidson HC. Imaging of the temporal bone. Neuroimaging Clin N Am 2004;14(4):721–760

Eisen MD, Yousem DM, Loevner LA, Thaler ER, Bilker WB, Goldberg AN. Preoperative imaging to predict orbital invasion by tumor. Head Neck 2000;22(5):456–462

Eisen MD, Yousem DM, Montone KT, et al. Use of preoperative MR to predict dural, perineural, and venous sinus invasion of skull base tumors. AJNR Am J Neuroradiol 1996;17(10):1937–1945

Fischbein NJ, A Assar OS, Caputo GR, et al. Clinical utility of positron emission tomography with 18F-fluorodeoxyglucose in detecting residual/recurrent squamous cell carcinoma of the head and neck. AJNR Am J Neuroradiol 1998;19(7):1189–1196

Ginsberg LE, De Monte F, Gillenwater AM. Greater superficial petrosal nerve: anatomy and MR findings in perineural tumor spread. AJNR Am J Neuroradiol 1996;17(2):389–393

Ginsberg LE. MR imaging of perineural tumor spread. Neuroimaging Clin N Am 2004;14(4):663–677

Goerres GW, Schmid DT, Bandhauer F, et al. Positron emission tomography in the early follow-up of advanced head and neck cancer. Arch Otolaryngol Head Neck Surg 2004;130(1):105–109, discussion 120–121

Goldman LW. Principles of CT and CT technology. J Nucl Med Technol 2007;35(3):115–128, quiz 129–130

Greenberg JJ, Oot RF, Wismer GL, et al. Cholesterol granuloma of the petrous apex: MR and CT evaluation. AJNR Am J Neuroradiol 1988;9(6):1205–1214

Greven KM, Williams DW III, McGuirt WF Sr, et al. Serial positron emission tomography scans following radiation therapy of patients with head and neck cancer. Head Neck 2001;23(11):942–946

Grossman RI, Yousem DM. Techniques in Neuroimaging In: Neuroradiology: The Requisites. 2nd ed. Philadelphia, PA: Mosby; 2003

Harnsberger HR, Dahlen RT, Shelton C, Gray SD, Parkin JL. Advanced techniques in magnetic resonance imaging in the evaluation of the large endolymphatic duct and sac syndrome. Laryngoscope 1995;105(10):1037–1042

Hasso AN, Lambert D. Magnetic resonance imaging of the paranasal sinuses and nasal cavities. Top Magn Reson Imaging 1994;6(4):209–223

Hermans R, Verwaerde L, De Schrijver T, Baert AL. CT and MR imaging in tumors of the tongue, tongue base, and floor of the mouth: a comparative study. J Belge Radiol 1994;77(2):78–83

Hounsfield GN. Computerized transverse axial scanning (tomography): 1. Description of system. Br J Radiol 1973;46(552):1016–1022

Ikeda K, Katoh T, Ha-Kawa SK, Iwai H, Yamashita T, Tanaka Y. The usefulness of MR in establishing the diagnosis of parotid pleomorphic adenoma. AJNR Am J Neuroradiol 1996;17(3):555–559

Ikeda M, Motoori K, Hanazawa T, et al. Warthin tumor of the parotid gland: diagnostic value of MR imaging with histopathologic correlation. AJNR Am J Neuroradiol 2004;25(7):1256–1262

Kapoor V, McCook BM, Torok FS. An introduction to PET-CT imaging. Radiographics 2004;24(2):523–543

Katzberg RW, Barrett BJ. Risk of iodinated contrast material—induced nephropathy with intravenous administration. Radiology 2007;243(3):622–628

Kau RJ, Alexiou C, Laubenbacher C, Werner M, Schwaiger M, Arnold W. Lymph node detection of head and neck squamous cell carcinomas by positron emission tomography with fluorodeoxyglucose F 18 in a routine clinical setting. Arch Otolaryngol Head Neck Surg 1999;125(12):1322–1328

Kim HS, Kim DI, Chung IH, Lee WS, Kim KY. Topographical relationship of the facial and vestibulocochlear nerves in the subarachnoid space and internal auditory canal. AJNR Am J Neuroradiol 1998;19(6):1155–1161

King AD, Ahuja AT, Yeung DKW, et al. Malignant cervical lymphadenopathy: diagnostic accuracy of diffusion-weighted MR imaging. Radiology 2007;245(3):806–813

King AD, Vlantis AC, Tsang RK, et al. Magnetic resonance imaging for the detection of nasopharyngeal carcinoma. AJNR Am J Neuroradiol 2006;27(6):1288–1291

Kostakoglu L, Agress H Jr, Goldsmith SJ. Clinical role of FDG PET in evaluation of cancer patients. Radiographics 2003;23(2):315–340, quiz 533

Kubota K, Yokoyama J, Yamaguchi K, et al. FDG-PET delayed imaging for the detection of head and neck cancer recurrence after radio-chemotherapy: comparison with MRI/CT. Eur J Nucl Med Mol Imaging 2004;31(4):590–595

Kuo PH, Kanal E, Abu-Alfa AK, Cowper SE. Gadolinium-based MR contrast agents and nephrogenic systemic fibrosis. Radiology 2007;242(3):647–649

Laszig R, Chang SO, Kubo T, et al. APSCI panel discussion 1: imaging and surgical issues. Ear Hear 2007;28(2, Suppl):119S–123S

Loevner LA, Sonners AI. Imaging of neoplasms of the paranasal sinuses. Neuroimaging Clin N Am 2004;14(4):625–646

Lufkin RB, Borges A, Villablanca P. Teaching Atlas of Head and Neck Imaging. New York: Thieme Medical Publishers; 2000

Maheshwari S, Mukherji SK. Diffusion-weighted imaging for differentiating recurrent cholesteatoma from granulation tissue after mastoidectomy: case report. AJNR Am J Neuroradiol 2002;23(5):847–849

McCollough CH, Bruesewitz MR, Kofler JM Jr. CT dose reduction and dose management tools: overview of available options. Radiographics 2006;26(2):503–512

McGuirt WF, Greven KM, Keyes JW Jr, et al. Positron emission tomography in the evaluation of laryngeal carcinoma. Ann Otol Rhinol Laryngol 1995;104(4 Pt 1):274–278

Mukherji SK, Mancuso AA, Kotzur IM, et al. CT of the temporal bone: findings after mastoidectomy, ossicular reconstruction, and cochlear implantation. AJR Am J Roentgenol 1994;163(6):1467–1471

Myers LL, Wax MK, Nabi H, Simpson GT, Lamonica D. Positron emission tomography in the evaluation of the N0 neck. Laryngoscope 1998;108(2):232–236

Powitzky ES, Hayman LA, Bartling SH, Chau J, Gupta R, Shukla V. High-resolution computed tomography of temporal bone: 3. Axial postoperative anatomy. J Comput Assist Tomogr 2006;30(2):337–343

Rao AG, Weissman JL. Imaging of postoperative middle ear, mastoid, and external auditory canal. Semin Ultrasound CT MR 2002;23(6):460–465

Rohren EM, Turkington TG, Coleman RE. Clinical applications of PET in oncology. Radiology 2004;231(2):305–332

Schmalfuss IM, Tart RP, Mukherji S, Mancuso AA. Perineural tumor spread along the auriculotemporal nerve. AJNR Am J Neuroradiol 2002;23(2):303–311

Schöder H, Yeung HW. Positron emission imaging of head and neck cancer, including thyroid carcinoma. Semin Nucl Med 2004;34(3):180–197

Schöder H, Yeung HW, Gonen M, Kraus D, Larson SM. Head and neck cancer: clinical usefulness and accuracy of PET/CT image fusion. Radiology 2004;231(1):65–72

Sharafuddin MJ, Diemer DP, Levine RS, Thomasson JL, Williams AL. A comparison of MR sequences for lesions of the parotid gland. AJNR Am J Neuroradiol 1995;16(9):1895–1902

Smith AB, Dillon WP, Gould R, Wintermark M. Radiation dose-reduction strategies for neuroradiology CT protocols. AJNR Am J Neuroradiol 2007;28(9):1628–1632

Som PM. The present controversy over the imaging method of choice for evaluating the soft tissues of the neck. AJNR Am J Neuroradiol 1997;18(10):1869–1872

Som PM, Curtin HD. Head and Neck Imaging. 4th ed. St. Louis, MO: Mosby; 2003

Som PM, Curtin HD. Lesions of the parapharyngeal space: role of MR imaging. Otolaryngol Clin North Am 1995;28(3):515–542

Som PM, Shapiro MD, Biller HF, Sasaki C, Lawson W. Sinonasal tumors and inflammatory tissues: differentiation with MR imaging. Radiology 1988;167(3):803–808

Srinivasan A, Dvorak R, Perni K, Rohrer S, Mukherji SK. Differentiation of benign and malignant pathology in the head and neck using 3T apparent diffusion coefficient values: early experience. AJNR Am J Neuroradiol 2008;29(1):40–44

Stambuk HE, Patel SG, Mosier KM, Wolden SL, Holodny AI. Nasopharyngeal carcinoma: recognizing the radiographic features in children. AJNR Am J Neuroradiol 2005;26(6):1575–1579

Sumi M, Kimura Y, Sumi T, Nakamura T. Diagnostic performance of MRI relative to CT for metastatic nodes of head and neck squamous cell carcinomas. J Magn Reson Imaging 2007;26(6):1626–1633

Sumi M, Sakihama N, Sumi T, et al. Discrimination of metastatic cervical lymph nodes with diffusion-weighted MR imaging in patients with head and neck cancer. AJNR Am J Neuroradiol 2003;24(8):1627–1634

Williams MT, Ayache D. Imaging of the postoperative middle ear. Eur Radiol 2004;14(3):482–495

Wong WL, Chevretton EB, McGurk M, et al. A prospective study of PET-FDG imaging for the assessment of head and neck squamous cell carcinoma. Clin Otolaryngol Allied Sci 1997;22(3):209–214

Yasumoto M, Shibuya H, Takeda M, Korenaga T. Squamous cell carcinoma of the oral cavity: MR findings and value of T1- versus T2-weighted fast spin-echo images. AJR Am J Roentgenol 1995;164(4):981–987

Yeung HW, Grewal RK, Gonen M, Schöder H, Larson SM. Patterns of (18)F-FDG uptake in adipose tissue and muscle: a potential source of false-positives for PET. J Nucl Med 2003;44(11):1789–1796

Yousem DM, Gad K, Tufano RP. Resectability issues with head and neck cancer. AJNR Am J Neuroradiol 2006;27(10):2024–2036

Yousem DM, Li C, Montone KT, et al. Primary malignant melanoma of the sinonasal cavity: MR imaging evaluation. Radiographics 1996;16(5):1101–1110

Yousem DM, Tufano RP. Laryngeal imaging. Neuroimaging Clin N Am 2004;14(4):611–624

8 Positron Emission Tomography–Computed Tomography for the Head and Neck

Lee A. Zimmer

Over the last 10 years, several technological advances have improved the treatment of patients in the realm of head and neck cancer and endoscopic cranial base surgery. Combining computed tomography (CT) with positron emission tomography (PET) has improved the medical management and posttreatment surveillance of patients with squamous cell carcinoma (SCCa) and other malignancies of the head and neck. This technology has the promise of accurately detecting response to nonsurgical therapies and identifying persistent or recurrent disease that is not detectable by physical examination alone.

◆ Positron Emission Tomography

Since the discovery that radioactive elements such as fluorine 18 (^{18}F) can be substituted in organic molecules, radioactive materials have been used in medical diagnosis and treatment. The fact that malignant tumors have increased glycolysis (the degradation of sugar for energy) allows the use of 2-fluoro-2-deoxy-D-glucose (^{18}F-FDG) as a marker for tumor activity. Since the early 1990s, researchers have used ^{18}F-FDG with PET for the identification of head and neck SCCa. Although excellent for identifying the presence of disease, PET does not allow a precise anatomical evaluation of the tumor site. In 2000, PET was combined with CT (PET-CT) images on a single acquisition platform to provide both tumor identification and anatomical detail (**Fig. 8.1**). PET-CT has multiple applications for the identification, staging, and treatment of head and neck SCCa; however, there are several limitations.

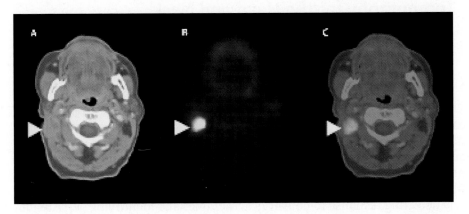

Fig. 8.1   **(A)** Axial computed tomography (CT) image without contrast at the level of the mandible showing a large right level II lymph node (*arrowhead*). **(B)** Axial positron emission tomography (PET) image at the level of the mandible in the same patient showing 2-fluoro-2-deoxy-D-glucose (FDG) uptake in the right level II lymph node (*arrowhead*). **(C)** Axial combined PET-CT image at the level of the mandible in the same patient showing FDG uptake in the right neck consistent with a metastatic level II lymph node.

◆ Evaluation and Treatment Planning

Patients presenting with a head and neck SCCa require appropriate staging for treatment planning. Staging requires a detailed evaluation of the primary tumor site (T stage), the nodes (N stage), and metastatic sites (M stage), such as the lungs and liver. The combination of T, N, and M staging allows the physician to formulate a treatment plan and to educate the patient as to the success of treatment.

A thorough history and physical examination, including imaging modalities, are required to stage SCCa. Multiple studies have shown that PET and PET-CT images have no advantage over traditional CT and magnetic resonance imaging (MRI) for evaluation of the primary tumor. The surgical oncologist gains little or no additional information about the primary tumor for surgical planning. However, a pretreatment PET allows the medical and radiation oncologist to follow tumor response to nonsurgical modalities (see discussion below).

PET and PET-CT may have a role in identifying local or distant spread of SCCa prior to treatment. This knowledge may alter treatment planning by including or excluding either surgical or nonsurgical treatment regimens. Recent studies have shown a superiority of PET in identifying local (neck) and distant metastasis compared with CT and MRI. Indeed, PET has on average a 10 to 20% better chance of identifying tumor spread to the neck or lungs than traditional imaging modalities. Furthermore, PET has a very low false-negative rate (< 10%). Thus, the lack of ^{18}F-FDG uptake in the neck, lungs, and liver is an accurate reflection that the primary tumor has not spread to other anatomical regions. The low false-negative rate of PET should be taken with caution, though, as PET cannot detect lesions < 5 mm, leaving room for false-negative results.

A difficult clinical situation is the patient with a large neck mass containing an SCCa with an unknown primary mucosal lesion in the head and neck. The majority of primary tumors in this scenario originate in the Waldeyer ring (base of tongue, tonsil, or nasopharynx), although one cannot discount the possibility of neck metastasis from a cutaneous malignancy on the scalp, ears, or face (**Fig. 8.2**). Although PET showed initial promise for identifying unknown primary tumors in the head and neck, more recent studies have shown little efficacy of PET in this clinical setting compared with a thorough physical examination and a direct laryngoscopy with tonsillectomy in the operating room. This may be attributed to the limited resolution of PET due to the high uptake of ^{18}F-FDG on PET in the Waldeyer ring.

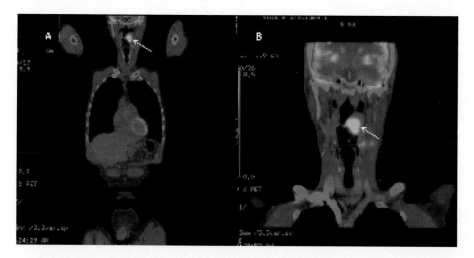

Fig. 8.2   **(A)** Coronal combined PET-CT whole-body image of a patient with squamous cell carcinoma (SCCa) of the left tonsil (*arrow*). **(B)** Higher magnification of the coronal image in **Fig. 8.2A** showing FDG uptake in the left tonsil (*arrow*).

◆ Positron Emission Tomography Use by the Medical and Radiation Oncologist

PET-CT can be used to plan radiation fields or conformational intensity-modulated radiation therapy (IMRT). IMRT allows the targeting of high-dose radiation to the primary tumor site, limiting radiation damage to normal tissues. PET-CT combines the identification of tumor with ^{18}F-FDG with the anatomical sensitivity of CT. Thus, if a tumor involves only a portion of the larynx, PET-CT would allow the radiation oncologist to target the diseased tissue. Recent studies have confirmed that PET-CT planning can limit the total exposure of tissues to high-dose radiation compared with CT imaging alone. Furthermore, the response of tumor to radiation can be followed closely with postradiation surveillance imaging. Although the timing of the posttreatment imaging is still in question, most studies agree that images can be obtained 8 to 12 weeks following radiation therapy.

For patients undergoing an organ-sparing protocol, a pretreatment FDG-PET may also allow the medical and radiation oncologist to monitor the primary tumor's response to chemotherapy and/or radiotherapy (**Fig. 8.3**). This information can be used in several ways. For patients receiving neoadjuvant chemotherapy, a PET scan performed after the first dose of chemotherapy may indicate tumor response. If a response is noted, further chemoradiation is provided. If not, the patient is shifted to a surgical protocol. A second PET is obtained 8 to 12 weeks after completion of chemoradiation to assess for a complete response. For concurrent chemoradiation, a posttreatment PET is obtained 8 to 12 weeks after the completion of therapy. Any persistent disease is then treated with surgery.

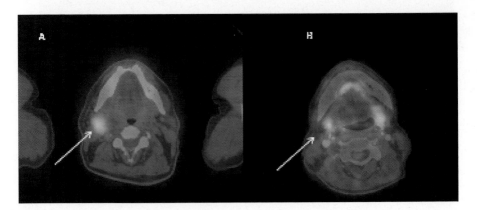

Fig. 8.3 **(A)** Axial PET-CT image at the level of the mandible showing FDG uptake in a right level II lymph node (*arrow*) prior to chemotherapy and radiation for a stage T1N2aMx SCCa of the left base of the tongue. **(B)** Axial PET-CT image at the level of the mandible in the same patient 8 weeks after the completion of chemotherapy and radiation. Note the absence of FDG uptake in the right neck (*arrow*).

There is considerable controversy concerning the role of routine neck dissection following definitive chemotherapy for patients with N2–N3-positive SCCa. Before PET, most surgeons and medical oncologists agreed that a therapeutic neck dissection should be performed following chemoradiation in this setting. Recent evidence suggests that PET has an excellent false-negative rate (5–10%) and reasonable false-positive rate (30–40%) in this scenario. PET therefore may be able to decrease the need for neck dissection in this population. Further prospective studies are currently under way to evaluate this possibility.

◆ General Surveillance

Surgical and radiologic treatment of SCCa of the head and neck causes tissue defects that distort normal anatomy and tissue planes. These changes can make the identification of tumor persistence or recurrence challenging with traditional imaging technologies. The specific uptake of ^{18}F-FDG by PET in this setting may increase the identification of tumor persistence or recurrence. Furthermore, the anatomical advantage of PET-CT may help guide further therapy. PET adds the promise of early tumor recurrence identification and the possibility of further surgical treatment. Studies have shown that PET can decrease the time for identifying recurrent disease within 14 months.

◆ Time Frame for ^{18}F-FDG–Positron Emission Tomography in Head and Neck Squamous Cell Carcinoma

Whenever a new technology is introduced to identify a cancer, questions arise as to when to use the modality, how often, and when to stop using it. PET is no exception. As noted above, a pretreatment PET-CT can help stage the initial tumor and allow the comparison of pre- and posttreatment therapies. It is clear from previous studies that a posttreatment PET-CT scan should be delayed for at least 8 weeks after medical or surgical treatment. This is due to the high false-positive rate that occurs with PET-CT in the first 8 weeks. The optimal time frame for the first posttreatment PET scan is 8 to 12 weeks.

An important point to evaluate is how often to use PET-CT imaging after definitive treatment. As mentioned above, the first imaging session should occur between 8 and 12 weeks of completing therapy. But then what? To date, there has been no definitive study evaluating the time frame for posttreatment PET surveillance. It is clear from the literature that most recurrences from head and neck SCCa occur in the first 24 months after treatment. Thus, the current recommendation is to obtain a PET surveillance study every 3 months until the 18th posttreatment month. It is assumed that PET would identify the majority of recurrences in this time frame. Further studies are warranted to test this protocol.

Suggested Reading

Beyer T, Townsend DW, Brun T, et al. A combined PET/CT scanner for clinical oncology. J Nucl Med 2000;41(8):1369–1379

Haberkorn U, Strauss LG, Reisser C, et al. Glucose uptake, perfusion, and cell proliferation in head and neck tumors: relation of positron emission tomography to flow cytometry. J Nucl Med 1991;32(8):1548–1555

Heron DE, Andrade RS, Flickinger J, et al. Hybrid PET-CT simulation for radiation treatment planning in head-and-neck cancers: a brief technical report. Int J Radiat Oncol Biol Phys 2004;60(5):1419–1424

Kole AC, Nieweg OE, Pruim J, et al. Detection of unknown occult primary tumors using positron emission tomography. Cancer 1998;82(6):1160–1166

Laubenbacher C, Saumweber D, Wagner-Manslau C, et al. Comparison of fluorine-18-fluorodeoxyglucose PET, MRI and endoscopy for staging head and neck squamous-cell carcinomas. J Nucl Med 1995;36(10):1747–1757

Myers LL, Wax MK, Nabi H, Simpson GT, Lamonica D. Positron emission tomography in the evaluation of the N0 neck. Laryngoscope 1998;108(2):232–236

Porceddu SV, Jarmolowski E, Hicks RJ, et al. Utility of positron emission tomography for the detection of disease in residual neck nodes after (chemo)radiotherapy in head and neck cancer. Head Neck 2005;27(3):175–181

Teknos TN, Rosenthal EL, Lee D, Taylor R, Marn CS. Positron emission tomography in the evaluation of stage III and IV head and neck cancer. Head Neck 2001;23(12):1056–1060

Terhaard CH, Bongers V, van Rijk PP, Hordijk GJ. F-18-fluoro-deoxy-glucose positron-emission tomography scanning in detection of local recurrence after radiotherapy for laryngeal/ pharyngeal cancer. Head Neck 2001;23(11):933–941

II Differential Diagnosis in Adult Otology and Neurotology

Section Editor: *Lawrence R. Lustig*

9 Unilateral Slowly Progressive Hearing Loss

Eric L. Slattery, Timothy E. Hullar, and Lawrence R. Lustig

Unilateral slowly progressive sensorineural hearing loss is perhaps one of the most common presentations of hearing loss. The key to differentiating the etiology is to determine how long hearing has been lost (days, weeks, months, or years), and whether or not there are any associated features, such as vertigo or other neurologic symptoms. Past history is important, particularly with regard to prior noise exposure. Radiographic evaluation is important for all cases of unilateral hearing loss to rule out a retrocochlear etiology, such as vestibular schwannoma.

◆ Sensorineural Hearing Loss: Inner Ear

Autoimmune Inner Ear Disease/Autoimmune Hearing Loss

Autoimmune hearing loss most commonly presents as a rapidly progressive (as opposed to sudden) hearing loss occurring over weeks to months. However, at times the hearing loss may be sudden. The sensorineural hearing loss may be associated with vestibular dysfunction and vertigo if the vestibular organs are also affected. There may also be symptoms or signs of a systemic autoimmune disorder, such as *relapsing polychondritis, rheumatoid arthritis, systemic lupus, Cogan syndrome,* or a *vasculitis.* Corticosteroids (systemic and/or parenteral) are used for treatment, and a beneficial response is also used to confirm the diagnosis. Laboratory testing for HSP (heat shock protein) 68 kD may be suggestive of the diagnosis but not pathognomonic. Although autoimmune hearing loss may be unilateral, it is usually bilateral.

Ototoxicity

The most common cochlear ototoxic medications are aminoglycoside and macrolide antibiotics, loop diuretics, quinine, and platinum chemotherapeutic compounds. Hearing loss from ototoxicity varies in its time course, depending on the offending ototoxic agent, and though usually slow and cumulative in onset, it may be sudden in some instances. With most aminoglycoside antibiotics, there is typically vestibular dysfunction before hearing loss. Otherwise, there are no other associated symptoms except tinnitus. Higher frequencies are affected first in ototoxicity, progressing to lower frequencies as the damage continues. As a result, screening for ototoxicity also involves testing of frequencies above 8 kHz. Although ototoxic sensorineural hearing loss may be unilateral, it is usually bilateral.

Meniere Disease

Patients with Meniere disease present with fluctuating, sudden, usually low-frequency sensorineural hearing loss in association with spells of vertigo, aural fullness, and roaring tinnitus. The diagnosis is made after excluding other potential etiologies, as there is no definitive test to identify the disease. In the early stages, the hearing will often be normal between spells, whereas in the later stages of the disease, there may be a permanent sensorineural hearing loss, which can occur gradually. Hearing loss may be unilateral or bilateral.

Radiation-Induced Inner Ear Injury

Radiation administered for nasopharyngeal, skull base, or intracranial pathologies may involve the inner ear. This can lead to both sensorineural hearing loss and tinnitus in one or both ears.

Hereditary Hearing Impairment

Most of the syndromic hereditary hearing impairments do not present as adults, and most are associated with comorbidities (this topic will be discussed further in section III). Nonsyndromic hereditary hearing loss, as seen in patients with connexin 26 anomalies, may present as adults. This is more commonly bilateral than unilateral.

Spirochetal Diseases

Both congenital and acquired *syphilis* may cause sensorineural hearing loss leading to deafness and tinnitus. One or both ears may be affected, with poor discrimination scores a hallmark in association with a progressive sensorineural hearing loss. Rarely, the hearing loss may present as a sudden deafness. Vestibular complaints are also commonly associated with the hearing loss. Diagnosis is based on the history and presence of associated symptoms of syphilis and suggested by serologic testing (the fluorescent treponemal antibody absorption test), but cerebrospinal fluid (CSF) analysis may be required. Similarly, *Lyme disease* may lead to vertigo and fluctuating sensorineural hearing loss. Lyme disease would be expected only in endemic areas.

Collagen Vascular Diseases

Collagen vascular diseases may lead to dizziness, tinnitus, and sensorineural hearing loss. Usually otologic symptoms are a relatively minor and late manifestation of disease. Specific disease entities include:

- *Rheumatoid arthritis*
- *Polyarteritis nodosa*
- *Temporal arteritis*
- *Nonsyphilitic interstitial keratitis (Cogan syndrome)*
- *Dermatomyositis*

- *Scleroderma*
- *Disseminated lupus erythematosus*
- *Wegener granulomatosis*
- *Rheumatic fever*
- *Relapsing polychondritis*
- Rare otic capsule bony diseases
  - *Paget disease*
  - *Fibrous dysplasia*

◆ Sensorineural Hearing Loss: Intracranial

Vestibular Schwannoma or Other Cerebellopontine Angle Tumor

A vestibular schwannoma (acoustic neuroma) may present as a slowly progressive hearing loss or sudden hearing loss. It is often present in association with vestibular dysfunction by testing, but not by symptoms. Patients usually report unilateral tinnitus. Other cranial neuropathies might also be evident, including, most commonly, cranial nerve (CN) V (trigeminal), in the form of facial hypoesthesia or paresthesia, and CN VII. The classic pattern of hearing loss is sensorineural and asymmetric, often with speech scores worse than expected given pure tone thresholds. Some patients complain of sound distortion, rather than hearing loss. Although hearing loss is usually gradual, sudden sensorineural hearing loss is not an infrequent audiologic presentation of vestibular schwannomas despite the fact that these are slow-growing lesions. Rapid deterioration is often thought to be due to further compression of a minimally patent internal auditory artery by tumor, thereby leading to cochlear ischemia. The clinical presentation may be similar in other cerebellopontine angle tumors, such as meningiomas. Patients with the rare syndrome of *neurofibromatosis* 2 have bilateral acoustic neuromas and auditory symptoms.

Demyelinating Diseases (Multiple Sclerosis)

Multiple sclerosis (MS) is a degenerative central nervous system (CNS) disease whose etiology is unknown. Only a small percentage of patients with MS will develop hearing loss. Hearing loss is usually bilateral and high frequency, and speech discrimination scores are often poorer than would be expected based on the level of hearing loss. Less commonly, the hearing loss is unilateral or sudden. The time course for the hearing loss is often slow, but there may be sudden deteriorations. Associated symptoms include visual disturbances (diplopia, blurry vision), extremity weakness, cognitive impairment, and other CNS symptoms. Diagnosis is confirmed through magnetic resonance imaging (MRI) and CSF analysis.

Rare Intracranial and Skull Base Lesions

These lesions can also cause sensorineural hearing loss, but other neurologic symptoms are often present, including:

- *Sarcoidosis*
- *Idiopathic pachymeningitis*
- *Superficial siderosis of the CNS*
- *Intra-axial tumors*
- *Endolymphatic sac tumor*
- *Petrous apex cholesterol granuloma*
- *Petrous apex mucocele*

◆ Conductive Hearing Loss: External Auditory Canal

Cerumen Impaction

Cerumen impaction rarely leads to a significant hearing loss, but if severe enough over time, a conductive hearing loss can arise in either one or both ears. Long-standing impaction may lead to aural pruritis and even otalgia. The diagnosis of cerumen impaction is easily made by inspection of the external auditory canal. Although accumulation of cerumen is a slow process, a patient may perceive a sudden hearing loss, often when getting the ear wet after swimming or bathing.

Exostosis and Osteoma

Osteomas and exostoses are slow-growing bony lesions of the external auditory canal that may be multiple. Typically, osteomas are single and have a narrow stalk. Exostoses are usually multiple, often bilateral, and have a broader base of attachment. Exostoses are often associated with swimming in cold water. If these lesions grow to an adequate size, a conductive hearing loss can develop. The lesions have a characteristic appearance and are covered with normal, uninflamed skin.

External Auditory Canal Cholesteatoma

In the case of external auditory canal cholesteatoma, purulent otorrhea may be admixed with keratin debris, and after suctioning, the external auditory canal skin may be found to be hyperkeratinized. Cholesteatomas may present anywhere in the ear canal, but they tend to occur in the inferior and posterior canal, just lateral to the annulus. Rarely, bloody otorrhea will be present. Patients may complain of pain, but this is not universal. There may be evidence of bony erosion of the external auditory canal as well. Hearing loss is due to debris accumulation and occurs slowly.

External Auditory Canal Tumors

External auditory canal tumors can arise from the skin of the external auditory canal, as in the case of:

- *Squamous cell carcinoma*
- *Basal cell carcinoma*
- *Melanoma*

In addition, tumors may arise from skin adnexal structures, such as:

- *Adenomatous tumor*
- *Adenocarcinoma*

The external auditory canal can be violated by regional tumors extending into this region, as in the case of a *glomus jugulare tumor* eroding through the floor of the external auditory canal. Any tumor in the external auditory canal can be fungating and produce purulent otorrhea. In addition, episodic bleeding from a tumor is not unusual. Tumors may be confined to the external auditory canal or may prolapse at the meatus. They may lead to hearing loss and facial paralysis over time.

Skull Base Osteomyelitis (Malignant or Necrotizing Otitis Externa)

Skull base osteomyelitis usually affects patients with diabetes mellitus or immunocompromised conditions. Patients will present with purulent or bloody otorrhea, otalgia, and often gradual onset hearing loss and tinnitus. If the osteomyelitis is more advanced, facial paresis may be present. In far advanced cases, lower cranial neuropathies could ensue, often followed by the patient's demise. On physical examination, granulation tissue and bony sequestrum may be present in the floor of the external auditory canal. Initial diagnosis can be further demonstrated on a radionuclide bone scan and by evidence of bone erosion on a high-resolution computed tomography (CT) scan of the temporal bones. MRI of the region may reveal regional enhancement with gadolinium.

◆ Conductive Hearing Loss: Middle Ear and Mastoid

Eustachian Tube Dysfunction

Eustachian tube dysfunction may lead to impaired mobility of the tympanic membrane and subsequent conductive hearing loss. Clinical manifestations usually include hearing loss in one or both ears. On physical examination, there may be retraction of the tympanic membrane or atelectasis onto the incus, stapes, or even the promontory. The evolution of these changes can take years, but acute eustachian tube dysfunction may be manifest after an upper respiratory infection or barotrauma associated with, for example, flying or scuba diving.

Tympanosclerosis

Tympanosclerosis is a chronic sclerosing process of the subepithelium of the middle ear, affecting the tympanic membrane and/or the ossicular chain in one or both ears. It is found in patients who have had recurrent otitis media. Other otologic symptoms of tinnitus, otorrhea, otalgia, or vertigo would not be expected. On examination, the tympanic membrane will become white and thickened, initially peripherally, and if progressive, the entire tympanic membrane can become involved. Tympanosclerotic plaques impairing the ossicular chain can only be well visualized through a tympanic membrane perforation.

Chronic Otitis Media

Chronic otitis media refers to a constellation of symptoms and signs resulting from chronic inflammation and infections of the middle ear and mastoid. The etiology is diverse, ranging from eustachian tube dysfunction to immune surveillance deficiencies. Symptoms may include recurrent purulent otorrhea that may be admixed with blood, hearing loss (conductive or mixed), otalgia, and aural fullness. In severe cases, facial nerve paralysis due to erosion of the fallopian canal or vertigo due to an inner ear fistula may also arise. Although the diagnosis is generally based on clinical presentation, it is supported by audiometric evaluation and high-resolution CT scanning.

Cholesteatoma

Cholesteatomas are slow-growing epithelial cysts that may be congenital or acquired. Though slow growing, they are destructive and may cause ossicular erosion and conductive hearing loss in one or both ears. Rarely, a cholesteatoma can lead to an otic capsule fistula and a sensorineural hearing loss. Cholesteatomas usually present with purulent otorrhea and hearing loss, but vertigo, tinnitus, and otalgia can occur as well. Bloody otorrhea can arise if concurrent granulation tissue is present. On physical examination, there is white keratinaceous debris that is characteristic in the external auditory canal. High-resolution CT scanning of the temporal bone can further define the extent of disease. Vertigo or disequilibrium can occur if the otic capsule structures become violated. Although cholesteatoma can erode the otic capsule at any site, this most frequently occurs with fistulization of the lateral semicircular canal. Facial paralysis can arise if there is erosion of the bone of the fallopian canal and neural compression and even degeneration.

Otosclerosis

Otosclerosis affects only the otic capsule and results in a slowly progressive conductive hearing loss as the oval window footplate becomes progressively more fixed from the otospongiotic changes that occur. Sensorineural hearing loss can occur if the process affects the bone surrounding the cochlea ("cochlear otosclerosis"). In either case, tinnitus may be present, and dizziness is rare. The pattern of hearing loss results in a characteristic bone conduction threshold "notch" at 2 kHz (Carhart notch), which deepens as the hearing loss progresses. Tympanometry typically demonstrates a type A shallow configuration and absent stapedial reflexes.

Middle Ear or Skull Base Tumor

Rarely, a middle ear tumor that blocks the eustachian tube or mastoid air cell system can lead to a secondary otitis media with resulting purulent otorrhea. In addition, these tumors may fungate and generate purulent or bloody otorrhea on their own. The presentation is typically a conductive hearing loss often with a tympanic membrane perforation and purulent otorrhea. With increased growth, facial paralysis may ensue. Diagnosis can be made before intervention in many cases based on the physical exam and radiographic features of the middle ear mass. Occasionally, however, the diagnosis is made unexpectedly during a mastoidectomy for chronic otitis media. These tumors may include:

- *Adenoma*
- *Carcinoid tumor*
- *Choristoma*
- *Glomus tympanicum tumor*
- *Eosinophilic granuloma (histiocytosis X)*
- *Schwannoma*
- *Rhabdomyosarcoma*
- *Leukemia*

In addition, tumors may arise from adjacent sites and extend into the middle ear and mastoid. From superiorly, these include:

- *Meningioma*
- *Facial nerve hemangioma*
- *Chondroblastoma*

From posteriorly:

- *Endolymphatic sac tumor*

From laterally:

- *Squamous cell carcinoma*
- *Basal cell carcinoma*
- *Melanoma*
- *Adenocarcinoma*

And from inferiorly:

- *Glomus jugulare tumor*
- *Jugular foramen schwannoma*
- *Jugular foramen meningioma*

◆ Conductive Hearing Loss: Inner Ear

Superior Semicircular Canal Dehiscence

Vertigo may result from superior canal dehiscence. Patients often present with pressure or noise-induced imbalance but can also have simply generalized imbalance. Other symptoms are autophony, conductive hearing loss, and conductive hypercusis. Symptoms are thought to be caused by the presence of a "third window." Vestibular evoked myogenic potential thresholds may be decreased in affected ears, and audiometric data often reveal a conductive hearing loss but hypernormal sensorineural hearing. Thin-slice CT often will detect a dehiscence, especially if custom sequences are performed in the plane of and orthogonal to the superior semicircular canal.

Suggested Reading

Brown SD, Hardisty-Hughes RE, Mburu P. Quiet as a mouse: dissecting the molecular and genetic basis of hearing. Nat Rev Genet 2008;9(4):277–290

Chen DA. Acoustic neuroma in a private neurotology practice: trends in demographics and practice patterns. Laryngoscope 2007;117(11):2003–2012

Cheng AG, Cunningham LL, Rubel EW. Mechanisms of hair cell death and protection. Curr Opin Otolaryngol Head Neck Surg 2005;13(6):343–348

Cureoglu S, Schachern PA, Ferlito A, Rinaldo A, Tsuprun V, Paparella MM. Otosclerosis: etiopathogenesis and histopathology. Am J Otolaryngol 2006;27(5):334–340

Ghossaini SN, Wazen JJ. An update on the surgical treatment of Ménière's diseases. J Am Acad Audiol 2006;17(1):38–44

Van Eyken E, Van Camp G, Van Laer L. The complexity of age-related hearing impairment: contributing environmental and genetic factors. Audiol Neurootol 2007;12(6):345–358

Yimtae K, Srirompotong S, Lertsukprasert K. Otosyphilis: a review of 85 cases. Otolaryngol Head Neck Surg 2007;136(1):67–71

10 Unilateral Sudden Hearing Loss

Eric L. Slattery, Timothy E. Hullar, and Lawrence R. Lustig

Unilateral sudden hearing loss is often dramatic and can cause the patient to urgently seek a medical consultation. Though often the result of benign disease, this symptom can nonetheless be the result of serious intracranial pathology, such as a tumor or acute vascular event. The associated symptoms and signs that may accompany the hearing loss will often provide clues to the diagnosis. In most cases, audiologic and imaging studies are required to pinpoint the diagnosis.

◆ Sensorineural Hearing Loss: Inner Ear

Idiopathic Sudden Sensorineural Hearing Loss

As the name implies, idiopathic sudden sensorineural hearing loss (ISSHL) presents with a sudden onset, unilateral sensorineural loss. By definition, the hearing loss should occur over three contiguous frequencies, in less than 3 days, with at least 30 dB of loss in each frequency. There are no other associated symptoms required for diagnosis, although patients often report concurrent or antecedent symptoms of an upper respiratory tract infection. A magnetic resonance imaging (MRI) scan is warranted, as rarely this presentation is caused by a skull base tumor, such as a vestibular schwannoma.

Barotrauma

Barotrauma may result from lifting a heavy weight, straining, scuba diving, flying in an unpressurized aircraft, or blunt trauma. It is also common in patients undergoing hyperbaric oxygen therapy. Barotrauma is more likely to occur in those with an acute upper respiratory infection. Otalgia is usually present, and if the tympanic membrane perforates, otorrhea may be present. Fluid and/or blood may also accumulate behind the drum, and the accumulation of blood (*hemotympanum*) will appear dark brown, purple, or red.

If a sensorineural hearing loss arises after one of these inciting pressure change events, several diagnoses must be entertained, including the presence of a *perilymphatic fistula* at the oval window, round window, or some other site. Dizziness and tinnitus will often accompany the sensorineural hearing loss. A fistula test with pneumatic otoscopy may be suggestive of this diagnosis, but there is no definitive diagnostic examination available, except for surgical exploration. Other possibilities *include inner ear membrane break* and *pneumolabyrinth* (usually from rapid ascent during diving).

Iatrogenic Injury

Iatrogenic middle and inner ear injury can result from minor surgeries (eg, myringotomy), middle ear and mastoid surgeries, and inner ear surgeries. Further iatrogenic injury can result from surgeries not directed toward the ear, including posterior and middle fossa craniotomies and regional head and neck surgeries, such as parotidectomies. If the trauma is limited to the external auditory canal, tympanic membrane, and/or ossicles, a sudden conductive hearing loss may ensue. If the trauma directly or indirectly injures the inner ear or auditory nerve, then sensorineural hearing loss would result. In either case, tinnitus, vertigo, otalgia, facial paralysis, and/or otorrhea could result as well.

Noise-Induced Hearing Loss

Unilateral sensorineural hearing loss is less common than bilateral hearing loss and implies that one ear was shielded from the offending noise. An example of this is a sudden sensorineural hearing loss associated with firing a rifle. In a right-handed individual, the right ear may be more protected because it is directly behind the blast noise arising from the muzzle of the rifle. Noise-induced hearing loss may be due to a single sudden event, or it may have a slow onset with less intense but frequently repeated noise insults to the inner ear.

Autoimmune Hearing Loss

Autoimmune hearing loss more commonly is slow and progressive, but it can be sudden (see Chapter 9).

Ototoxicity

Hearing loss caused by ototoxicity is usually bilateral, but it can be unilateral and sudden (see Chapter 9).

Meniere Disease

Hearing loss caused by Meniere disease more commonly is slow and progressive, but it can be sudden (see Chapter 9).

Spirochetal Diseases

Hearing loss caused by spirochetal diseases is often bilateral, but it can be unilateral (see Chapter 9).

Collagen Vascular Diseases

Hearing loss caused by collagen vascular diseases is often bilateral, but it can be unilateral (see Chapter 9).

◆ Sensorineural Hearing Loss: Intracranial

Meningitis

A common complication of meningitis is hearing loss.

Stroke (Cerebrovascular Accident)

An acute infarction of the anteroinferior cerebellar artery may result in a sudden and profound sensorineural hearing loss. There will nearly always be associated vertigo as well as other significant findings of central nervous system dysfunction. In cases of a transient ischemic attack, the loss may be temporary. In other cases of a cerebrovascular accident involving the central auditory pathways or centers, auditory perception or speech discrimination may be impaired in the setting of intact threshold detection.

Demyelinating Diseases

For information on hearing loss caused by demyelinating disease (eg, *multiple sclerosis*), see Chapter 9.

Vestibular Schwannoma or Other Cerebellopontine Angle Tumor

Hearing loss caused by a vestibular schwannoma or other cerebellopontine angle tumor is usually slow and progressive, but it may be sudden (see Chapter 9).

◆ Conductive Hearing Loss: External Auditory Canal

Cerumen Impaction

For a discussion on hearing loss resulting from cerumen impaction, refer to Chapter 9.

External Auditory Canal Foreign Body

A foreign body in the external auditory canal will typically cause otalgia, conductive hearing loss, and purulent or possibly bloody otorrhea. The presentation is most common in children and the mentally handicapped. Foreign bodies can range from small toys, to food (eg, peas), to insects, to hearing aid batteries. The diagnosis is made on otoscopy.

◆ Conductive Hearing Loss: Middle Ear and Mastoid

Eustachian Tube Dysfunction

See Chapter 9 for information on hearing loss that is caused by eustachian tube dysfunction.

Acute Otitis Media

The source of acute otitis media may be an upper respiratory infection arising from the nasal cavity. This can lead to eustachian tube dysfunction and middle ear effusion. If grossly infected, the effusion may be purulent, and increased middle ear pressure may result in a tympanic membrane rupture with subsequent otorrhea. When the tympanic membrane is intact, there is a hearing loss due to a decrease in the vibratory capacity of the tympanic membrane caused by the middle ear fluid. Associated symptoms include aural pressure, a crackling and popping sensation in the ear (particularly with swallowing), autophony, and otalgia. Examination reveals an opaque tympanic membrane and middle ear effusion. Audiometry demonstrates a conductive hearing loss and type B tympanogram.

If the tympanic membrane ruptures, there is a release of purulent otorrhea that may be admixed with blood. Patients often report relief of pain once the tympanic membrane perforates, relieving the pressure. Diagnosis is based on purulent drainage from a perforation in the tympanic membrane.

Facial paralysis due to acute otitis media may occur as a result of direct involvement of the nerve through preformed anatomical pathways.

Trauma

Depending on the mechanism of injury, the hearing loss from trauma may be conductive secondary to *ossicular disruption, hemotympanum* and impaired tympanic membrane mobility, or *a traumatic rupture of the tympanic membrane*; sensorineural hearing loss develops in the setting of a severe trauma, resulting in an *otic capsule concussion* or a *temporal bone fracture* involving the otic capsule. Trauma will be obvious on physical examination, with scalp ecchymosis or laceration. Bloody otorrhea, hemotympanum, and even a fracture line in the posterosuperior external auditory canal may be visible. With either conductive or sensorineural hearing loss, there may be associated vertigo or facial nerve paralysis. High-resolution computed tomography scanning of the temporal bone can aid in diagnosis with characteristic findings of incus subluxation in the case of conductive hearing loss and otic capsule fracture in the case of sensorineural hearing loss.

Suggested Reading

Banerjee A, Parnes LS. Intratympanic corticosteroids for sudden idiopathic sensorineural hearing loss. Otol Neurotol 2005;26(5):878–881

Conlin AE, Parnes LS. Treatment of sudden sensorineural hearing loss: 1. A systematic review. Arch Otolaryngol Head Neck Surg 2007;133(6):573–581

Lee H. Sudden deafness related to posterior circulation infarction in the territory of the nonanterior inferior cerebellar artery: frequency, origin, and vascular topographical pattern. Eur Neurol 2008;59(6):302–306

Myrseth E, Pedersen PH, Møller P, Lund-Johansen M. Treatment of vestibular schwannomas: why, when and how? Acta Neurochir (Wien) 2007;149(7):647–660, discussion 660

Ruben R. Bacterial meningitic deafness: historical development of epidemiology and cellular pathology. Acta Otolaryngol 2008;128(4):388–392

Yehudai D, Shoenfeld Y, Toubi E. The autoimmune characteristics of progressive or sudden sensorineural hearing loss. Autoimmunity 2006;39(2):153–158

11 Bilateral Slow-Onset Hearing Loss

Eric L. Slattery, Timothy E. Hullar, and Lawrence R. Lustig

Bilateral slow-onset hearing loss is one of the most common reasons patients visit an otolaryngologist. Often a thorough history, physical examination, and audiogram are all that is necessary to arrive at a working diagnosis.

◆ Sensorineural Hearing Loss: Inner Ear

Presbycusis

Presbycusis, or age-associated hearing loss, is the most common cause of bilateral slow-onset sensorineural hearing loss. It is prevalent over the age of 65 and becomes more common with increasing age. There may be tinnitus but no other associated symptoms. History and physical examination are otherwise normal.

Hereditary Hearing Impairment

See Chapter 9 for a discussion of hearing loss as a result of hereditary hearing impairment.

Noise-Induced Hearing Loss

See Chapter 10 for a discussion of noise-induced hearing loss.

Ototoxicity

See Chapter 9 for a discussion of hearing loss caused by ototoxicity.

Barotrauma

Hearing loss as a result of barotrauma may be unilateral (see Chapter 10).

Meniere Disease

Hearing loss resulting from Meniere disease has other associated symptoms and is rarely bilateral (see Chapter 9).

Autoimmune Hearing Loss

Autoimmune hearing loss is often unilateral (see Chapter 9).

Radiation-Induced Inner Ear Injury

Hearing loss resulting from radiation-induced inner ear injury is often unilateral (see Chapter 9).

Spirochetal Diseases

See Chapter 9 for a discussion of hearing loss caused by spirochetal diseases.

Collagen Vascular Disease

See Chapter 9 for a discussion of hearing loss that is caused by collagen vascular disease.

Rare Otic Capsule Bony Diseases

Rare otic capsule bony diseases, such as *Paget disease*, can result in hearing loss as well.

◆ Sensorineural Hearing Loss: Intracranial

Vestibular Schwannoma or Other Cerebellopontine Angle Tumor

Hearing loss caused by a vestibular schwannoma or other cerebellopontine angle tumor very rarely is bilateral (see Chapter 9).

Demyelinating Disease

See Chapter 9 for a discussion of hearing loss caused by a demyelinating disease, such as multiple sclerosis.

Meningitis

See Chapter 9 for information on hearing loss resulting from meningitis.

Rare Intracranial and Skull Base Lesions

Hearing loss can be symptomatic of rare intracranial and skull base lesions, such as

- *Sarcoidosis*
- *Idiopathic pachymeningitis*
- *Superficial siderosis of the central nervous system*

◆ Conductive Hearing Loss: External Auditory Canal

Cerumen Impaction

See Chapter 9 for information on hearing loss caused by cerumen impaction.

Exostosis and Osteoma

Chapter 9 includes information on hearing loss caused by exostoses and osteomas.

◆ Conductive Hearing Loss: Middle Ear and Mastoid

Tympanosclerosis

See Chapter 9 for a discussion of hearing loss resulting from tympanosclerosis.

Otosclerosis

Hearing loss from otosclerosis may be unilateral or bilateral (see Chapter 9).

Eustachian Tube Dysfunction

See Chapter 9 for information on hearing loss that is caused by eustachian tube dysfunction.

Cholesteatoma

Hearing loss resulting from a cholesteatoma is often unilateral (see Chapter 9).

Chronic Otitis Media

Hearing loss caused by chronic otitis media is often unilateral (see Chapter 9).

Trauma

Hearing loss brought on by trauma is often unilateral (see Chapter 10).

Suggested Reading

Chen DA. Acoustic neuroma in a private neurotology practice: trends in demographics and practice patterns. Laryngoscope 2007;117(11):2003–2012

Cheng AG, Cunningham LL, Rubel EW. Mechanisms of hair cell death and protection. Curr Opin Otolaryngol Head Neck Surg 2005;13(6):343–348

Cureoglu S, Schachern PA, Ferlito A, Rinaldo A, Tsuprun V, Paparella MM. Otosclerosis: etio-pathogenesis and histopathology. Am J Otolaryngol 2006;27(5):334–340

Ghossaini SN, Wazen JJ. An update on the surgical treatment of Ménière's diseases. J Am Acad Audiol 2006;17(1):38–44

Van Eyken E, Van Camp G, Van Laer L. The complexity of age-related hearing impairment: contributing environmental and genetic factors. Audiol Neurootol 2007;12(6):345–358

Yimtae K, Srirompotong S, Lertsukprasert K. Otosyphilis: a review of 85 cases. Otolaryngol Head Neck Surg 2007;136(1):67–71

12 Purulent Otorrhea

Eric L. Slattery, Timothy E. Hullar, and Lawrence R. Lustig

Purulent otorrhea may be the result of a variety of pathologies arising in the ear canal or middle ear. Although most of these causes are primarily due to an acute or chronic infectious problem, they may rarely be secondary to a more worrisome clinical entity, such as a tumor. As a result, a thorough investigation of the patient with purulent otorrhea is always warranted.

◆ External Auditory Canal Origin

External Auditory Canal Foreign Body

See Chapter 10 for a discussion of purulent otorrhea resulting from a foreign body in the external auditory canal.

Noninfectious Otitis Externa: Eczema, Psoriasis, and Seborrheic Dermatitis

Eczema, psoriasis, and *seborrheic dermatitis* are dermatologic conditions of the ear canal. Affected patients are often at risk for similar dermatitis on other parts of the body, although the ear canal may be the only region affected. Presenting symptoms are chronic aural pruritis, otorrhea, and, at times, otalgia. The ear canal skin may appear dry and flaky, and the external auditory meatus often appears thickened and narrowed. There can be acute bacterial otitis externa secondary to skin breakdown. There is often a complete absence of cerumen. If the cause is a contact dermatitis from the use of ear drops, then you may see a reddish streak along the front of the pinna, to the lobule, and onto the neck, where drops have drained out the ear.

Infectious Otitis Externa: Bacterial, Fungal, or Atypical Mycobacterium

Otitis externa is a common cause of purulent otorrhea and otalgia, and, at times, hearing loss. Examination reveals purulent otorrhea alone or, in the case of otomycosis, admixed with characteristic fungal hyphae. The otorrhea may be sent for culture, but regardless, it should be suctioned. This reveals edematous and erythematous external auditory canal skin with a normal-appearing tympanic membrane. The infections may be acute or chronic.

Radiation-Induced Chronic Otitis Externa

Radiation to the nasopharynx, skull base, or intracranial targets may damage the skin of the external auditory canal and the tympanic bone, resulting in a chronic state of infection and necrosis. Bone may be exposed on the floor of the external auditory canal, and there may be chronic bloody purulent otorrhea. There is usually no otalgia.

Skull Base Osteomyelitis: Malignant or Necrotizing Otitis Externa

Malignant or necrotizing otitis externa usually causes pain and hearing loss, although purulent otorrhea can be part of the presentation (see Chapter 9).

External Auditory Canal Cholesteatoma

See Chapter 9 for information on purulent otorrhea resulting from an external auditory canal cholesteatoma.

External Auditory Canal Tumor

Rarely, a tumor in the external auditory canal causes purulent otorrhea (see Chapter 9).

◆ Middle Ear and Mastoid Origin

Myringitis

Myringitis (inflammation or infection of the tympanic membrane) can lead to purulent otorrhea. Otalgia is typically the most common presentation. Otomicroscopy will demonstrate an inflamed tympanic membrane with increased vascularity and a granular appearance with associated purulent covering. It is distinguished from an acute otitis media by the presence of a normal middle ear, if this is visible through a portion of the tympanic membrane. Otorrhea may be purulent or bloody.

A variation of this entity is *bullous myringitis*, in which blisters form on the tympanic membrane; this is felt to be of viral origin. Bullous myringitis usually causes significant otalgia. Diagnosis of either entity is based on the physical examination and, if necessary, high-resolution computed tomography (CT) of the temporal bones, confirming a normal aerated middle ear.

Acute Otitis Media with Perforation

See Chapter 10 for information on purulent otorrhea resulting from acute otitis media with perforation.

Chronic Otitis Media

See Chapter 9 for information on purulent otorrhea caused by chronic otitis media.

Cholesteatoma

See Chapter 9 for information on purulent otorrhea that is caused by a cholesteatoma.

Middle Ear Tumor

See Chapter 9 for information on purulent otorrhea that results from a middle ear tumor.

Barotrauma

Barotrauma causes tympanic membrane perforation, intratympanic hemorrhage, middle ear effusion, or hemotympanum (see Chapter 10).

Encephalocele

A temporal lobe encephalocele into the middle ear or mastoid blocking the mastoid antrum can lead to mastoiditis. Furthermore, if the encephalocele begins to leak cerebrospinal fluid (CSF), the CSF otorrhea can become secondarily infected, again leading to purulent otorrhea, but with the added risk of meningitis. Rarely, the CSF may be bloody as well. Diagnosis is based on radiographic findings (both CT and magnetic resonance imaging), as well as a positive β_2-transferrin test of the otorrhea.

Suggested Reading

Bardanis J, Batzakakis D, Mamatas S. Types and causes of otorrhea. Auris Nasus Larynx 2003;30(3):253–257

Dohar JE. All that drains is not infectious otorrhea. Int J Pediatr Otorhinolaryngol 2003;67(4):417–420

Haynes DS, Rutka J, Hawke M, Roland PS. Ototoxicity of ototopical drops—an update. Otolaryngol Clin North Am 2007;40(3):669–683, xi

Heim SW, Maughan KL. Foreign bodies in the ear, nose, and throat. Am Fam Physician 2007;76(8):1185–1189

Isaacson G. Diagnosis of pediatric cholesteatoma. Pediatrics 2007;120(3):603–608

Neilson LJ, Hussain SS. Management of granular myringitis: a systematic review. J Laryngol Otol 2008;122(1):3–10

Osguthorpe JD, Nielsen DR. Otitis externa: review and clinical update. Am Fam Physician 2006;74(9):1510–1516

Papanikolaou V, Bibas A, Ferekidis E, Anagnostopoulou S, Xenellis J. Idiopathic temporal bone encephalocele. Skull Base 2007;17(5):311–316

Smith JA, Danner CJ. Complications of chronic otitis media and cholesteatoma. Otolaryngol Clin North Am 2006;39(6):1237–1255

13 Bloody Otorrhea

Eric L. Slattery, Timothy E. Hullar, and Lawrence R. Lustig

For most patients, bloody otorrhea is particularly frightening. Fortunately, it is usually due to a benign process. As with other pathologies within the head and neck, though, it can be the harbinger of a more serious diagnosis; thus, prompt examination is warranted. Clinical examination will usually distinguish between one of the many pathologies that give rise to bloody otorrhea.

◆ External Auditory Canal Origin

Trauma: External

See Chapter 10 for information on bloody otorrhea resulting from trauma to the external ear canal.

Iatrogenic Injury

Bloody otorrhea can be the result of an iatrogenic injury, such as that caused by an inserted foreign body (see Chapter 10).

Radiation-induced Chronic Otitis Externa

See Chapter 12 for information on radiation-induced chronic otitis externa.

Skull Base Osteomyelitis: Malignant or Necrotizing Otitis Externa

See Chapter 9 for a discussion of malignant or necrotizing otitis externa.

Foreign Body in the External Auditory Canal

See Chapter 10 for a discussion of otorrhea caused by a foreign body in the external auditory canal.

External Auditory Canal Cholesteatoma

See Chapter 9 for information on cholesteatoma in the external auditory canal.

External Auditory Canal Tumors

See Chapter 9 for a discussion of tumors in the external auditory canal.

◆ Middle Ear and Mastoid Origin

Myringitis

Bloody otorrhea can be symptomatic of inflammation of the tympanic membrane, or myringitis (see Chapter 12).

Acute Otitis Media

Acute otitis media is associated with otorrhea only if there is perforation of the tympanic membrane (see Chapter 10).

Chronic Otitis Media

Chronic otitis media is associated with otorrhea only if there is perforation of the tympanic membrane (see Chapter 9).

Cholesteatoma

Otorrhea as the result of a cholesteatoma is usually purulent and foul-smelling, but it may be bloody (see Chapter 9).

Barotrauma

Bloody otorrhea can be caused by perforation of the tympanic membrane, or perhaps myringitis or intratympanic hemorrhage (see Chapter 10).

Middle Ear Tumor

Otorrhea is rare in the case of tumor of the middle ear (see Chapter 9).

Encephalocele

Otorrhea is rare in the case of encephalocele, and it may be only watery cerebrospinal fluid (see Chapter 12).

Suggested Reading

Bardanis J, Batzakakis D, Mamatas S. Types and causes of otorrhea. Auris Nasus Larynx 2003;30(3):253–257

Conoyer JM, Kaylie DM, Jackson CG. Otologic surgery following ear trauma. Otolaryngol Head Neck Surg 2007;137(5):757–761

Lasak JM, Van Ess M, Kryzer TC, Cummings RJ. Middle ear injury through the external auditory canal: a review of 44 cases. Ear Nose Throat J 2006;85(11):722, 724–728

Little SC, Kesser BW. Radiographic classification of temporal bone fractures: clinical predictability using a new system. Arch Otolaryngol Head Neck Surg 2006;132(12):1300–1304

Neilson LJ, Hussain SS. Management of granular myringitis: a systematic review. J Laryngol Otol 2008;122(1):3–10

Okada K, Ito K, Yamasoba T, Ishii M, Iwasaki S, Kaga K. Benign mass lesions deep inside the temporal bone: imaging diagnosis for proper management. Acta Otolaryngol Suppl 2007;559(559):71–77

Rubin Grandis J, Branstetter BF IV, Yu VL. The changing face of malignant (necrotising) external otitis: clinical, radiological, and anatomic correlations. Lancet Infect Dis 2004;4(1):34–39

14 Itchy Ear

Eric L. Slattery, Timothy E. Hullar, and Lawrence R. Lustig

Aural pruritis, or itchy ear, is a chronic, indolent problem for many patients. It rarely is caused by serious pathology, but more commonly is the result of an irritative dermatitis or self-inflicted instrumentation of the canal (eg, use of cotton swabs). Scratching the ear canal in response to the itching will lead to more irritation and continued itching, resulting in a vicious scratch/itch cycle.

◆ Noninfectious Otitis Externa: Eczema, Psoriasis, and Seborrheic Dermatitis

See Chapter 12 for a discussion of noninfectious otitis externa.

◆ Cerumen Impaction

With cerumen impaction, the patient will experience fullness and perhaps the sensation of muffled hearing (see Chapter 9).

◆ Infectious Otitis Externa: Bacterial, Fungal, or Atypical Mycobacterium

In addition to itching as with that caused by noninfectious otitis externa, the patient will have pain, swelling, and perhaps hearing loss (see Chapter 12).

◆ Radiation-Induced Chronic Otitis Externa

See Chapter 12 for information on radiation-induced chronic otitis externa.

Suggested Reading

Breau RL, Gardner EK, Dornhoffer JL. Cancer of the external auditory canal and temporal bone. Curr Oncol Rep 2002;4(1):76–80

Djalilian HR, Memar O. Topical pimecrolimus 1% for the treatment of pruritic external auditory canals. Laryngoscope 2006;116(10):1809–1812

Heim SW, Maughan KL. Foreign bodies in the ear, nose, and throat. Am Fam Physician 2007;76(8):1185–1189

McCarter DF, Courtney AU, Pollart SM. Cerumen impaction. Am Fam Physician 2007;75(10):1523–1528

Osguthorpe JD, Nielsen DR. Otitis externa: review and clinical update. Am Fam Physician 2006;74(9):1510–1516

Yeung P, Bridger A, Smee R, Baldwin M, Bridger GP. Malignancies of the external auditory canal and temporal bone: a review. ANZ J Surg 2002;72(2):114–120

15 Auricular Mass or Skin Change of the Auricle

Eric L. Slattery, Timothy E. Hullar, and Lawrence R. Lustig

An auricular mass is a common reason for referral to the otolaryngologist. A variety of entities can present in this fashion, ranging from infectious to benign to malignant processes. Although differentiating between a malignant and benign tumor requires a biopsy, often a diagnosis of nontumor causes can be achieved by a simple examination.

◆ Mass without Significant Skin Change

Keloid or Hypertrophic Scar

In susceptible individuals, the auricle or meatus can develop a keloid or hypertrophic scar. A common scenario is keloid formation following ear piercing of the auricle. Such scars are firm and fleshy, originating from the site of an incision or region of trauma. Keloids will extend beyond the boundaries of the original wound, whereas hypertrophic scars usually do not extend beyond the original wound boundary.

Auricular Trauma: Auricular Hematoma and Cauliflower Ear

If the vascular perichondrial lining of the auricle becomes separated from the underlying cartilage, a subperichondrial auricular hematoma can develop. This injury is particularly prevalent in boxers and wrestlers; there is invariably a history of trauma. The hematoma will present as a painful bulging auricular mass with loss of the normally delicate auricular landmarks. Failure to drain a hematoma or a history of repeated auricular hematomas may result in remodeling of the cartilage, which thickens and deforms the architecture of the auricle. The resultant deformity is known as a cauliflower ear.

Benign Idiopathic Cystic Chondromalacia (Pseudocyst of the Auricle)

Pseudocysts of the auricle occur inside the cartilage of the pinna, usually along the antihelical fold, or scaphoid fossa. These cysts have no epithelial lining and are fluid-filled. They are asymptomatic except for the visible mass and may be related to trauma, although usually no such history is noted. Auricular pseudocysts may resemble *relapsing polychondritis* or *chondrodermatitis nodularis chronica helicis*; however, pseudocysts are painless. Pseudocysts can be bilateral.

Chondrodermatitis Nodularis Helicis (Winkler Disease)

This is an exquisitely tender nodule that presents on the posterior superior helix and may be related to recurrent trauma or perhaps pressure to the auricle. Typically, the skin over the nodule is normal. These lesions are more common in younger men and can be bilateral.

Kimura Disease

Kimura disease is an immune-modulated disorder that presents with a non-tender mass or nodules that may occur on or behind the pinna or elsewhere in the head or neck. Auricular lesions may be accompanied by significant lymphadenopathy. This entity is most common in Asian populations. Kimura disease does not have malignant potential. Biopsy of the affected area reveals endothelial proliferation with fibrosis in the dermal or subdermal tissue and follicular hypertrophy of lymphatic tissue. Patients may have eosinophilia and an increased sedimentation rate. Kimura disease has a similar presentation to *angiolymphoid hyperplasia with eosinophilia (ALHE)* but is a distinct entity. ALHE consists of smaller, more superficial lesions and may be a neoplasm related to epithelioid angiosarcoma.

Rheumatoid (Arthritis) Nodules

Rheumatoid nodules occur in patients who have rheumatoid arthritis; therefore, history of joint pain and deformity is important. These nodules may be tender, and with time they may break down and become necrotic.

Gouty Tophus

Gout is a disease that results from abnormal uric acid metabolism and deposition. Painful gouty tophus nodules are often found at the auricular helical rim. Characteristic urate crystals can be identified on biopsy.

◆ Mass with Skin Change

Auricular Tumors

The sun-exposed auricle is at significant risk for developing various types of skin cancers, including

- *Squamous cell carcinoma*
- *Basal cell carcinoma*
- *Melanoma*

These lesions may be exophytic or endophytic and may cause pain. Bloody or purulent drainage may be present as well.

Leprosy

Mycobacterium leprae is the causative organism for leprosy, a rare disease in most developed countries. This presents with infiltrating nodules of the auricle usually interspersed with skin ulcerations.

◆ Skin Change without Mass

Ramsay Hunt Syndrome

Ramsay Hunt syndrome is characterized by painful vesicles, which may ulcerate, in the concha bowl and external auditory canal. Patients usually present with sensorineural hearing loss and facial paresis. It is caused by herpes reactivation (see Chapter 16).

Chondritis

With chondritis, the skin will be warm and red because of underlying infection (see Chapter 16).

Wegener Granulomatosis

Wegener granulomatosis rarely presents with auricular manifestations alone; the most common otologic manifestations are chronic middle ear effusion and sensorineural hearing loss. However, affected patients may develop erythema, edema, and tenderness of the auricle.

Discoid Lupus Erythematosus

Discoid lupus can involve the auricle. These autoimmune cutaneous lesions are plaquelike, erythematous, and clearly defined. Over time, scarring of the skin can develop, as can changes in pigmentation. The lesions most often occur in a sun-exposed region.

◆ Draining Sinus

Preauricular Sinus or Pit

A preauricular sinus or pit is a remnant from auricular fetal development, originating from a small sinus tract at the root of the auricular helix. It usually presents in an area anterior to the superior attachment of the auricle or tragus. A preauricular sinus may travel deep to an area anterior to the tragal cartilage, ending in a blind pouch. It can become infected repeatedly, causing a preauricular cyst and an intermittently draining sinus.

Branchial Cleft Sinus

Another fetal developmental remnant, the branchial cleft sinus, can present as an ear canal or periauricular mass. A *first branchial cleft sinus* can drain into the external auditory canal (EAC) and can appear to cause a mass along the anteroinferior portion of the EAC. Any portion of the sinus can become blocked, leading to swelling and drainage. External drainage is usually through a sinus just inferior to the lobule.

Suggested Reading

de Ru JA, Lohuis PJ, Saleh HA, Vuyk HD. Treatment of chondrodermatitis nodularis with removal of the underlying cartilage alone: retrospective analysis of experience in 37 lesions. J Laryngol Otol 2002;116(9):677–681

Devaney KO, Boschman CR, Willard SC, Ferlito A, Rinaldo A. Tumours of the external ear and temporal bone. Lancet Oncol 2005;6(6):411–420

Effat KG. Angiolymphoid hyperplasia with eosinophilia of the auricle: progression of histopathological changes. J Laryngol Otol 2006;120(5):411–413

Elgart ML. Cell phone chondrodermatitis. Arch Dermatol 2000;136(12):1568

Froelich K, Staudenmaier R, Kleinsasser N, Hagen R. Therapy of auricular keloids: review of different treatment modalities and proposal for a therapeutic algorithm. Eur Arch Otorhinolaryngol 2007;264(12):1497–1508

Giles WC, Iverson KC, King JD, Hill FC, Woody EA, Bouknight AL. Incision and drainage followed by mattress suture repair of auricular hematoma. Laryngoscope 2007;117(12):2097–2099

Gumbs MA, Pai NB, Saraiya RJ, Rubinstein J, Vythilingam L, Choi YJ. Kimura's disease: a case report and literature review. J Surg Oncol 1999;70(3):190–193

House JW, Fayad JN. External auditory canal polyp. Ear Nose Throat J 2005;84(3):124

Jahn V, Breuninger H, Garbe C, Moehrle M. Melanoma of the ear: prognostic factors and surgical strategies. Br J Dermatol 2006;154(2):310–318

Kopera D, Soyer HP, Smolle J, Kerl H. "Pseudocyst of the auricle," othematoma and otoseroma: three faces of the same coin? Eur J Dermatol 2000;10(6):451–454

Kung IT, Gibson JB, Bannatyne PM. Kimura's disease: a clinico-pathological study of 21 cases and its distinction from angiolymphoid hyperplasia with eosinophilia. Pathology 1984;16(1):39–44

Lazar RH, Heffner DK, Hughes GB, Hyams VK. Pseudocyst of the auricle: a review of 21 cases. Otolaryngol Head Neck Surg 1986;94(3):360–361

Letko E, Zafirakis P, Baltatzis S, Voudouri A, Livir-Rallatos C, Foster CS. Relapsing polychondritis: a clinical review. Semin Arthritis Rheum 2002;31(6):384–395

Martinez Del Pero M, Majumdar S, Bateman N, Bull PD. Presentation of first branchial cleft anomalies: the Sheffield experience. J Laryngol Otol 2007;121(5):455–459

Moore MG, Deschler DG, McKenna MJ, Varvares MA, Lin DT. Management outcomes following lateral temporal bone resection for ear and temporal bone malignancies. Otolaryngol Head Neck Surg 2007;137(6):893–898

16 Primary Otalgia

Eric L. Slattery, Timothy E. Hullar, and Lawrence R. Lustig

This chapter covers primary otalgia, which is ear pain caused by otologic disease. Many patients with ear pain have referred otalgia from another site, a topic which is covered in Chapter 17.

◆ Auricular Origin

Chondritis

Chondritis is usually related to trauma or an inflammatory or infectious process. Traumatic chondritis is a common complication of burns and ear piercing, and the originating cause is usually obvious. Inflammatory chondritis may be related to an autoimmune disease, for example, *relapsing polychondritis*. It presents as part of a constellation of symptoms, with episodic hyperemia and edema of the auricle, nasal septum, and other cartilages (eg, larynx and trachea), and is associated with ocular inflammation, chronic malaise, arthropathy, and fever. Other inflammatory causes of chondritis are *rheumatoid arthritis* and *polyarteritis*. Infectious chondritis is often caused by penetrating trauma and is usually bacterial and caused by *Pseudomonas*. The lobule of the auricle is made up of fibrofatty tissue and skin, but has no cartilage; it thus is spared in patients with chondritis.

Cellulitis

Cellulitis of the auricle may be due to a specific traumatic event, or it may arise without a definable cause. An inciting cause could include a *laceration, contusion, burn*, or even *frostbite*. The skin of the auricle, including the lobule, may be edematous and erythematous, and the auricle is painful. Regional lymphadenopathy can also develop.

Herpes Zoster Oticus (Ramsay Hunt Syndrome)

This is a painful reactivation of the herpes varicella (chickenpox) virus, affecting the ear. It is more common in elderly and immunocompromised patients. Pain or itching typically precedes visible signs, which may include erythema, vesicles, and drainage. Herpes zoster oticus is associated with hearing loss, imbalance, and facial nerve weakness. A polycranial neuropathy may arise as well. Diagnosis can usually be made on history and physical examination, although serologic tests and viral culture can be confirmatory. Patients are contagious and should be isolated from pregnant women.

Preauricular Sinus, Branchial Cleft Sinus, Auricular Trauma, Chondrodermatitis Nodularis Helicis

See Chapter 15 for details on these conditions.

◆ External Auditory Canal Origin

Infectious Otitis Externa

Infectious otitis externa is probably the most common etiology of ear pain. Patients will have significant pain with palpation of the tragus or auricle (see Chapter 12).

External Auditory Canal Abscess

Abscesses of the external auditory canal (EAC) typically arise from hair follicles in the lateral EAC and are usually caused by skin flora such as *Staphylococcus*. They can be confused with tumor, and recurrent cases must be biopsied. An abscess may communicate with the parotid space through the fissures of Santorini in the cartilaginous EAC and can cause anterior cellulitis or parotitis. On examination, an abscess will be swollen, erythematous, ballotable, and painful, and may preclude visualization of the tympanic membrane.

Skull Base Osteomyelitis: Malignant or Necrotizing Otitis Externa

Otalgia is a key part of this presentation (see Chapter 9).

Trauma

Usually etiology is easy to determine, and pain is almost always present (see Chapter 10).

Foreign Body in the External Auditory Canal

Foreign bodies can range from small toys to hearing aid batteries. The diagnosis is made on otoscopy (see Chapter 10).

Noninfectious Otitis Externa - Eczema, Psoriasis, Seborrheic Dermatitis

Usually itching and irritation are more significant than pain (see Chapter 12).

Radiation-Induced Chronic Otitis Externa

Radiation treatment may cause chronic skin infection and necrosis in the external auditory canal (see Chapter 12).

External Auditory Canal Tumors

External auditory canal tumors usually are not painful, but they may lead to hearing loss and facial paralysis (see Chapter 9).

◆ Middle Ear Origin

Myringitis

Myringitis, an inflammation or infection of the tympanic membrane, is quite painful (see Chapter 12).

Eustachian Tube Dysfunction

In eustachian tube dysfunction, the patient experiences ear pressure and pain (see Chapter 9).

Acute Otitis Media

Pain is associated with distention of the tympanic membrane. Otitis media may present with hearing loss and fever, without ear pain, however (see Chapter 10).

Barotrauma

The patient will report pressure and pain and may have associated symptoms, such as vertigo and hearing loss (see Chapter 10).

Acute Mastoiditis

Acute mastoiditis arises from acute otitis media. The patient may be febrile and ill with postauricular pain. There is usually postauricular erythema and edema and mastoid tenderness. Examination of the tympanic membrane usually reveals erythema and purulent middle ear fluid. This is a medical or surgical emergency.

Middle Ear Tumor

A middle ear tumor rarely causes pain and can be diagnosed on physical exam and x-ray (see Chapter 9).

Suggested Reading

Ely JW, Hansen MR, Clark EC. Diagnosis of ear pain. Am Fam Physician 2008;77(5):621–628

Ho T, Vrabec JT, Yoo D, Coker NJ. Otomycosis: clinical features and treatment implications. Otolaryngol Head Neck Surg 2006;135(5):787–791

Mirza S, Richardson H. Otic barotrauma from air travel. J Laryngol Otol 2005;119(5):366–370

Rubin Grandis J, Branstetter BF IV, Yu VL. The changing face of malignant (necrotising) external otitis: clinical, radiological, and anatomic correlations. Lancet Infect Dis 2004;4(1):34–39

Stone KE. Otitis externa. Pediatr Rev 2007;28(2):77–78, discussion 78

Sweeney CJ, Gilden DH. Ramsay Hunt syndrome. J Neurol Neurosurg Psychiatry 2001;71(2):149–154

17 Referred Otalgia

Eric L. Slattery, Timothy E. Hullar, and Lawrence R. Lustig

Referred otalgia is more vexing to diagnose and treat than primary otalgia because its source is often not obvious. It may require imaging, endoscopy, or a trial of empiric treatment. It is crucial not to miss a pharyngeal cancer presenting as referred otalgia.

◆ Dental Sources

Pathologic processes affecting the teeth and gums are a common cause of referred otalgia. Examples include *dental caries, periodontal infection, impacted teeth, dental injury,* and *ill-fitting dentures.*

◆ Pharyngeal Sources

The vagus nerve innervates a portion of the auricle, as well as the pharynx and larynx, so that pathologies in the pharynx and larynx may lead to referred otalgia. In fact, in some cases, a patient will have almost no symptoms at the site of the primary problem and will have only ear pain. Refer to the specific chapters on the oral cavity and throat pain for additional discussion of the pathologies listed below, all of which can present with significant referred otalgia:

- *Pharyngitis*
- *Peritonsillar abscess*
- *Laryngitis*
- *Gastroesophageal reflux disease*
- *Neoplasms: oral cavity, pharynx, and larynx (see sections VI and VII)*

Tonsil neoplasm is particularly known as a common source of referred otalgia

◆ Temporomandibular Joint Dysfunction

Temporomandibular joint (TMJ) disorders can cause otalgia because the posterior boundary of the TMJ is the same as the anterior wall of the bony external auditory canal. Referred pain from the TMJ may sometimes be localizable to the ear, or it may be a more general sensation of a headache, often unilateral. Radiating pain may occur along the muscles of mastication, including the m. temporalis above the ear and the m. masseter anterior to the ear. *Myofascial pain disorder* is a common variant, with typical demographics: patients are middle-aged and women are more commonly affected than men. Patients tend to have multiple sites of pain with tender muscle "trigger points." Pain may occur suddenly and sharply with opening or closing of the jaw, or it may be a more chronic aching feeling. Patients often have a history of bruxism. The TMJ, palpated just in front of the tragus, is often tender, which may be worsened by opening and closing the jaw. Malocclusion or worn tooth facets may also be noted.

Radiology evaluation of the TMJ (usually magnetic resonance imaging is the best study) may not show internal joint derangement, but that does not rule out TMJ-associated problems as the source of referred otalgia. Even without cartilage erosion or other internal problems, the joint capsule can be inflamed, with surrounding muscle spasm and trigger points. This usually responds to joint rest, heat, massage, and intermittent use of a mouth guard.

Clicking or popping of the TMJ with mouth opening or closing is not necessarily a sign of disease, but is in fact a normal finding in many patients.

◆ Neuralgia

Otalgia may be due to primary neurologic processes. The ear is innervated by cranial nerves V, VII, IX, and X and by branches of the cervical plexus. Neuralgias in these distributions may also lead to referred otalgia. The patient's physical examination and imaging studies may be normal with the exception of possible trigger points. Specific diagnoses include:

- *Trigeminal neuralgia*: the primary pain is unilateral facial.
- *Glossopharyngeal neuralgia*: the primary pain is unilateral pharyngeal.

Eagle Syndrome

Eagle syndrome, or otalgia related to ossification of the stylomastoid ligament, may be associated with prior tonsillectomy or upper neck surgery. The pain may be exacerbated by swallowing or by turning the head. Palpation of the neck may indicate an enlarged styloid process just inferior and anterior to the mastoid tip. Transoral palpation lateral to the upper molars may reveal a tender, hard mass. Noncontrast computed tomography scan of the skull base and neck usually reveals an extremely long styloid process or a calcified stylohyoid ligament.

Suggested Reading

Charlett SD, Coatesworth AP. Referred otalgia: a structured approach to diagnosis and treatment. Int J Clin Pract 2007;61(6):1015–1021

Laurens MB, Becker RM, Johnson JK, Wolf JS, Kotloff KL. MRSA with progression from otitis media and sphenoid sinusitis to clival osteomyelitis, pachymeningitis and abducens nerve palsy in an immunocompetent 10-year-old patient. Int J Pediatr Otorhino-laryngol 2008;72(7):945–951

Martin TJ, Friedland DR, Merati AL. Transcervical resection of the styloid process in Eagle syndrome. Ear Nose Throat J 2008;87(7):399–401

Thaller SR, De Silva A. Otalgia with a normal ear. Am Fam Physician 1987;36(4):129–136

Thoeny HC, Beer KT, Vock P, Greiner RH. Ear pain in patients with oropharynx carcinoma: how MRI contributes to the explanation of a prognostic and predictive symptom. Eur Radiol 2004;14(12):2206–2211

Yanagisawa K, Kveton JF. Referred otalgia. Am J Otolaryngol 1992;13(6):323–327

18 Vertigo and Disequilibrium

Eric L. Slattery, Timothy E. Hullar, and Lawrence R. Lustig

Vertigo and disequilibrium can be due to otologic, neurologic, psychiatric, metabolic, and cardiac etiologies, so patients with these symptoms may require evaluation by multiple clinicians. A thorough clinical history is sufficient to diagnose a majority of patients presenting with imbalance, although imaging can also be indicated.

Vertigo is often described as an acute intense rotary spinning sensation, whereas disequilibrium, dizziness, and giddiness are often thought of as less intense chronic sensations of imbalance. Rather than being separate entities, however, vertigo and disequilibrium may be part of a continuum of movement sensations and may be present in the same patient suffering from a single diagnostic entity.

Medications that can cause vertigo and disequilibrium are listed in **Table 18.1.** Eye movements seen on neurovestibular examination are listed in **Table 18.2.**

◆ Vertigo and Disequilibrium: Inner Ear

Labyrinthitis

Labyrinthitis is a common cause of vertigo that usually arises during or after a viral upper respiratory infection. Symptoms of vertigo may be intense, and there may be associated sensorineural hearing loss and/or tinnitus. Nystagmus is typical; however, other neurologic findings would not be expected. A change in any position can worsen dizziness symptoms, but the symptoms do not arise in a specific inciting position.

Alcohol-Induced Vestibulopathy

Alcohol ingestion can cause acute nausea and can exacerbate preexisting vestibular conditions. It affects both the peripheral vestibular system and the central nervous system. Examination will often reveal obvious signs of alcohol use, as well as nystagmus. Chronic alcohol usage can lead to cerebellar atrophy with resulting ataxia. Gait is often more affected than limb and ocular control.

Benign Paroxysmal Positional Vertigo

Benign paroxysmal positional vertigo is a common cause of peripheral vertigo. Canalithiasis, with free-floating otoconia in the endolymph of the membranous labyrinth, is the most commonly accepted etiology, occurring mainly in the posterior semicircular canal, but in some patients affecting the lateral semicir-

Table 18.1 Medications Known to Cause Dizziness

Drug	Type of Dizziness	Mechanism
Aminoglycosides Platinum compounds (cisplatinum)	Vertigo, Disequilibrium	Damage to vestibular hair cells
Antiepileptics Carbamazepine Phenytoin Primidone	Disequilibrium	Cerebellar toxicity
Tranquilizers Barbiturates Antihistamines Tricyclic amines	Intoxication	CNS depression
Antihypertensives, diuretics	Near-syncope	Postural hypotension, reduced cerebral blood flow
Amiodarone (Cordarone)	Disequilibrium	Unknown
Alcohol	Intoxication, disequilibrium, positional vertigo	CNS depression Cerebellar toxicity Change in cupula-specific gravity
Methotrexate (Rheumatrex)	Disequilibrium	Brainstem and cerebellar toxicity
Anticoagulants	Vertigo	Hemorrhage into inner ear or CNS

Abbreviation: CNS, central nervous system.

cular canal. Posterior canal symptoms include vertigo of brief duration, with associated rotational geotropic (toward the ground) torsional nystagmus, which is fatigable and precipitated by head movement. Diagnosis is made by inducing fatigable nystagmus with the Dix-Hallpike maneuver, which entails taking the patient from the sitting position to the lying position with the neck extended and head hanging and turned to one side or the other.

Superior Semicircular Canal Dehiscence

A superior semicircular canal dehiscence is associated with pressure- or noise-induced dizziness, with conductive hearing loss (see Chapter 9).

Table 18.2 Functional Classes of Eye Movements

Class of Eye Movement	Main Function
Visual fixation	Holds the image of a stationary object on the fovea
Vestibular	Holds images of the visual world steady on the retina during brief head rotations
Optokinetic	Holds images of the visual world steady on the retina during sustained head rotations
Smooth pursuit	Holds the image of a moving target on the fovea
Nystagmus (quick phase)	Resets the eyes during prolonged rotation and direct gaze toward the oncoming visual scene
Saccades	Brings images of objects of interest onto the fovea
Vergence	Movements of the eyes in opposite directions (ie, toward each other—convergence—or away—divergence) so that images of a single object are placed simultaneously on both foveas

Ototoxicity

Aminoglycosides cause vestibulotoxicity more than cochleotoxicity. Vestibulotoxicity is usually bilateral; therefore, it does not typically cause vertigo (see Chapter 9).

Meniere Disease

Patients with Meniere disease have spells of vertigo and usually low-frequency sensorineural hearing loss (see Chapter 9).

Barotrauma

Barotrauma usually has a clear event history, with a pressure change or audible "pop" (see Chapter 10).

External Trauma/Iatrogenic Injury

Associated history of external trauma/iatrogenic injury is very important (see Chapter 10).

Cholesteatoma with Lateral Semicircular Canal Fistula

A cholesteatoma can erode the otic capsule; most often it occurs with fistulization of the lateral semicircular canal, causing vertigo and disequilibrium (see Chapter 9).

Autoimmune Inner Ear Disease/Autoimmune Hearing Loss

If the vestibular organs are affected as a result of an autoimmune disease, vertigo and vestibular disequilibrium may result (see Chapter 9).

Spirochetal Diseases

Lyme disease may lead to vertigo and fluctuating sensorineural hearing loss (see Chapter 9).

Collagen Vascular Diseases

Collagen vascular diseases may lead to dizziness, tinnitus, and sensorineural hearing loss. See Chapter 9 for a listing of specific disease entities.

◆ Vertigo and Disequilibrium: Intracranial

Vestibular Neuronitis

Like labyrinthitis, vestibular neuronitis is thought to arise from an upper respiratory infection, but its time course is usually longer, lasting weeks, and hearing loss and tinnitus are not characteristic. In fact, some make the distinction between vestibular neuronitis and labyrinthitis—labyrinthitis has hearing loss, whereas vestibular neuronitis does not—but not all use the terminology that way. Apart from nystagmus early in the course, the rest of the neurotologic evaluation is benign. A change in any position can worsen dizziness symptoms, but the symptoms do not arise in a specific inciting position.

Migraine

The mechanism of migraine is poorly understood but is thought to be neurovascular in origin. If an initial aura, such as visual symptoms, parageusia, or vertigo, is present, these symptoms are thought to be due to a vasoconstrictive phase. It is posited that the subsequent intense unilateral headache is due to intracranial vascular dilatation or aminergic brainstem ion channel dysfunction. Migraines most commonly occur in women of child-bearing age. It is estimated that 25% of migraine sufferers develop vertigo at some time during their course. In addition, some have the vertigo aura but will not go on to have a headache. A history of migraine should be elicited in all patients with vertigo and disequilibrium. The symptom duration during an episode can range from minutes to days.

Complex Partial Seizures

Complex partial, temporal lobe seizures may result in dizziness for several minutes, possibly associated with sensory or cognitive deficits. A history of a seizure disorder can often be elicited.

Vertebrobasilar Ischemia

Vertebrobasilar ischemia usually presents in an elderly patient with a history of arteriosclerosis. In this case, the arteriosclerosis has narrowed the vertebral artery, so that head motion can further kink the offending vessel, leading to brief episodes of central ischemia, which may be manifest as vertigo, hypesthesias, and dysarthria.

Vestibular Schwannoma or Other Cerebellopontine Angle Tumor

Lesions are usually so slow-growing that vertigo is not a common symptom (see Chapter 9).

Demyelinating Disease

Protean manifestations, which can include vertigo, are associated with demyelinating disease (see Chapter 9).

Rare Intracranial and Skull Base Lesions

Such lesions include the following:

- *Sarcoidosis*
- *Idiopathic pachymeningitis*
- *Superficial siderosis of the central nervous system*
- *Intra-axial tumors*
- *Endolymphatic sac tumor*
- *Petrous apex cholesterol granuloma*
- *Petrous apex mucocele*

Suggested Reading

Schwaber MK. Transtympanic gentamicin perfusion for the treatment of Meniere's disease. Otolaryngol Clin North Am 2002;35(2):287–295, vi

Staab JP. Chronic dizziness: the interface between psychiatry and neuro-otology. Curr Opin Neurol 2006;19(1):41–48

Zhou G, Gopen Q, Poe DS. Clinical and diagnostic characterization of canal dehiscence syndrome: a great otologic mimicker. Otol Neurotol 2007;28(7):920–926

19 Tinnitus

Eric L. Slattery, Timothy E. Hullar, and Lawrence R. Lustig

Tinnitus is an extraordinarily common condition, yet its etiology is not well understood. Present theories posit that inner ear hypofunction decreases input to the auditory nerve, leading to a form of neural plasticity manifest as a compensatory hyperactivity or upregulation of central nuclei of the ascending auditory pathways.

Tinnitus may be unilateral, bilateral, or not localized. It may be pulsatile or nonpulsatile. Pulsatile tinnitus may be objective, in that a clinician can auscultate a bruit, or subjective. Most often there is no definable cause, and in cases for which a cause can be defined, there is often no intervention that leads to a cure. The most common form of tinnitus, which is nonpulsatile and subjective, usually presents in a healthy patient with a benign examination who may or may not have some degree of hearing loss. There is a strong correlation between chronic tinnitus and a diathesis of depression.

◆ Objective, Vascular, and Pulsatile Tinnitus

Objective tinnitus may be heard by the examiner, although it is not a requirement for the diagnosis. Most objective tinnitus is classified as either arterial or venous. Venous tinnitus can be decreased with pressure to the internal jugular vein, whereas arterial tinnitus is unchanged by this maneuver.

Carotid Bruit

Pulsatile tinnitus can arise from bruits transmitted from the carotid artery. Often it is simply a transmitted flow murmur. Auscultation of the neck can suggest the diagnosis.

Aortic Valve Bruit

Pulsatile tinnitus can arise from bruits transmitted from the cardiac aortic valve with organic valvular disease. Auscultation of the thorax can suggest the diagnosis.

Dural Arteriovenous Malformation

Approximately 15% of intracranial arteriovenous malformations (AVMs) are dural. Pulsatile tinnitus reported by patients with dural AVM is arterial and often worse at night. Dural AVM is thought to be acquired following sinus thrombosis, most commonly in the transverse and sigmoid sinuses. Usually, a loud bruit is audible over the involved sinus. Patients may present with other neurologic manifestations if cortical hypertension results secondary to the AVM. Sudden change in tinnitus may herald impending cortical hypertension following venous outflow thrombosis.

Glomus Tumors

Pulsatile tinnitus caused by a paraganglioma may be due to *glomus tympanicum* or *glomus jugulare* tumors. Tinnitus is classically unilateral, and patients may also have a conductive hearing loss. A tumor found on the cochlear promontory may be seen behind the tympanic membrane as a purplish mass on otoscopy. If the lesion is a glomus jugulare, additional jugular foramen symptoms may be present, including hoarseness, dysphagia, aspiration, and vocal cord paresis. Computed tomography (CT) and magnetic resonance imaging reveal a middle ear lesion in the case of a glomus tympanicum, and in the case of a jugulare, erosion into the jugular bulb and often beyond.

Benign Intracranial Hypertension (Pseudotumor Cerebri)

Benign intracranial hypertension is often seen in overweight women. Tinnitus, along with hearing loss, has been reported as presenting symptoms for benign intracranial hypertension. More common symptoms are headache and blurred vision. Tinnitus often can be auscultated and is venous in origin. Both tinnitus and low-frequency hearing loss may be lessened with internal jugular vein compression. Papilledema is almost always present on physical examination. The pathophysiology is not well known, with poor absorption of cerebrospinal fluid likely. The differential diagnosis includes an *intracranial mass*, an *AVM*, and *venous sinus thrombosis*. Increased opening pressure with lumbar puncture is necessary to confirm the diagnosis.

◆ Objective, Vascular, and Nonpulsatile Tinnitus

Venous Hum

A venous hum is caused by turbulence in the sigmoid sinus or jugular vein; though not pulsatile, the sound may have a repetitive, machinelike quality. It often gets worse with head turns or in particular positions. Pressure on the jugular vein usually lessens the sound. Treatment is limited to observation and postural changes.

Dehiscent Jugular Bulb

Tinnitus that changes with exercise or with external pressure on the internal jugular vein may be due to a dehiscent jugular bulb. The tinnitus is usually not pulsatile, but it can have a repetitive, machinelike quality. A bluish discoloration of the posteroinferior quadrant of the tympanic membrane may be seen. Encountering an unanticipated dehiscent jugular bulb, which can be obscured if transmandibular retraction is present, during middle ear surgery can lead to inadvertent injury. CT of the temporal bone will clearly delineate this abnormality.

High-Flow State: Pregnancy, Anemia, Thyrotoxicosis, and Paget Disease

Conditions that lead to increased cardiac output, including pregnancy, anemia, increased thyroid hormone, and Paget disease, can lead to tinnitus. Paget disease can also cause tinnitus due to increased blood flow in the temporal bone itself, supporting increased bony turnover.

◆ Objective Tinnitus: Nonvascular

Myoclonus of the Stapedius, Tensor Tympani, and Levator Palatini Muscles

Objective tinnitus may occur with myoclonus of the stapedius, tensor tympani, and levator palatini muscles. Contractions usually occur 10 to 240 times per minute, and symptoms most commonly occur in young patients. Patients complain of a repetitive clicking sound. Oral cavity examination may reveal rapid soft palate contractions. If the stapedius muscle is the cause of myoclonus, stapedial reflex testing will be diagnostic. These conditions may coincide with other neurologic findings, such as prior brainstem infarct, multiple sclerosis, and trauma.

Patulous Eustachian Tube

Patients with a patulous eustachian tube often present with autophony and a sensation of "noise in the ear." The perception of a patient's own voice or breathing is annoying and makes it more difficult to hear external sounds. Inspiration–expiration variations of a type A tympanometric tracing may be obvious. Direct visualization can document motion of the tympanic membrane with respiration.

◆ Subjective Tinnitus: Definable Etiologies

External Auditory Canal

Lesions of the external auditory canal (EAC) rarely cause tinnitus. Instead, the tinnitus may be caused by:

- *Cerumen impaction*
- *Foreign body in the EAC*

- *EAC cholesteatoma*
- *Skull base osteomyelitis*
- *EAC tumor*

Middle Ear and Mastoid

More commonly, lesions in the middle ear and mastoid cause tinnitus, but they also usually have other, more prominent symptoms:

- *Eustachian tube dysfunction*
- *External trauma*
- *Acute otitis media*
- *Chronic otitis media*
- *Cholesteatoma*
- *Barotrauma*
- *Otosclerosis*
- *Middle ear tumor*

Inner Ear

Lesions in the inner ear often present with subjective tinnitus:

- Sensorineural hearing loss, all etiologies
  - *Hereditary*
  - *Congenital*
  - *Presbycusis*
- Sudden
  - *Noise-induced*
  - *Ototoxicity (see Chapter 9)*
  - *Meniere disease (see Chapter 9)*
  - *Iatrogenic injury (see Chapter 10)*
  - *Radiation-induced inner ear injury (see Chapter 9)*
  - *Herpes zoster oticus (see Chapter 15)*
  - *Autoimmune inner ear disease (see Chapter 9)*
  - *Spirochetal disease (see Chapter 9)*
  - *Collagen vascular disease (see Chapter 9)*

◆ Subjective Tinnitus: Definable Etiologies

Intracranial/Intratemporal Bone

Lesions of the intracranial/intratemporal bone often present with tinnitus.

Vestibular Schwannoma or Other Cerebellopontine Angle Tumor

Patients with a vestibular schwannoma usually report unilateral tinnitus with hearing loss (see Chapter 9).

Demyelinating Disease

Patients with multiple sclerosis usually report fluctuating tinnitus, which is associated with other neurologic symptoms (see Chapter 9).

Meningitis

If tinnitus is chronic after meningitis, it is usually associated with hearing loss (see Chapter 10).

Stroke

Tinnitus as an isolated finding is very rare in stroke cases (see Chapter 10).

Sarcoidosis

See Chapters 9 and 11.

Idiopathic Pachymeningitis

See Chapters 9 and 11.

Superficial Siderosis of the Central Nervous System

See Chapter 11.

Petrous Apex Cholesterol Granuloma

See Chapters 9 and 18.

Petrous Apex Mucocele

See Chapters 9 and 18.

Endolymphatic Sac Tumor

See Chapters 9 and 18.

Fibrous Dysplasia

See Chapter 9.

Suggested Reading

Anderson JE, Teitel D, Wu YW. Venous hum causing tinnitus: case report and review of the literature. Clin Pediatr (Phila) 2009;48(1):87–88

de Felício CM, Melchior MdeO, Ferreira CL, Da Silva MA. Otologic symptoms of temporomandibular disorder and effect of orofacial myofunctional therapy. Cranio 2008;26(2):118–125

Mattox DE, Hudgins P. Algorithm for evaluation of pulsatile tinnitus. Acta Otolaryngol 2008;128(4):427–431

Penner MJ. Audible and annoying spontaneous otoacoustic emissions: a case study. Arch Otolaryngol Head Neck Surg 1988;114(2):150–153

Poe DS. Diagnosis and management of the patulous eustachian tube. Otol Neurotol 2007;28(5):668–677

Sismanis A. Otologic manifestations of benign intracranial hypertension syndrome: diagnosis and management. Laryngoscope 1987;97(8 Pt 2, Suppl 42):1–17

Sutbas A, Yetiser S, Satar B, Akcam T, Karahatay S, Saglam K. Low-cholesterol diet and antilipid therapy in managing tinnitus and hearing loss in patients with noise-induced hearing loss and hyperlipidemia. Int Tinnitus J 2007;13(2):143–149

Xenellis J, Nikolopoulos TP, Felekis D, Tzangaroulakis A. Pulsatile tinnitus: a review of the literature and an unusual case of iatrogenic pneumocephalus causing pulsatile tinnitus. Otol Neurotol 2005;26(6):1149–1151

20 Facial Nerve Dysfunction

Eric L. Slattery, Timothy E. Hullar, Lawrence R. Lustig, and Thuy-Anh Melvin

Dysfunction of the facial nerve can occur anywhere along the length of the nerve, from the pontomedullary root exit zone to the arborizing branches distal in the parotid gland. In addition to segmental lesions, diffuse facial nerve inflammation may occur. Although hyperkinetic dysfunction in the form of a tic or spasm can occur, the most common dysfunction is weakness. No perfect clinical facial nerve grading scale exists, however, so the House-Brackmann system is widely used as a common language to define dysfunction objectively as best as possible.

Facial paralysis may be caused by a wide array of disorders and heterogeneous etiologies, including congenital, traumatic, infectious, neoplastic, and metabolic causes. The clinician must identify a history of diabetes, pregnancy, autoimmune disorders, cancer, prior surgery, or trauma as a potential etiology. Facial nerve dysfunction often occurs in the context of other clinical deficits, such as hearing loss, tinnitus, otorrhea, otalgia, facial mass, and facial hypesthesia, to name a few. Facial nerve dysfunction may certainly result from pathology in the temporal bone, but it may also arise secondary to intracranial and even extratemporal processes. A focused neurologic examination and assessment of the parotid gland are essential components of a clinical evaluation. Radiologic imaging may be helpful in localizing the site of the lesion or injury. If otologic disease is present, then formal audiologic testing is indicated.

◆ Facial Paralysis: Site of Origin, Primarily within the Temporal Bone

Bell Palsy

Less sophisticated clinicians may refer to any facial paralysis as a Bell palsy, when in fact 30% of facial paralyses are due some definable cause. Bell palsy is defined as idiopathic facial palsy, with some recovery. The etiology of Bell palsy is increasingly understood to result from a herpes simplex virus geniculate ganglionitis that causes edema and ischemia at the narrow meatal foramen in the labyrinthine segment of the fallopian canal; this nerve edema causes swelling and compression of the nerve with resultant weakness. Bell palsy is a diagnosis of exclusion and usually presents quickly over hours or a few days in the absence of other clinical findings, such as otitis media or a parotid mass. Subtle associated findings can be present, such as periauricular hypesthesia or discomfort. Lyme titers and, if appropriate, evaluation for human immunodeficiency virus (HIV) are part of the diagnostic evaluation. If facial nerve recovery does not begin within 1 month, then magnetic resonance imaging (MRI) with gadolinium of the internal auditory canal and temporal bone is appropriate as well. Bell palsy may be recurrent.

Infectious Etiologies

Infectious etiologies related to facial nerve dysfunction include:

- *Acute otitis media*
- *Chronic otitis media*
- *Skull base osteomyelitis*
- *Herpes zoster oticus (Ramsay Hunt syndrome)*: herpes zoster infection
- *Rare infectious etiologies*
    - *Spirochetal infection*
    - *Mumps*
    - *Rubella*
    - *Mononucleosis*
    - *Tuberculosis*
    - *Lyme disease*
    - *HIV*

Neoplasms

Facial nerve schwannomas are benign, slow-growing lesions that may arise anywhere along the length of the nerve. If one arises in the middle ear, the first symptom may even be a conductive hearing loss. Lesions are rarely multiple. The onset of facial weakness may be very slow. Other neoplasms not intrinsic to the facial nerve are:

- Middle ear neoplasm, such as *adenoma* or *glomus tumor*
- External auditory canal neoplasm, such as *squamous cell carcinoma, basal cell carcinoma, melanoma, sebaceous gland carcinoma, adenoid cystic carcinoma, mucoepidermoid carcinoma,* or *sarcoma*

Trauma

Blunt and penetrating external trauma to the temporal bone can cause facial nerve injury.

Iatrogenic Injury

Typically, during otologic surgery; the most common location for injury is to a dehiscent portion of the tympanic segment during middle ear dissection, not the mastoid segment during drilling, as might be expected.

Other Temporal Bone Diseases

These other processes can cause facial nerve paresis, from direct invasion or from compression:

- *Cholesteatoma*
- *Osteopetrosis*
- *Petrous apex cholesterol granuloma*

◆ Facial Paralysis: Site of Origin, Primarily Intracranial

Meningitis

Other findings are reported in cases of meningitis besides facial paralysis.

Cerebrovascular Accident

Isolated facial paralysis would be rare in the case of a cerebrovascular accident, but possible.

Intracranial Neoplasm

An intracranial neoplasm is most likely the cause of facial paralysis when the mass is present in the cerebellopontine angle. Examples include *facial schwannoma*, *acoustic schwannoma*, and *meningioma*. Facial paralysis may also be caused by *metastatic disease* to the brain.

Multiple Sclerosis

Multiple sclerosis classically presents as multiple episodic neurologic lesions over time, with recovery of function between episodes. Facial nerve paralysis can be a manifestation.

Möbius Syndrome

Möbius syndrome is a neuromuscular condition that includes congenital bilateral or unilateral palsies of the facial and abducens cranial nerves, as well as a broad scope of multisystem abnormalities.

Congenital Absence of the Facial Nerve

This obviously presents at birth.

◆ Facial Paralysis: Site of Origin, Primarily Extracranial

Parotid Neoplasm

It is exceedingly rare for a benign parotid tumor such as a *pleomorphic adenoma* to cause facial paralysis. Parotid malignancies, such as *mucoepidermoid carcinoma, adenoid cystic carcinoma, carcinoma ex pleomorphic adenoma, adenocarcinoma*, and *malignant mixed tumor* cause facial paresis or paralysis far more frequently. These tumors usually present initially with the finding of a parotid mass, which might also be painful or show skin ulceration, although the first presentation may be facial weakness, with the parotid mass only discovered later. The facial weakness may involve selected branches of the nerve, or the entire nerve may be paralyzed if the main trunk has tumor.

Blunt and Penetrating Facial Trauma

Diagnosis of this etiology is usually not a problem. However, with some cases of blunt trauma, the facial paralysis can be delayed (caused by edema) for 24 hours or more, which might make the facial paralysis appear to be due to a secondary etiology rather than the blunt trauma.

Infectious Parotitis

Facial paralysis is a rare complication of parotitis, which presents with unilateral pre- and infra-auricular pain, edema, and erythema. Elderly, dehydrated patients, and patients with sialolithiasis have a diathesis for infections at this site. Purulent intraoral drainage from the Stensen duct during palpation of the parotid gland is diagnostic of parotitis.

Guillain-Barré Syndrome

Guillain-Barré syndrome is an acute inflammatory demyelinating polyneuropathy. It is autoimmune in etiology and often follows an infection. The syndrome often starts in the lower extremities and spreads to involve the upper extremities and face.

Melkersson-Rosenthal Syndrome

This disease is characterized by recurring facial paralysis, swelling of the face and lips (usually the upper lip), and the development of folds and furrows in the tongue. Onset is in childhood or early adolescence.

◆ Hyperkinetic Facial Nerve Dysfunction

Hemifacial Spasm

Hemifacial spasm may be due to vascular compression of the facial nerve near the root entry zone. This may also be a primary neurologic condition.

Suggested Reading

Adour KK, Byl FM, Hilsinger RL Jr, Kahn ZM, Sheldon MI. The true nature of Bell's palsy: analysis of 1,000 consecutive patients. Laryngoscope 1978;88(5):787–801

Brown JS. Bell's palsy: a 5 year review of 174 consecutive cases: an attempted double blind study. Laryngoscope 1982;92(12):1369–1373

House JW, Brackmann DE. Facial nerve grading system. Otolaryngol Head Neck Surg 1985;93(2):146–147

Isaacson B, Telian SA, McKeever PE, Arts HA. Hemangiomas of the geniculate ganglion. Otol Neurotol 2005;26(4):796–802

Kvestad E, Kvaerner KJ, Mair IW. Otologic facial palsy: etiology, onset, and symptom duration. Ann Otol Rhinol Laryngol 2002;111(7 Pt 1):598–602

Peitersen E. The natural history of Bell's palsy. Am J Otol 1982;4(2):107–111

Perez R, Chen JM, Nedzelski JM. Intratemporal facial nerve schwannoma: a management dilemma. Otol Neurotol 2005;26(1):121–126

Siddiq MA, Hanu-Cernat LM, Irving RM. Facial palsy secondary to cholesteatoma: analysis of outcome following surgery. J Laryngol Otol 2007;121(2):114–117

III Differential Diagnosis in Pediatric Otology and Neurotology

Section Editors: *Max M. April and Robert F. Ward*

21 Otalgia in Children

Margaret A. Kenna

The symptom of ear pain can be unilateral or bilateral, constant or intermittent, and mild to severe. It may present alone or in conjunction with hearing loss, aural fullness, vertigo, or otorrhea. This chapter outlines the causes of otalgia in children.

Otitis Media

Otitis media is the most common cause of otalgia in children. It is also the most common inflammatory otolaryngologic disorder in children and involves inflammation of the middle ear and mastoid spaces. Two thirds of children have had at least one episode, and one third of children have had more than three episodes of acute otitis media (AOM) by the age of 3 years. The diagnosis of AOM is defined by rapid onset, presence of middle ear effusion, and signs and symptoms of inflammation of the middle ear. The most common symptoms of AOM are rapid onset of otalgia, irritability, fever, lethargy, and otorrhea. Patients with AOM may present with severe otalgia that quickly improves after spontaneous perforation of the tympanic membrane (TM).

Otitis media with effusion (OME) is experienced by > 50% of children during the first year of life, with a peak incidence at ~24 months. In young children having a single episode of AOM, OME is present 50% of the time after 1 month, 30% after 2 months, and 10% after 3 months. Although most cases of OME are asymptomatic (except for hearing loss), many children with OME have mild intermittent *otalgia*, especially at night, and may occasionally experience imbalance.

Complications of otitis media, including intratemporal complications, include chronic suppurative otitis media (chronic drainage through a nonintact TM), acquired cholesteatoma, acute or chronic TM perforation, mastoiditis, labyrinthitis, petrous apicitis, cholesterol granuloma, facial paralysis, and external otitis, as well as intracranial complications: meningitis, lateral sinus thrombosis, otitic hydrocephalus, and extradural/subdural abscess, or brain abscess, may all present with, or be associated with, otalgia. Depending on the duration and type of complication, otalgia may be sudden onset or chronic, severe or just persistent, and may be hard to localize, especially when associated with an intracranial complication. In cases of intracranial complications, the pain may be severe and difficult to distinguish from headache (which may be present as a separate set of symptoms due to the intracranial process). If otalgia persists and/or is severe, and even if the physical examination of the TM is not extremely abnormal (eg, "only" serous middle ear effusion or very retracted TM is seen), the patient requires attention and probable imaging to rule out some of these complications. Additionally, some of the intracranial complications will present with otalgia and neurologic or visual changes; in these cases, the middle ear and mastoid need to be investigated until disease of these structures has been ruled out or addressed.

Otitis Externa

Otitis externa is inflammation of the soft tissue structures of the external auditory canal (EAC) that may spread to involve the pinna and posterior auricular area; severe cases may involve the periosteum and perichondrium of the EAC and mastoid. Pain can be severe and out of proportion to the physical findings, especially in early otitis externa. Persistent otalgia after what is thought to be adequate local or systemic therapy may herald soft tissue extension of the otitis externa and should be investigated further.

Eustachian Tube Dysfunction

Although most patients with eustachian tube dysfunction are asymptomatic, some will describe intermittent otalgia, popping, and cracking, even if there are no other signs or symptoms of otitis media. Children with significant negative middle ear pressure seen on tympanometry or with pneumatic otoscopy may be more likely to have otalgia, which is often characterized as "deep inside" the ear or behind the ear over the mastoid.

Cholesteatoma

Cholesteatoma of the middle ear and/or mastoid may cause otalgia. Congenital cholesteatomas are generally asymptomatic unless associated with obstruction of the eustachian tube or secondary otitis media. Acquired cholesteatoma is often associated with *chronic suppurative otitis media* and may therefore cause otalgia, but pain is usually not a principal component.

Preauricular Cysts/Tracts/Pits

These often become infected, resulting in localized otalgia, erythema, and drainage. Children with *microtia/atresia*, often in association with preauricular pits or cysts, may present with otalgia, edema, and erythema. These symptoms may represent infection alone, or they may occur if there is trapped squamous debris (cholesteatoma). Because the EAC and middle ear in children with stenotic or atretic ear canals cannot be adequately examined, imaging in these cases is essential if a complication is suspected.

Foreign Bodies

Foreign bodies of the EAC, including toys (modeling clay, plastic pieces, etc.), vegetable matter (peas, beans, corn, etc.), insects, and other objects (eg, sponge, tissue, or cotton ball) will often cause otalgia, especially if the otalgia is associated with a secondary otitis externa or cerumen impaction. Earrings or other jewelry that become infected, resulting in perichondritis, will also cause otalgia.

Trauma

Trauma to the pinna or ear canal often causes otalgia, and the pain may be present with even minimal edema or erythema. Trauma to the pinna resulting in hematoma or localized perichondritis may be associated with severe otalgia, requiring surgical drainage of the hematoma and systemic antimicrobial therapy.

Neoplastic and Hyperplastic Processes

Neoplastic and hyperplastic processes are an uncommon cause of otalgia in children. Benign/hyperplastic processes include *exostoses, fibrous dysplasia,* and *ossifying fibroma. Hemangioma, vascular anomalies,* and *lymphatic malformations* involving the temporal bone or neck may all cause otalgia. Head and neck neurofibromas are common in children with *neurofibromatosis 1 (NF1),* although otalgia is relatively uncommon unless the neurofibromas involve the pinna or middle ear/mastoid itself or involve a sensory nerve supplying the pinna or other ear structures. Eighth nerve tumors that occur in children with *NF2* rarely present with otalgia; hearing loss, vertigo, or facial paralysis would be more common. Malignant lesions include *Langerhans cell histiocytosis, rhabdomyosarcoma, lymphoma, leukemia, squamous cell carcinoma, adenocarcinoma, sarcoma,* and *melanoma.*

Referred Otalgia

Otalgia that originates from processes outside the ear—referred otalgia—is not infrequent. It is a common complaint with *pharyngitis* or *after tonsillectomy.* Other nonotologic causes of referred otalgia are temporomandibular joint *dysfunction, teething,* or *other dental sources; parotid disease* (either referred or by direct extension); *inflammatory lesions* of the head and neck (including the nasopharynx); and intracranial processes. Lesions involving other cranial nerves can also cause referred otalgia (**Table 21.1**).

Table 21.1 Causes of Referred Otalgia in Children

Trigeminal Nerve	Vagus Nerve
Dental	Larynx
Jaw	Hypopharynx
TMJ	Esophagus (includes GER)
Oral cavity (tongue)	Thyroid
Infratemporal fossa masses	
Facial Nerve	**Cervical Nerves**
Bell palsy	Lymph nodes
Ramsay Hunt (herpes zoster)	Cysts/masses
Tumors	Neck infection
	Cervical spine
Glossopharyngeal Nerve	**Miscellaneous**
Tonsil	Migraine
Pharynx	Paranasal sinus disease
Eustachian tube	CNS
Posterior one third of tongue	Neuralgias
Parotid	Munchausen syndrome

Abbreviation: CNS, central nervous system; GER, gastroesophageal reflux; TMJ, temporomandibular joint.

Source: Adapted from Dolitsky, J. Otalgia. In: Bluestone CD, Stool SE, Alper CM, Casselbrant ML, Dohar JE, Yellon RF, eds. Pediatric Otolaryngology. 4th ed. Philadelphia, PA: WB Saunders; 2003:287–295.

Suggested Reading

Dolitsky J. Otalgia. In: Bluestone CD, Stool SE, Alper CM, Casselbrant ML, Dohar JE, Yellon RF, eds. Pediatric Otolaryngology. 4th ed. Philadelphia, PA: WB Saunders; 2003:287–295

22 Otorrhea or Bleeding from the Ear in Children

Margaret A. Kenna

Ear drainage may be continuous or intermittent, can be thin or thick, and may be clear, cloudy, frankly purulent, or have the consistency of cottage cheese.

Purulent otorrhea may be associated with *acute otitis media* with either a perforated tympanic membrane (TM) or indwelling tympanostomy tube, *chronic suppurative otitis media (CSOM)* through a tympanostomy tube or TM perforation, or *otitis externa.*

Clear otorrhea may be due to cerebrospinal fluid (CSF) leak after a temporal bone fracture, *perilymphatic fistula* (usually traumatic but occasionally congenital), or *otitis media.*

White cheesy otorrhea is often caused by *fungal infection* of either the external auditory canal (EAC) or middle ear.

Foreign bodies in the EAC, including retained tympanostomy tubes, which develop secondary otitis externa or granulation tissue may also present with otorrhea.

Bleeding from the ear is most commonly caused by *acute otitis media* (through a nonintact TM) or an *acutely perforated TM,* or it is associated with *granulation tissue* secondary to a tympanostomy tube, foreign body, or other cause of localized infection. *Trauma* to the EAC or TM may cause bleeding. *Neoplasia,* though rare in children, may also present with bleeding from the ear. Very rarely, inflammatory or neoplastic lesions involving the nasopharynx or upper pharynx may have reflux of secretions and blood through the eustachian tube and a nonintact TM, presenting as bleeding from the ear.

Suggested Reading

Dohar J. *Otorrhea.* In: Bluestone CD, Stool SE, Alper CM, Casselbrant ML, Dohar JE, Yellon RF, eds. Pediatric Otolaryngology. 4th ed. Philadelphia, PA: WB Saunders; 2003

23 Vertigo and Disequilibrium in Children

Margaret A. Kenna

Dizziness in children may present as a sensation of motion (if the child is old enough to talk and articulate the sensation), but in very young children, it may be manifested by imbalance, delayed or clumsy walking, or falling more often than expected. Symptoms may last a few seconds or last several minutes or hours, may occur infrequently or often, and can be debilitating.

Common causes of vestibular dysfunction in young children include *otitis media* and anatomical abnormalities of the inner ear structures (*enlarged vestibular aqueduct, dehiscent posterior or superior semicircular canal*, etc.). Otitis *media–related imbalance* generally resolves rapidly after the otitis media has resolved (after placement of tympanostomy tubes or resolution of middle ear effusion).

Older children may have *migraine-equivalent vertigo*, vertigo associated with *sensorineural hearing loss, vestibular (viral) neuronitis*, and *benign paroxysmal positional vertigo. Meniere disease* (or other causes of endolymphatic hydrops) does occur in children and is often associated with vertigo, either with or without other associated Meniere symptoms (tinnitus and hearing loss). Traumatic causes of vertigo include *brain concussion, inner ear concussion, temporal bone fracture, traumatic endolymphatic hydrops*, and *perilymphatic fistula*. Although rare in children, *vestibular schwannoma* (seen in neurofibromatosis 2) or other congenital or acquired abnormalities of the eighth cranial nerve, brain, or brainstem may rarely present with vertigo.

Suggested Reading

Casselbrant M, Furman J. Balance disorders. In: Bluestone CD, Stool SE, Alper CM, Casselbrant ML, Dohar JE, Yellon RF, eds. Pediatric Otolaryngology. 4th ed. Philadelphia, PA: WB Saunders; 2003

Furman J, Casselbrant M, Whitney S. Vestibular evaluation. In: Bluestone CD, Stool SE, Alper CM, Casselbrant ML, Dohar JE, Yellon RF, eds. Pediatric Otolaryngology. 4th ed. Philadelphia, PA: WB Saunders; 2003

24 Hearing Loss in Children

Margaret A. Kenna

Hearing loss is a common symptom in children. It may be congenital or acquired and is classified as conductive hearing loss (CHL), sensorineural hearing loss (SNHL), and mixed hearing loss (MHL).

CHL is very common in *otitis media, otitis externa, cerumen impaction, ossicular abnormalities* (both acquired and congenital), and *middle ear cholesteatoma.* CHL, MHL, or SNHL may be a presenting symptom of inner ear structural abnormalities, such as *enlarged vestibular aqueduct or superior semicircular canal dehiscence.*

The most frequently identified causes of SNHL are infectious, anatomical, and genetic. Infectious causes include *congenital cytomegalovirus and postnatal bacterial meningitis.* The most common anatomical cause of SNHL is *enlarged vestibular aqueduct* (EVA); EVA and other inner ear anomalies often have a genetic basis. The most common genetic causes are mutations in the gap junction β 2 gene (*GJB2*) encoding the connexin 26 (Cx26) protein. In many countries, > 50% of the SNHL is genetic, with 30% being syndromic and the remainder nonsyndromic. Of the nonsyndromic causes, ~80% are autosomal recessive, 15 to 17% are autosomal dominant, 2 to 3% are X-linked, and ~1% are mitochondrial. Of the nonsyndromic autosomal recessive causes, approximately half are due to mutations in *GJB2*.

Auditory dyssynchrony is a recently identified subset of SNHL. Causes include *extreme prematurity, hyperbilirubinemia,* anatomical abnormalities of the inner ear structures and the eighth cranial nerve, and genetic causes. Auditory dyssynchrony presents and evolves on a spectrum. Some children will have significant spontaneous improvement, developing useful hearing that supports spoken language development. Auditory dyssynchrony associated with anatomical anomalies is generally permanent. Children with the bilateral variety who have generally normal temporal bone anatomy but who do not develop significant usable hearing that supports spoken language may benefit from cochlear implants.

Suggested Reading

Grundfast K, Siparsky N. Hearing loss. In: Bluestone CD, Stool SE, Alper CM, Casselbrant ML, Dohar JE, Yellon RF, eds. Pediatric Otolaryngology. 4th ed. Philadelphia, PA: WB Saunders; 2003

25 Tinnitus in Children

Margaret A. Kenna

Ringing in the ears is an uncommon complaint in children, but it may be under-appreciated, as children are frequently not asked or are too young to describe it. Tinnitus may be unilateral or bilateral, soft or loud, intermittent or continuous.

Common causes of tinnitus are *otitis media, cerumen impactions, a foreign body in the external auditory canal, hearing loss* (both conductive and sensorineural), and *Meniere disease*. In patients with acquired causes of sensorineural hearing loss, including noise or ototoxic drugs, tinnitus may be present before obvious changes in the audiogram.

If hearing loss is not present or there is no obvious otologic cause of tinnitus, other diagnoses need to be considered. Vascular etiologies include *venous causes*, often associated with head position, and other, less common vascular causes, including *arteriovenous fistula* of the head and neck (often secondary to head trauma). Head and neck masses, including arteriovenous malformations, may be associated with tinnitus or an audible bruit. Myogenic causes of tinnitus include *palatal myoclonus*, as well as *contractions of tensor tympani or stapedius muscles*. Dental causes of tinnitus include *dysfunction of the temporomandibular joint* and *bruxism*. Finally, the underlying cause of some tinnitus remains idiopathic, despite extensive evaluation.

Suggested Reading

Black O, Lilly D. Tinnitus in children. In: Bluestone CD, Stool SE, Alper CM, Casselbrant ML, Dohar JE, Yellon RF, eds. Pediatric Otolaryngology. 4th ed. Philadelphia, PA: WB Saunders; 2003

26 Facial Paralysis in Children

Margaret A. Kenna

Facial paralysis is much less common in children than adults. The most common cause of **acquired** facial paralysis in children is *otitis media*; other causes are *temporal bone trauma, Lyme disease, Bell palsy, Ramsay Hunt syndrome*, and *neoplasia* (especially of the parotid). **Congenital** paralysis/paresis is often associated with anatomical and temporal bone abnormalities, including *hemifacial microsomia, Möbius syndrome*, and *CHARGE (coloboma, heart defect, atresia choanae, retarded growth and development, genital abnormality, and ear abnormality) association*, but it may occur in isolation. *Birth trauma* may also result in facial paresis or paralysis of one or more branches. *Tumors of the eighth cranial nerve and brainstem* may have facial paresis/paralysis as their presenting symptom.

Sudden onset of facial paralysis (if not due to obvious trauma) is often due to infectious causes, including *otitis media, Bell palsy*, and *Lyme disease*.

Gradual onset of facial paralysis or recurrent paralysis is often due to neoplasia. Abnormalities of taste, tearing, or salivary flow may accompany facial paralysis, helping to localize the lesion. Onset of facial paralysis in association with otalgia without onset of a new mass (eg, in the parotid) is often infectious. Persistent otalgia in association with facial paresis/paralysis despite adequate therapy for otitis media, Lyme disease, or viral causes (Bell palsy or Ramsay Hunt syndrome) should prompt investigation for neoplasia or other less common causes. Recurrent facial paralysis is characteristic of *Melkersson-Rosenthal syndrome* in association with fissured tongue and recurrent facial swelling.

Suggested Reading

Shapiro A, Schaitkin B, May B. Facial paralysis in children. In: Bluestone CD, Stool SE, Alper CM, Casselbrant ML, Dohar JE, Yellon RF, eds. Pediatric Otolaryngology. 4th ed. Philadelphia, PA: WB Saunders; 2003

IV Differential Diagnosis in Adult Rhinology and Sinus Disease

Section Editor: *Bradley F. Marple*

27 Nasal Obstruction

Suman Golla

The complaint of nasal airway obstruction arguably shares the most overlap between normal relatively mild and common disease states and more significant pathologic conditions. It therefore serves as an ideal example of the type of complaint that may require a thorough understanding of anatomical variances, physiology, and available diagnostic modalities required to differentiate its varied potential causes.

◆ Anatomy Pertinent to Nasal Airway Obstruction

The nasal cavity consists of a rigid or fixed framework that includes the bony lateral walls, cartilaginous septum, bony septum, and bony portions of the turbinate (**Fig. 27.1**). The narrowest portion of the nose is the anterior section from the nostrils to the piriform aperture. Any obstruction in the narrowest part of the nose will further the resistance to airflow and lead to nasal obstruction. There is also a significant dynamic component that may contribute to nasal blockage. The mucosal surfaces and the vasculature associated with these surfaces contribute to this variable portion. The nose, in particular, the turbinates, is lined by highly vascular mucosa, including the Kiesselbach plexus on the septum and cavernous tissue of the turbinates. Physiologic congestion, under the

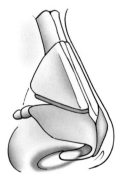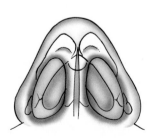

Fig. 27.1 Cartilages of the nose. The upper and lower lateral cartilages are noted along the lateral nasal wall. Note that the medial crura of the lower lateral cartilages extend medially along the caudal septum, where they lie adjacent to the quadrangular cartilage.

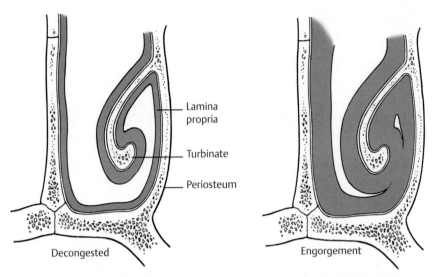

Fig. 27.2 Nasal cycle. Physiologic congestion, under the control of the autonomic nervous system, causes the nasal mucosa to congest and decongest in a cyclical side-to-side fashion; at any time, one side might be more congested than the opposite side.

control of the autonomic nervous system, causes the nasal mucosa to congest and decongest in a cyclical side-to-side fashion. At any time, one side might be more congested than the opposite side; this is known as the nasal cycle (**Fig. 27.2**). The nasal cycle is also affected by changes in posture, temperature, humidity, and sleep. The internal valve is defined as the area between the caudal end of the upper lateral cartilages and the cartilaginous septum. The external nasal valve consists primarily of the fibrofatty tissues of the alar lobule and, to a lesser extent, the lower lateral cartilages, the caudal septum, and the piriform aperture.

◆ Important Aspects of Assessment Pertinent to Nasal Airway Obstruction

History

- Fixed versus intermittent: early determination of this piece of information provides for a logical initial branching point for development of a differential diagnosis.

- Associated factors or complaints
  - Sneezing
  - Rhinorrhea
  - Epistaxis
  - Headache
  - Nasal pain
- Past trauma or surgery
- Exposures
  - Environmental
  - Infectious
  - Medications

Physical Examination

- Otoscopy
  - Middle ear effusion may indicate pathology in the nose and/or paranasal sinuses or cerebrospinal fluid (CSF).
  - Negative middle ear pressure (eustachian tube dysfunction): naso-pharynx pathology
- Nasal examination
  - Anterior rhinoscopy
    - Nasal vestibule
    - Anterior aspect of the inferior turbinate
    - Anterior nasal septum
    - Visualization of the midportion or posterior nasal cavity can be challenging.
  - Nasal endoscopy
    - Provides a detailed and complete examination of the more posterior aspect of the nasal cavity
    - Middle and superior turbinates and meatus
    - Posterior septum
- Nasopharyngeal examination
  - Indirect technique with mirror; may provide a limited view.
- Endoscopic evaluation

◆ Differential Diagnosis of Fixed Obstruction

Nasal

- *Nasal septal deformity* may be the most common source of nasal obstruction. This obstruction is usually unilateral; however, at times it may affect both sides. Patients may have a known history of trauma; occasionally, an insult to the nose may be occult, or the deflection may be developmental in nature. Patients may experience increased sensitivity to the nasal cycle and complain of symptoms that worsen at night. The physical examination often reveals an anterior deflection of the septum with a compensatory hypertrophy of the contralateral or open side. Posterior deflections or septal spurs usually are not as symptomatic as anterior deflections. Septal deviations may also exacerbate or accentuate obstruction in the setting of nasal valve collapse.
- *Internal nasal valve collapse* results from a lack of support to the lateral elements of the nasal vestibule and cavity. It can be divided into mucocutaneous or skeletal/structural disorders. The degree to which lateral wall movement occurs depends on the intrinsic stability of the skeletal and soft tissue support and on the pressure changes the nasal valve is subjected to during quiet and forced inspiration. According to the Bernoulli principle, as the flow velocity of inspired or expired air increases, the pressure inside the nasal vault decreases relative to atmospheric pressure. At a threshold flow velocity, the disparity between pressures inside and outside the nasal vault overcomes the stability of the lateral nasal wall, and collapse occurs. This intrinsic stability derives from the rigidity of the unaltered nasal anatomy or from the support provided by the skeletal and soft tissue elements that remain after rhinoplasty.

  Because ventilation involves pressure changes, the nasal airways must be stable both at rest and under the negative pressures created during quiet and forced inspiration. The internal and external nasal valves depend on satisfactory skeletal stability of the upper and lower lateral cartilages, respectively. When either the skeletal or the soft tissue component is congenitally deficient or has been compromised by surgery or trauma, the patient experiences a dynamic collapse of the valve during inspiration, with resultant airway obstruction. The normal nasal valves collapse with vigorous respiratory effort; however, a patient with dynamic nasal valve dysfunction may have a lateral nasal wall that is so weakened that it collapses even during normal nasal breathing. In most instances, the mucocutaneous and skeletal components and the static and dynamic components contribute in varying degrees to the overall nasal valvular dysfunction.

  - The mucocutaneous component refers to the mucosal swelling (secondary to allergic, vasomotor, or infectious rhinitis) that can significantly decrease the cross-sectional area of the nasal valve and thus reduce nasal airway patency.
  - The skeletal/structural component refers to any abnormalities in the structures that contribute to the nasal valve area. This includes the nasal septum, upper and lower lateral cartilage, fibroareolar lateral tissue, piri-

form aperture, head of the inferior turbinate, and floor of the nose. The skeletal component can be further divided into static and dynamic nasal dysfunction.

— Static dysfunction is secondary to continuous obstruction at the level of the nasal valve due to deformities such as a deviated septum, inferior turbinate hypertrophy, or inferomedially displaced upper lateral cartilage.
— Dynamic dysfunction is obstruction that varies in severity with respiratory effort and is usually related to deficiencies in the structural support of the lateral nasal wall, including the cartilaginous, fibroareolar, and muscular components. The lateral nasal wall caudal to the bony arch is mobile and responds variably to pressure changes.

- *Nasal fracture* as a source of obstruction will be obtained by history. Nasal airway obstruction occurs as a result of decreased cross-sectional area of the nasal cavity due to either soft tissue or nasal skeletal disruption.
- *Septal hematoma/abscess* will be responsible for sudden onset nasal obstruction. Patients will usually have an antecedent history of nasal trauma or fracture. Usually, impressive pain accompanies an examination, which demonstrates a pale, purplish, or erythematous fluctuant mass in the anterior portion of the septum. Clinical examination with anterior rhinoscopy or endoscopy may be more beneficial than imaging studies in the diagnosis of this entity.
- *Turbinate hypertrophy* may be physiologic or pathologic. It is related to an increase in vascular inflow and engorgement of the parenchyma or soft tissue of the inferior turbinates. Rarely, a concha bullosa or air cell in the middle turbinate area will lead to obstruction complaints. Techniques to measure the obstruction objectively may include rhinostereometry or acoustic rhinomanometry; however, most specialists will base the diagnosis on the patient's history and clinical evaluation.
- *Nasal polyposis* may lead to obstruction, which is unilateral or bilateral. The etiology is related to chronic inflammation of the mucosal lining of the nose and paranasal sinuses. Polyps present as clear or bluish masses of tissue arising from the mucosa of the nasal cavity. There is often some vasculature present on the surface of these structures that is best visualized with an endoscope. Polyposis is often associated with *chronic rhinosinusitis, allergic fungal sinusitis*, or *recurrent acute rhinosinusitis*. There is a strong association between polyps and *allergic rhinitis*, both of which can lead to nasal obstruction. In addition to causing nasal airway obstruction, polyps can be associated with hyposmia or anosmia. Patients with polyposis can also have asthma, allergies, or *Samter triad*.

  o Bilateral polyps are most common. Occasionally, they are seen on anterior rhinoscopy; however, they are best visualized by endoscopy. Further delineation with radiologic imaging is often warranted.
  o Unilateral polyps are less common, and this finding may represent a nasal neoplasm masquerading as polyposis. As such, a high index of suspicion should guide management of this condition. More extensive evaluation should be considered.

- ○ *Antrochoanal polyps* present symptomatically as unilateral nasal obstruction. Often there is a simple-appearing polyp extruding through an accessory ostia or in the middle meatus. Radiologic imaging defining the confines of this mass to within the maxillary and extending into the nasal cavity and eventually into the nasopharynx may narrow the diagnosis. Pathologic analysis is also critical to exclude a malignant unilateral process.
- ○ *Cystic fibrosis* is an autosomal recessive disorder that is often associated with nasal polyposis, as well as other systemic disorders. The mutation in the cystic fibrosis transmembrane regulator (CFTR) protein is thought to effect abnormalities in chloride channel transport. This eventually leads to ciliary function abnormalities within the paranasal sinuses. The heterozygous (chromosome 7) mutation within the CFTR protein is thought to be associated with chronic rhinosinusitis. Ninety percent of patients are affected within the first year of life. In addition to sinusitis and nasal polyposis, affected individuals exhibit pulmonary problems, pancreatic insufficiency, and biliary cirrhosis. This is the most common lethal inherited disorder within the Caucasian population, with a high prevalence in those of Northern European descent. Diagnosis is confirmed by sweat chloride testing of > 80 nmol/mL of chloride noted on the skin. Other diagnostic tests are genotyping and semen analysis, which reveals obstructive azoospermia.

- • *Synechia*, or *scarring* leading to obstructions, is usually diagnosed based on a history of previous surgery or trauma. Anterior rhinoscopy, in addition to endoscopic evaluation, is essential for diagnosis.
- • *Ciliary immotility* syndromes may also lead to chronic nasal obstructive symptoms. This may be related to *primary ciliary dyskinesia (PCD)* or *Kartagener syndrome*. Patients with PCD may also exhibit chronic otitis media, bronchitis, and bronchiectasis. Those with Kartagener syndrome exhibit sinusitis, situs inversus, bronchiectasis, and male infertility. Like cystic fibrosis, PCD is an autosomally recessively inherited genetic disorder that is heterogeneous in its presentation. Difficulty lies in differentiating between primary ciliary disease and changes associated with cilia during a simple viral infection. Saccharine tests can only exclude PCD if they are negative. Levels of nasal nitric oxide concentrations may prove to be the most sensitive test because they are extremely low in patients with PCD. Examination under electron microscopy of the ciliary microtubular structure can also be diagnostic. The defect lies in the inner or outer microtubules of the 9 + 2 microtubular structure, presenting as a partial or total dynein arm defect or absence.
- • Neoplasms are usually unilateral and slowly progressive. Often they are associated with epistaxis (see Chapter 29) or nasal mass (see Chapter 30). There may be polypoid mucosal changes overlying or anterior to the mass, so suspicion for neoplasm in any unilateral polyp is important.

- ○ Benign neoplasms include *respiratory papilloma, inverted papilloma, angiofibroma, hemangiopericytoma, osteoma, chondroma, hemangioma,* and *pyogenic granuloma*.

- Malignant neoplasms leading to obstruction include *squamous cell carcinoma, lymphoma, nasopharyngeal carcinoma, sinonasal undifferentiated carcinoma, esthesioneuroblastoma, mucosal melanoma,* and minor salivary gland malignancy, such as *adenoid cystic carcinoma, mucoepidermoid carcinoma,* or *adenocarcinoma,* or *metastasis.*
- Midline destructive lesions have been given several names throughout the years. The former *"idiopathic lethal midline destructive disease"* is now recognized as *lymphoma* in many cases, requiring special stains and markers for definitive diagnosis. Other midline destructive processes are either inflammatory or traumatic.

- *Encephalocele/meningocele*
- *Atrophic rhinitis* involves paradoxical complaints of obstruction associated with loss of intranasal tissue. It can be associated with a disease process (granulomatous diseases, aggressive invasive fungal infections) or be iatrogenic, with over-resection of nasal tissue or excessive stripping of nasal mucosa and its associated ciliary transport system. It is also known as "open nose" or "empty nose" syndrome.

Nasopharyngeal

- *Adenoid hypertrophy* is perhaps the most common cause of obstruction in children. The classic feature of open mouth breathing, constant purulent rhinorrhea, and disordered sleeping patterns may support this diagnosis. Diagnosis is confirmed if the patient will allow an endoscopic nasopharyngeal examination. Occasionally, an uncooperative patient may be diagnosed with a lateral neck x-ray.
- *Tornwaldt cyst* is a centrally located cyst within the nasopharynx. Occasionally, it can enlarge to encompass the entire nasopharynx and lead to obstruction. Imaging studies may be essential to exclude intracranial connections or involvement.
- *Choanal atresia* usually presents in childhood, but a unilateral case may present in the adult.
- Neoplasm

  - Benign neoplasms include *juvenile angiofibroma,* which affects pubertal boys. Patients may present with nasal obstruction as well as epistaxis. A computed tomography (CT) scan and angiography can be helpful in this diagnosis.
  - Malignant lesion or *nasopharyngeal carcinoma* can be either *squamous cell carcinoma* or *lymphoepithelioma.* This lesion commonly originates in the fossa of Rosenmüller and can cause otologic symptoms of ear fullness and/or serous otitis media with effusion. It often presents with cervical lymphadenopathy, usually bilateral. Nasopharyngeal carcinoma is associated with Epstein-Barr virus exposure and with Chinese heritage. *Lymphoma* and *hemangiopericytoma* can also present in the nasopharynx.

◆ Differential Diagnosis of Fluctuating Obstruction

Nasal

- Inflammatory rhinitis/rhinosinusitis
  - *Allergic rhinitis* is perhaps the most common cause of nasal obstruction. This condition affects up to 20% of the adult population and ~40% of the pediatric population. Family history is imperative in the diagnosis of allergic rhinitis, as this disease is heritable. Thirty-five percent of the offspring of a single allergic parent will have some form of allergy; this number increases to 65% if both parents have allergy. The majority of patients with allergic rhinitis will have nasal congestion. In addition to obstruction or congestion, characteristic symptoms include repetitive sneezing; rhinorrhea (runny nose); postnasal drip; pruritic (itchy) eyes, ears, nose, or throat; and generalized fatigue. Symptoms can also include wheezing, eye tearing, sore throat, and impaired smell. A chronic cough may be secondary to postnasal drip but should not be mistaken for asthma. Sinus headaches, facial pressure, clogged ears, and muffled hearing are also common. Allergic triggers may be seasonal or perennial, outdoors or indoors.
    - Seasonal
      - Tree, grass, and ragweed pollens are primarily seasonal outdoor allergens. Seasonal pollens depend on wind for cross-pollination. These seasonal pollens, which include trees in the spring months, grasses in the summer months, and weeds in the fall, are common sources for allergies.
    - Perennial
      - Dust mites, cockroaches, molds, and animal dander are examples of year-round allergens.
      - Mold spores grow in warm, damp environments. The highest counts occur in early spring, late summer, and early fall, but mold spores can be measured indoors year-round.
      - Animal allergens are also important indoor allergens. The major cat allergen is secreted through the sebaceous glands of the animal's skin. These small, light proteins are capable of staying suspended in the air for up to 6 hours and can be measured for several months after a cat is removed from an indoor environment.
  - *Nonallergic rhinitis* can be elicited through questioning during the initial evaluation. Questions should include symptom exacerbations with outdoor irritants, smoke, perfumes/odors, exposure to foods, and lack of a family history of allergic disease. Patients may often have symptoms regardless of exposure to animals. Although nonallergic rhinitis can have an inflammatory component (*nonallergic rhinitis with eosinophilia syndrome, NARES*), the vast majority of this type is noninflammatory and is termed vasomotor rhinitis or perennial nonallergic rhinitis. Triggers can

include environmental and respiratory irritants (eg, cigarette smoke and dust), weather changes (cold, dry air), spicy food, alcohol, strong odors, and bright lights. Other forms of nonallergic rhinitis are *rhinitis medicamentosa, atrophic rhinitis, gastroesophageal reflux disease (GERD)–induced rhinitis, drug-induced rhinitis,* and hormonal variations, especially in pregnancy. Like allergic rhinitis, nonallergic rhinitis can be the result of an occupational exposure. In contrast to allergic rhinitis, 70% of nonallergic rhinitis develops in adulthood, and women comprise > 70% of those affected.

- *Nasal polyposis* can fluctuate in size, particularly with medical treatment, and may cause fluctuating or fixed nasal obstruction. Any etiology can cause either symptom pattern.
- *Allergic fungal sinusitis (AFS)* is an intense inflammatory reaction to colonization with *Aspergillus* and dematiaceous fungi (*Alternaria, Bipolaris, Curvularia,* etc.). Imaging reveals heterogeneous areas of signal intensity on CT scan with occasional remodeling or expansion of the involved paranasal sinuses. On magnetic resonance imaging, there is a decrease in signal intensity on both the T1- and T2-weighted images secondary to the high protein content of the allergic mucin. The combination of nasal polyposis with radiologic findings and intraoperative retrieval of thick, tenacious mucin is highly suggestive of the diagnosis. The pathologic findings of Charcot-Leyden crystals and noninvasive fungal hyphae within eosinophilic mucus confirm the diagnosis. Recent guidelines have listed eosinophilic mucin, histologic evidence of noninvasive fungus, and fungal-specific immunoglobulin E with in vivo or in vitro testing to be diagnostic of AFS.
- *Sarcoidosis* is a systemic granulomatous disorder characterized by varying degrees of involvement of noncaseating granulomata within structures of the head and neck. Although lymphadenopathy is the most common presentation, nasal obstruction can also occur. Nasal sarcoidosis can present as nasal obstruction, with rhinorrhea and nasal bleeding; the nasal mucosa of the patients usually shows small submucosal nodules, with some synechia formation also possible. Biopsy of abnormal lesions can be diagnostic.
- *Wegener granulomatosis* is a rare granulomatous disease affecting ~1 in 100,000 people per year. It is characterized pathologically by necrotizing granulomatous vasculitis and clinically by the triad of vasculitis, necrotizing granulomas of the upper and lower airway, and glomerulonephritis. This disease process often affects men and women equally, with a Caucasian predominance. Patients often have elevated levels of cytoplasmic antineutrophil cytoplasmic antibody on serologic testing. Often patients manifest with nasal obstruction, crusting, septal perforation, epistaxis, or sinusitis as the primary or initial symptom(s) of their disease. Eventually, 90% of patients will develop at least some nasal symptoms. Diagnosis may require biopsy, but nasal biopsy is notoriously unreliable in establishing the diagnosis; typically only acute and chronic inflammation are seen, and the characteristic necrotizing granulomatous vasculitis is almost never seen in nasal biopsy specimens. The biopsy sites with the highest yield are the lung and kidney.
- *Churg-Strauss syndrome* is yet another vasculitis that may present with fluctuating nasal obstruction (up to 70% of patients). This systemic process

is characterized by a triad of bronchial asthma, systemic vasculitis, and eosinophilia. Patients may have systemic eosinophilia with tissue infiltration or vasculitis as the primary process leading to symptoms. Characteristic pathologic findings include necrotizing vasculitis and extravascular necrotizing granulomas, usually with eosinophilic infiltrates; these lesions are known as allergic granulomas.

Drug Induced

- *Rhinitis medicamentosa* is a frequent iatrogenic cause of fluctuating nasal obstruction. The most common offending medication is topical nasal decongestants. The sympathomimetic amines mimic the action of the sympathetic nervous system and lead to the stimulation of the α receptors, resulting in vasoconstriction. They also are mild β receptor agonists and cause rebound nasal vasodilation after the α effect has waned. In addition, some α receptors become refractory, which leads to further obstruction, requiring more stimulation (more medication use) for continued effect. The reason for continued fluctuating nasal obstruction is actually the use of the topical decongestant. The preservative benzalkonium chloride has also been incriminated as potentially part of the problem. There is no correlation between the extent of topical decongestant use and symptoms. Immediate discontinuation of sprays, however, causes increased congestion.
- Other drugs can cause fluctuating nasal obstruction (*drug-induced rhinitis*), including aspirin, antihypertensives, erectile dysfunction drugs, hormones, nonsteroidal antiinflammatory drugs, and psychotropic drugs. Discontinuation of the offending medication will result in rapid congestion relief.

Infectious

- *Viral infection* is the most common etiology of rhinitis, which is a frequent cause of fluctuating or short-lived nasal obstruction.
- *Bacterial rhinitis* or *sinusitis* is the next most common cause of fluctuating or short-lived nasal obstruction. The most common organisms involved are *Streptococcus pneumoniae, Haemophilus influenzae,* and *Moraxella catarrhalis.*
- *Rhinoscleroma* is an unusual chronic granulomatous disease of the upper airways with an infectious etiology. Synonymous with Mikulicz disease, it commonly affects the nasal cavity, as well as the nasopharynx, larynx, trachea, and bronchi. It is caused by *Klebsiella rhinoscleromatis,* a gram-negative bacteria, and is usually contracted directly by droplets or by contamination of material that is subsequently inhaled; it is rare in the United States. The disease is present in three stages: catarrhal/atrophic, granulomatous, and sclerotic/cicatricial. The catarrhal stage begins with a nonspecific rhinitis, which evolves into purulent, fetid rhinorrhea and crusting, lasting for weeks or months. The granulomatous stage leads to the nasal mucosa becoming bluish red and granular with intranasal rubbery nodules or polyps.

Epistaxis is common, and nasal enlargement, deformity, and destruction of the nasal cartilage are also frequently noted (this is called the "Hebra nose"). The symptoms may progress to anosmia, anesthesia of the soft palate, enlargement of the uvula, dysphonia, and various degrees of airway obstruction. In the cicatricial stage, obstruction can be fixed.

- *Syphilis* is another, less commonly considered bacterial infection that can lead to nasal obstruction. Nasal disease secondary to infection by the spirochete *Treponema pallidum* can occur at any age, including in the neonate. Primary, secondary, and tertiary syphilis can all cause intranasal disease. Congenital syphilis is the most common infection associated with nasal manifestations. This infection is characterized by marked rhinitis, with nasal obstruction and a bloody, mucopurulent discharge. The ulcerative lesions can lead to chondritis, osteitis, and a saddle nose deformity. The diagnosis of nasal syphilis can be confirmed through serologic testing (rapid plasma regain or Venereal Disease Research Laboratory) or direct treponemal testing (fluorescent treponemal antibody–absorption [FTA-ABS]).

- *Rhinosporidiosis* is a rare infection that needs to be considered especially in patients with a history of an international background, particularly from Central Europe, Central America, and India. Rhinosporidiosis is a chronic granulomatous infectious process that involves the mucous membranes of the septum, turbinates, and structures of the eyes. The primary manifestation of the disease is formation of vascular friable polyps. The responsible etiologic agent is *Rhinosporidium seeberi,* which has never been successfully cultured in vitro and is thought to represent a mold.

- *Mycobacterium leprae* is an acid-fast bacillus that causes leprosy, an extremely rare disease that causes granulomatous nasal obstruction. Infection can lead to plaquelike thick lesions in the anterior nasal septum or the anterior end of the inferior turbinate. Progression of the infection can lead to obstruction, ulceration, and nasal collapse.

- **Fungal infections** can cause fluctuating nasal obstruction, but more commonly they cause progressive nasal obstruction.

  ○ *Fulminant invasive fungal sinusitis* results in massive tissue destruction, epistaxis, crusting, and obstruction. This is usually associated with poorly controlled diabetes mellitus or states of significant immunocompromise. Mucormycosis (*Zygomycetes* sp.) and *Aspergillus* sp. are the most common etiologies.

  ○ *Indolent invasive fungal sinusitis* is similar to that of more fulminant forms of the disease, but its progression is slower. As with the more fulminant forms of this disease, indolent invasive fungal sinusitis is typically associated with diabetes mellitus or immunocompromise. *Zygomycetes* and *Aspergillus* are also the most common species.

  ○ *Chronic granulomatous invasive fungal sinusitis* is most common in Northern Africa and the Middle East. Unlike other forms of invasive fungal sinusitis, the host is frequently immunocompetent. The disease is characterized by the combination of tissue invasion by fungus and formation of granulomata; it tends to be slowly progressive in its course.

Physiologic or Anatomical Factors

- *Nasal cycle* is a normal phenomenon: a fluctuation in nasal patency that is related to alternating congestion and decongestion phases in the right and left nostril. This cycle may be involved in the mucociliary clearance and humidification of the nose.
- *Nasal septal perforation* can cause fluctuating or fixed obstruction; this is usually caused by inflammatory or infectious disease or trauma. The perforation itself may not lead to obstruction; however, the buildup of crust or blood can cause obstruction. Most traumatic or iatrogenic perforations result from (1) mucosal lacerations on corresponding sides of the septum with exposure of the underlying cartilage or (2) a fracture of the cartilaginous septum. Perforation occurs because the cartilage relies on the overlying mucoperichondrium for its blood supply and nutrients. Iatrogenic causes include nasal surgical procedures and nasal intubation or nasogastric tube placement; prior septal surgery is the most common cause of septal per-

Table 27.1 Nasal Obstruction: Differential Diagnosis Based on Symptoms

Symptom	Time Course	Etiologies
Nasal obstruction	Constant	Septal deviation Nasal fracture Turbinate hypertrophy Choanal atresia Septal hematoma/ abscess Nasal polyposis Neoplasm Nasopharyngeal mass Nasal valve collapse Nasal synechia Atrophic rhinitis

Nasal obstruction	Intermittent/fluctuating	Allergic rhinitis
		Rhinitis medicamentosa
		Hormonal/pregnancy
		Nonallergic rhinitis
		Sarcoidosis
		Wegener granulomatosis
		Viral rhinitis or
		  rhinosinusitis
		Bacterial rhinitis or
		  rhinosinusitis
		Allergic fungal sinusitis
		Mucormycosis
		Nasal cycle
		Nasal septal perforation

forations. Infectious and inflammatory etiologies, including *tuberculosis, syphilis, Wegener granulomatosis,* and *sarcoidosis,* should always be considered in the differential diagnosis as the cause of septal perforations. *Abuse of nasal inhalants* is often implicated in septal perforation, the most common of which is cocaine. Rarely, vasoconstrictive and steroid nasal sprays have been implicated (**Table 27.1**).

Suggested Reading

Baptista P, Carlos GV, Carlos GV, et al. Acquired nasopharyngeal stenosis: surgical treatment for this unusual complication after chemoradiation for nasopharyngeal carcinoma. Otolaryngol Head Neck Surg 2007;137(6):959–961

Corey JP, Houser SM, Ng BA. Nasal congestion: a review of its etiology, evaluation, and treatment. Ear Nose Throat J 2000;79(9):690–693, 696, 698

Farmer SE, Eccles R. Chronic inferior turbinate enlargement and the implications for surgical intervention. Rhinology 2006;44(4):234–238

Grymer LF, Hilberg O, Elbrønd O, Pedersen OF. Acoustic rhinometry: evaluation of the nasal cavity with septal deviations, before and after septoplasty. Laryngoscope 1989;99(11):1180–1187

Lockey RF. Rhinitis medicamentosa and the stuffy nose. J Allergy Clin Immunol 2006;118(5):1017–1018

Moinuddin R, Mamikoglu B, Barkatullah S, Corey JP. Detection of the nasal cycle. Am J Rhinol 2001;15(1):35–39

Schlosser RJ, Park SS. Surgery for the dysfunctional nasal valve: cadaveric analysis and clinical outcomes. Arch Facial Plast Surg 1999;1(2):105–110

Settipane RA, Lieberman P. Update on nonallergic rhinitis. Ann Allergy Asthma Immunol 2001;86(5):494–507, quiz 507–508

28 Rhinorrhea

Stephanie A. Joe

As with many nasal symptoms, rhinorrhea is a common complaint offered by patients. Its presentation can vary widely over several different descriptive parameters, with each providing some potential information that can be used to better diagnosis its underlying cause.

◆ Nasal Sources of Rhinorrhea

- The unique anatomy of the nasal cavities with the mucosa-lined turbinates and meatus allows for maximal contact of inspired air with the mucosal surface area within a small space. The effects on inspired air include:
  - Temperature regulation
  - Humidification
  - Filtration
  - Lubrication
  - Odor detection
  - Protection against airborne pathogens
  - Preparation of inspired air for the lower airways
- Components of the nasal lining (mucosa)
  - The nasal vestibule is lined with keratinized, stratified, squamous epithelium containing the vibrissae, sweat glands, and sebaceous glands.
  - At the mucocutaneous junction is the limen vestibule, pseudostratified respiratory epithelium that lines the entire nasal cavity and is composed of three major cell types:
    - Ciliated columnar cells are the predominant cell type found in this epithelium. These cells contain cilia and microvilli that project in the mucus blanket.
    - Goblet cells have a characteristic shape and lie between the columnar cells. Their cytoplasm is packed with mucus droplets extending up to the mucosal surface.
    - Basal cells lie deeper in the epithelium and assist with anchoring columnar cells to the basement membrane.
  - The cells of the respiratory mucosa rest on a basement membrane that overlies a connective tissue layer referred to as the lamina propria.
  - The submucosa is thin and adherent to the periosteum and perichondrium. It contains venous plexus, blood vessels, sensory nerves, immune cells, and glands.
  - Glands of mucosa and submucosa

- Serous glands are located at the nasal vestibule and are a small contribution to overall mucus production.
- Seromucous glands lie in the submucosa, with ~100,000 lining the nasal cavities, where they produce most of the mucus. Their acini are either serous or mucous, with 4 to 8 times more serous acini.
- Intraepithelial glands are few in number.

○ Critical to mucociliary flow, cilia can number up to 100 per cell and beat 1000 times or more a minute. They are composed of microtubules in the "9 + 2" pattern, with two microtubules surrounded by nine interconnected pairs of microtubules. The nine outer pairs of microtubules are linked by dynein arms. Ciliary movement is accomplished in a biphasic pattern: a rapid phase in which cilia straighten and contact the mucous blanket, followed by the relaxation and a recovery stroke. Ciliary function can be adversely affected by pathologic processes such as inflammation or infection.

- The mucous blanket

○ The nasal cavity produces 1 to 2 L of mucus per day.
○ Mucus is highly acidic (pH ~ 6.0) and contains:

- Water
- 1–2% salts
- 2–3% glycoproteins
- Immunoglobulins

○ After secretion, mucus forms a bilayer consisting of a thicker, more viscous gel layer on the surface. This overlies the more serous sol layer.
○ Mucus is swept from posterior to anterior by cilia toward the nasal vestibule.

- Autonomic control

○ Innervation of the nasal cavity glands and vasculature is under sympathetic and parasympathetic control.

- From the cervical sympathetic ganglion, fibers travel along the internal carotid artery and form the deep petrosal nerve. This merges with the greater superficial petrosal nerve to form the vidian nerve. This travels to the pterygopalatine fossa and contributes to the sphenopalatine ganglion. Fibers pass through without synapsing and join the second branch of the trigeminal nerve (V2) for distribution throughout the nasal mucosa.
- Parasympathetic fibers travel with the facial nerve to the geniculate ganglion. Without synapsing, the fibers exit as the greater superficial petrosal nerve. These then join with the sympathetic nerves to form the vidian nerve. These fibers synapse in the sphenopalatine ganglion and join V2 for distribution.
- Goblet cell production is at a steady rate that is independent of autonomic input.

◆ Intracranial Source of Rhinorrhea

Cerebrospinal fluid (CSF) is continually produced to keep the total volume in an adult at ~100 to 150 mL. Its rate of formation is 350 to 500 mL/day or 20 mL/hour (or 0.35 mL/min). This total volume is turned over four or five times a day. The consistency of CSF is a thin, watery liquid that is clear and has a salty and/or metallic taste. The normal intracranial CSF pressure is ~8 to 18 cm water pressure, and the following activities increase CSF pressure: sneezing, laughing, Valsalva maneuver, rapid eye movement (REM) sleep, and orthostatic position changes (ie, from supine to sitting, pressure can increase to 40 cm water pressure).

CSF can escape into the nasal cavity and represent a source of rhinorrhea at sites of weakness or when the integrity of the skull base is breached. Sites of natural weakness include the cribriform plate, ethmoidal artery canal, optic nerve sheath, sellar diaphragm, and other congenitally weak areas of the skull base. The etiologies of skull base defect and a CSF leak are surgical dissection, external trauma, inflammatory disease, and neoplasms. CSF rhinorrhea can also be caused by CSF otorrhea draining through the eustachian tube.

Spontaneous CSF leakage associated with benign intracranial hypertension can occur. Patients are frequently middle-aged, obese, and female. Associated complaints include imbalance, pulsatile tinnitus, and pressure headaches. Radiographic evidence of empty, expanded sella has been noted in this population of patients.

◆ Pertinent History

- Duration
- Laterality
- Viscosity
- Fetid smell
- Timing to significant events, exacerbating and/or relieving events, and antecedent events
- History of head trauma
- History of prior sinus surgery
- History of meningitis
- History of sinonasal neoplasm
- History of polyposis, mucocele, or complex rhinosinusitis

◆ Physical Examination

- Anterior rhinoscopy
- Nasal endoscopy

- Otoscopy (middle ear effusion indicates possible CSF otorrhea)
- Provocation (head hanging/straining that induces rhinorrhea may indicate CSF rhinorrhea)

◆ Diagnostic Testing

- Allergy testing
- Computed tomography (CT) scan of the sinuses
- Magnetic resonance imaging (MRI) scan
- Evaluation for CSF leak
  - ○ Beta-2 transferrin is a protein found in CSF and the aqueous and vitreous humor of the eye. Nasal fluid is collected and sent for laboratory examination. Electrophoresis is performed to separate proteins and detect beta-2 transferrin. When present, CSF leak is confirmed; however, a negative test result does not exclude the diagnosis of CSF leak.
  - ○ Radionuclide study is a highly sensitive test for detecting a CSF leak. It involves the intrathecal injection of a radioactive tracer, indium 111 DTPA (pentetate). Intranasal pledgets are placed and left for several hours. These are then removed and placed in a radioactive counter to detect the tracer. The patient's serum levels are drawn for comparison counts.

◆ Differential Diagnosis of Anterior Rhinorrhea

Bilateral

Laterality offers a differentiating point separating a more global nasal process from focal problems. Bilateral rhinorrhea renders focal causes of rhinorrhea, such as CSF fistula, to a lower probability on the differential diagnosis. Inflammatory and infectious conditions, nasal manifestations of systemic processes, and medication side effects are most common.

It is also helpful to distinguish the characteristics of the rhinorrhea in formulating a differential diagnosis.

- Watery and thin rhinorrhea
  - ○ Inflammatory
    - — *Allergic rhinitis* will have clear mucoid rhinorrhea, which can be watery and thin, or also somewhat sticky and tenacious, but always clear. It is associated with nasal congestion, sneezing, itchy nose and eyes, and epiphora. Other symptoms of generalized allergy are generalized pruritis, itchy ears, and dark circles under the eyes. On nasal examination, typical findings include edematous mucosa throughout the nasal cavities bilaterally; pale, bluish, hypertrophic turbinates; clear, thin, mu-

coid nasal drainage; and hyperreactive mucosa associated with sneezing during endoscopy.

- ○ Infectious

    - *Viral rhinitis and sinusitis* usually cause clear, thin, mucoid nasal rhinorrhea. Bacterial rhinitis and rhinosinusitis usually cause thick, purulent rhinorrhea

- ○ Autonomic

    - *Vasomotor rhinitis* is associated with clear, mucoid rhinorrhea in the absence of inhalant allergies. Rhinorrhea can be exacerbated by exercise, cold temperatures, or eating.

- ○ Medications

    - *Antihypertensives* (eg, α- and β-adrenergic antagonists)
    - *Oral contraceptives*
    - *Psychotropic agents* (eg, amitriptyline, thioridazine, and alprazolam)
    - Runoff from nasally applied medications

- ○ Systemic conditions with associated sinonasal manifestations and possibly rhinorrhea

    - Autoimmune disorders (eg, *systemic lupus erythematosus*)
    - Vasculitides (eg, *Wegener granulomatosis*)
    - *Ciliary dyskinesias* (associated with mucus stasis, thick mucus, and crusting)
    - Hormonal imbalances (eg, *pregnancy*) are associated with mucoid drainage and congestion. Pregnancy can also exacerbate underlying rhinitis, such as allergic rhinitis.
    - *Sarcoidosis:* lesions are submucosal, giving the mucosa a characteristic nodular appearance. Crusting and thick mucus may be present.

- ○ *CSF rhinorrhea* is less likely to be bilateral unless the skull base defect spans bilateral sinonasal cavities or multiple defects are present.
- ○ Mechanical drainage problems

    - *Recirculation* from an accessory maxillary sinus ostia, or an iatrogenic ostia, can cause clear, watery rhinorrhea, but mucus is more often thick and tenacious.

- ○ *Neoplasms* may cause rhinorrhea due to obstruction.

- ● Thick, viscous rhinorrhea

- ○ Inflammatory

    - *Inflammatory rhinosinusitis* with or without polyps: drainage can be thick and tenacious, caused by impaired mucociliary clearance, and mechanical obstruction of nose and sinuses. In *allergic fungal rhinosinusitis*, drainage can be very thick and dark, almost of a peanut butter consistency.
    - *Allergic rhinitis* will have clear mucoid rhinorrhea, which can be watery and thin, or also somewhat sticky and tenacious, but always clear.

○ Infectious

— *Infectious rhinosinusitis*

- *Acute rhinosinusitis* lasts less than 3 weeks and is characterized by thick rhinorrhea, with nasal congestion, sinus pressure, and cough. It also can have associated symptoms: fever, epistaxis, and headache. Bacterial and viral rhinosinusitis can have discolored rhinorrhea caused by white blood cell infiltration. The presence of white or yellow mucus does not always indicate a bacterial infection.
- *Subacute rhinosinusitis:* symptoms are the same as acute rhinosinusitis but last 3 to 12 weeks.
- *Chronic infectious rhinosinusitis:* at least 12 weeks of purulent rhinorrhea, with congestion, cough, postnasal drainage, and often a sensation of chronic fatigue or malaise. Usually patients do not have headache or pain.

○ Systemic conditions with associated sinonasal manifestations

— Autoimmune disorders (eg, *systemic lupus erythematosus*)
— Vasculitides (eg, *Wegener granulomatosis*)
— *Ciliary dyskinesias* (see above)
— Hormonal imbalances (eg, *pregnancy*) (see above)
— *Sarcoidosis* (see above)

○ Iatrogenic

— *Recirculation* from an iatrogenic ostia or an accessory maxillary ostia
— *Foreign body:* thick mucoid drainage associated with a bilateral foreign body, such as nasal packing. Usually this is unilateral and not bilateral.

○ *Neoplasms* may cause rhinorrhea due to obstruction.

Unilateral

This is more suggestive of focal pathology.

- Watery and thin rhinorrhea

○ *CSF rhinorrhea* must be considered.

— Past history of prior trauma or surgery
— Patients will report watery rhinorrhea exacerbated by the Valsalva maneuver or bending forward.
— Beta-2 transferrin test to distinguish CSF from nasal fluid
— Evaluation to identify the site of the leak

- Nasal endoscopy using an angled telescope. To increase possible leak detection, the patient can be asked to perform a Valsalva maneuver. A stream of clear fluid may be seen. If there is a larger bony defect or an encephalocele, transmitted pulsations from the dura may be seen, along with a smooth, gray-pink pulsatile mass.
- High-resolution CT scan of sinuses and temporal bones are critical to evaluating for sinus and mastoid disease, tumors, and the presence of skull base defects.

- CT cisternogram involves the intrathecal injection of a water-soluble contrast agent, such as iohexal. The patient is placed in the prone position for coronal views to encourage leakage from the intracranial cavity into the sinonasal cavity. An active leak must be present for detection with passage of contrast into the sinonasal cavity. Contrast remains in the intrathecal space for up to 24 hours, and delayed images can be obtained to detect an intermittent leak.
- MRI is helpful for distinguishing mucosal edema from encephalocele, meningoencephalocele, or aggressive arachnoid granulation.
- Intrathecal fluorescein with endoscopy can be used to detect an active CSF leak and is often used during surgical repair of CSF leaks for localization. This is not approved by the U.S. Food and Drug Administration, but there are some reports in the literature documenting the safe use of diluted fluorescein in large series.

o Infectious

— *Infectious rhinosinusitis* is rarely watery, but it can be unilateral.

o Inflammatory

— *Allergic rhinitis* rarely presents with unilateral rhinorrhea.
— *Inflammatory rhinosinusitis* is rarely watery or unilateral.

o Autonomic rhinorrhea (*vasomotor rhinitis*) is usually watery but rarely unilateral.
o *Foreign body or rhinolith:* foul smell from nose; rarely, thin rhinorrhea
o Mechanical drainage problem

— *Recirculation* can be unilateral.

- Thick, viscous rhinorrhea

o Infectious

— Infectious rhinosinusitis can be unilateral.

- *Acute rhinosinusitis*
- *Subacute rhinosinusitis*
- *Chronic rhinosinusitis*

o Inflammatory

— *Allergic rhinitis* rarely presents with unilateral rhinorrhea.
— *Inflammatory rhinosinusitis* can be unilateral, although it more commonly is bilateral; associated rhinorrhea is usually thick and viscous.

o *Foreign body or rhinolith:* foul smell and thick, purulent rhinorrhea. This is usually unilateral.
o *Neoplasms* can cause thick rhinorrhea due to obstruction.
o *Systemic conditions* with associated sinonasal manifestations very rarely cause unilateral rhinorrhea.
o Mechanical drainage problem

— *Recirculation* can be unilateral.

— *Choanal atresia* is rare in adults, but it can present as unilateral, thick rhinorrhea.

◆ Differential Diagnosis of Posterior Rhinorrhea

Laterality is less reliable in the evaluation of posterior nasal drainage.

- Watery, thin rhinorrhea
  - *CSF rhinorrhea,* particularly if associated with salty or sweet taste. CSF rhinorrhea that drains posteriorly is more likely to be from the sphenoid or posterior ethmoid area.
  - Can be *CSF otorrhea,* draining down the eustachian tube
  - *Vasomotor rhinitis*
- Thick, viscous rhinorrhea
  - Essentially, the same differential diagnosis as thick anterior rhinorrhea (see above)
  - *Infectious rhinosinusitis*
  - *Inflammatory rhinosinusitis*
  - *Foreign body*
  - *Neoplasm* causing obstruction and aberrant drainage
  - *Recirculation*
  - *Laryngopharyngeal reflux:* symptoms can mimic postnasal rhinorrhea—cough, throat clearing, and sensation of thick mucus. If there is no evidence of postnasal rhinorrhea, but the patient has persistent symptoms, then consider laryngopharyngeal reflux. Characteristic physical examination findings on laryngoscopy include arytenoid and interarytenoid edema and erythema, postcricoid edema, and pachydermia of the postcricoid area of the pharynx and esophageal inlet.

See **Table 28.1** for an outline of the differential diagnosis of rhinorrhea based on symptoms.

Table 28.1 Rhinorrhea: Differential Diagnosis Based on Symptoms

	Bilateral	Unilateral
Watery and thin	Allergic rhinitis Viral rhinosinusitis Vasomotor rhinitis Medications Systemic condition with nasal manifestation CSF Mechanical drainage problem	CSF Allergic rhinitis Infectious rhinosinusitis Inflammatory rhinosinusitis Vasomotor rhinitis Foreign body Recirculation
Thick and viscous	Inflammatory rhinosinusitis Infectious rhinosinusitis Systemic condition with nasal manifestation Recirculation Foreign body Neoplasm	Infectious rhinosinusitis Inflammatory rhinosinusitis Foreign body Neoplasm Systemic condition with nasal manifestation Recirculation Choanal atresia

Abbreviation: CSF, cerebrospinal fluid.

Suggested Reading

Joe S, Benson A. Nonallergic rhinitis. In: Cummings CW, Flint PW, Haughey BH, et al, eds. Otolaryngology: Head and Neck Surgery. 4th ed.

Lane AP. Nasal anatomy and physiology. Facial Plast Surg Clin North Am 2004;12(4):387–395, v

Meltzer EO, Hamilos DL, Hadley JA, et al; American Academy of Allergy, Asthma and Immunology; American Academy of Otolaryngic Allergy; American Academy of Otolaryngology–Head and Neck Surgery; American College of Allergy, Asthma and Immunology; American Rhinologic Society. Rhinosinusitis: establishing definitions for clinical research and patient care. Otolaryngol Head Neck Surg 2004;131(6, Suppl):S1–S62

Schlosser RJ, Bolger WE. Nasal cerebrospinal fluid leaks: critical review and surgical considerations. Laryngoscope 2004;114(2):255–265

29 Epistaxis

Samuel D. Cohen and James W. Mims

◆ Anatomy

The blood supply of the nose comes from branches of both the internal and external carotid artery systems, and there are multiple anastomoses between the two systems. Knowledge of the nasal cavity's blood supply affects how epistaxis is diagnosed and treated.

- Lateral nasal wall (**Fig. 29.1**)
  - Anterior ethmoidal artery: The anterior ethmoidal artery branches off the ophthalmic, which is the first branch of the internal carotid artery. The anterior ethmoidal artery enters the anterior ethmoidal foramen, which is ~14 to 22 mm posterior to the anterior crest of the lacrimal fossa. This is usually at the horizontal plane of the cribriform plate. The vessel then passes just under the skull base across the roof of the anterior ethmoid sinuses. The lateral branch supplies the anterior aspect of the lateral nasal wall. The anterior ethmoidal artery is absent in 7 to 14% of the population.
  - Posterior ethmoidal artery: The posterior ethmoidal artery is also a branch of the ophthalmic artery. It enters the posterior ethmoidal canal, which is usually located in the frontoethmoid suture, ~10 mm posterior to the anterior ethmoidal canal. The posterior ethmoidal artery has a lateral branch supplying the superior aspect of the lateral nasal wall. The posterior ethmoidal artery is absent in ~31% of the population.

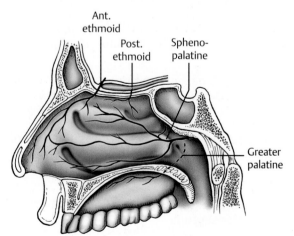

Fig. 29.1 Arterial supply of the lateral nasal wall.

- ○ Sphenopalatine artery (SPA): The external carotid artery supplies the nasal mucosa via several branches. The maxillary artery is a terminal branch of the external carotid artery. After passing through the lateral pterygoid muscles, the maxillary artery passes through the pterygomaxillary fissure tenter the pterygopalatine fossa. Here it terminally branches into the sphenopalatine, descending palatine, pharyngeal, pterygoid canal, infraorbital, and posterior superior alveolar arteries. The SPA enters the nasal cavity via the sphenopalatine foramen, located posterior to the middle turbinate.

  - — Lateral branches of the SPA (or posterior nasal artery): These are terminal branches of the SPA supplying the lateral nasal wall and the middle and inferior turbinates.
  - — Septal branch of the SPA: This branch crosses the anterior face of the sphenoid (inferior to the ostia) before branching onto the posterior septum.

- ○ Ascending pharyngeal artery branches: The ascending pharyngeal artery is a branch of the maxillary artery and supplies the inferoposterior lateral nasal wall.
- ○ Superior labial artery: Another branch by which the external carotid artery provides blood to the lateral nasal wall is the superior labial artery, which is a branch of the facial artery. It provides several nasal branches supplying the anterolateral nasal wall.
- ○ Vascular regions

  - — Woodruff region: Throughout the nose there are several areas of anastomosis between the many arteries that supply the mucosa. The Woodruff region, also known as the nasopharyngeal plexus, lies on the posterolateral nasal wall in the region of the inferior meatus (between the inferior turbinate and nasal floor). It comprises vessels from the pharyngeal and posterior nasal arteries.

- ● Nasal septum (**Fig. 29.2**)

  - ○ Anterior ethmoidal artery: The anterior ethmoidal artery gives off medial and lateral branches. The medial branch supplies the anterosuperior nasal septum.
  - ○ Posterior ethmoidal artery: The posterior ethmoidal artery has medial and lateral branches. The medial branch supplies the superior septum.
  - ○ Sphenopalatine artery (SPA)

    - — Septal branch of SPA: After the SPA has entered the nasal cavity and given off branches to the lateral nasal wall, the septal branch then continues across the sphenoid face to become the major blood supply to the posterior septum.
    - — Greater palatine artery: The descending palatine artery is a branch of the SPA and passes through the palatine canal where it becomes the greater palatine artery. It then passes through the incisive canal to supply the nasal floor and anteroinferior septum.

  - ○ Superior labial artery: Nasal branches from the superior labial artery enter the nose to supply the anterior septum.

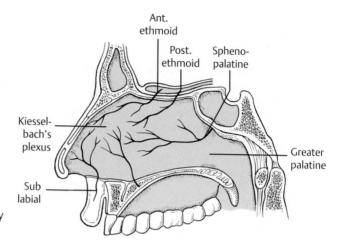

Ant.
ethmoid

Post.   Spheno-
ethmoid   palatine

Kiessel-
bach's
plexus

Greater
palatine

Sub
labial

Fig. 29.2 Arterial supply
of the septum.

- Vascular regions
  - Little area: The Little area, also known as the Kiesselbach plexus, is an area of anastomosis on the anterior nasal septum. It is the major area of anastomosis between the external and internal carotid artery blood supply to the nose. The vessels in Little's area come from the SPA, greater palatine, anterior ethmoidal, posterior ethmoidal, and nasal branches of the superior labial arteries.
  - Woodruff plexus of the posterior septum: Some authors consider the Woodruff plexus as a region of the posterior septum where ethmoid artery branches anastomose with the septal branches of the SPA.

◆ Diagnostic Factors to Consider in Epistaxis

- Location
  - Anterior: Anterior epistaxis often originates from Little area (Kiesselbach plexus) on the nasal septum.
  - Posterior
  - Hemoptysis can be the presenting sign of epistaxis, particularly posterior epistaxis.
  - Hematemesis can also be the presenting sign of epistaxis, particularly posterior epistaxis. Patients with neurological disease involving a decreased gag reflex may be more prone to ingesting large quantities of blood, and patients who are supine for a long period of time (eg, an intubated patient in the intensive care unit) is at increased risk of ingesting or aspirating blood from epistaxis.

- Severity
- Frequency
- Other factors in history
  - Other bleeding sites: A history of other bleeding, especially mucosal bleeding, can be indicative of a systemic cause of epistaxis.
  - Family history of bleeding
  - Medications: There are numerous medications that are associated with epistaxis. Antiplatelet drugs such as aspirin and clopidogrel, warfarin, and nasal sprays may play a role in epistaxis.
  - Illicit intranasal drug use
  - Trauma: external (eg, blunt trauma, fracture) and internal (eg, finger manipulation)
  - Recent nasal surgery
- Physical examination
  - Airway, breathing, and circulation: always important first steps in any patient with active bleeding or trauma
  - Nasal exam
    - Always use personal protective equipment (eye protection, gloves, mask, etc.).
    - Anterior rhinoscopy
      - Remove all blood clots.
      - Use topical decongestant for visualization and to slow or stop bleeding. Placement of a cotton pledget with a topical vasoconstrictor may be needed to allow visualization.
      - The Kiesselbach plexus is the most likely area to bleed.
    - Nasal endoscopy may be required, particularly to see behind deviations in the nasal septum or to see the posterior nasal cavity.
  - Laboratory evaluation
    - Prothrombin time (PT)
      - Warfarin use
      - Liver disease
      - Malnutrition or malabsorption
    - Partial thromboplastin time (PTT)
      - Heparin use
      - Von Willebrand disease
      - Factor VIII and factor IX deficiencies
    - Bleeding time
      - Decreased platelet aggregation
      - Von Willebrand disease
    - Platelet count
      - Hemoglobin and hematocrit

○ Radiography: There is no indication for routine imaging in the diagnosis of epistaxis. There are certain situations, though, when imaging may be useful.

　— Computed tomography: If there is a suspicion of a nasal or sinus mass, then computed tomography (CT) with intravenous contrast may help in locating the source of bleeding, for example, in juvenile nasopharyngeal angiofibroma (JNA).
　— Magnetic resonance imaging: for improved soft tissue definition
　— Angiography: This is useful for both diagnosis and potential treatment, if embolization is available.

◆ Differential Diagnosis of Local Etiologies of Epistaxis

● **Trauma**: Trauma is the most common local cause of epistaxis. It can be minimal and subtle or massive and obvious.

○ *Digital (finger)*: Digital trauma is common in adults and children. Frequent localized trauma, usually to the anterior septum, can devitalize the perichondrium leading to increased risk of epistaxis. Prolonged exposure to digital trauma can eventually lead to septal perforation with resultant turbulent airflow, drying of the mucosa, and epistaxis.
○ *Fracture*: Fracture of the nasal bony framework or nasal septum will usually present with epistaxis, as well as airway obstruction, external deformity, or swelling.
○ *Surgery*: Epistaxis can occur after nasal and sinus surgery.
○ *Arterial pseudoaneurysm*: Posttraumatic pseudoaneurysm is rare and can present weeks to months after maxillofacial trauma.

● **Environmental factors**

○ *Low humidity*
○ *Elevated altitude*, including airplane travel
○ *Cold air*
○ *Continuous positive airway pressure (CPAP) or nasal oxygen use*: Both can cause turbulent airflow and mucosal drying through the nose, which leads to drying of the mucosa.

● **Rhinitis**: The inflammation associated with any rhinitis causes increased nasal mucosal blood flow and can cause epistaxis.

○ *Allergic rhinitis*
○ *Infectious rhinitis and rhinosinusitis*
○ *Inflammatory rhinitis and rhinosinusitis*

● **Anatomical**

○ *Septal spur/deviation*: Septal spurs and deviations create turbulent airflow in the nasal cavity, which leads to localized mucosal drying, and sometimes crusting, with the area more prone to bleeding.

- ○ *Septal perforation*: Septal perforations also cause turbulent airflow with localized drying and crusting with subsequent bleeding, especially from the posterior edge.
- **Nasal foreign body**: Unilateral epistaxis in a child or cognitively impaired patient, associated with unilateral foul-smelling nasal discharge may indicate a nasal foreign body.
- **Intranasal medications and drugs**
  - ○ *Topical decongestants*: When used excessively topical decongestants can cause mucosal trauma and bleeding. Nasal steroid sprays can also cause epistaxis.
  - ○ *Intranasal use of drugs*: Drugs such as cocaine, hydrocodone, and oxycodone cause significant damage to the nasal mucosa and epistaxis. They can also cause septal perforation.
- **Nasal/sinus neoplasm** (see Chapter 30): Epistaxis accompanied by nasal obstruction, nasal drainage, and/or epiphora may indicate a nasal, sinus, or nasopharyngeal tumor.
  - ○ *Benign neoplasms* include *respiratory papilloma, inverted papilloma, angiofibroma, osteoma, chondroma, hemangioma, pyogenic granuloma,* and *hemangiopericytoma.*
  - ○ *Malignant neoplasms* leading to obstruction include *squamous cell carcinoma, lymphoma, nasopharyngeal carcinoma, sinonasal undifferentiated carcinoma, esthesioneuroblastoma, mucosal melanoma,* or *minor salivary gland malignancy* such as *adenoid cystic carcinoma, mucoepidermoid carcinoma,* or *adenocarcinoma,* or *metastasis.*

◆ Differential Diagnosis of Systemic Causes of Epistaxis

- **Vascular and cardiovascular disease**
  - ○ *Hypertension*: Although most hypertensive patients do not develop epistaxis, many patients with epistaxis are hypertensive. Debate exists over whether hypertension is an independent cause.
  - ○ *Atherosclerotic disease*: Vascular changes, along with mucosal dryness, are thought to be related to the increased incidence of posterior epistaxis observed in adults over 50 years old. It renders vessels unable to constrict to stop bleeding.
  - ○ *Hereditary hemorrhagic telangiectasia (HHT)*: Formerly, Osler-Weber-Rendu syndrome. Autosomal dominant with varying penetrance. HHT is caused by a defect in Alk-1 or endoglin proteins, which are normally highly expressed in vascular endothelial cells. This results in the development of mucocutaneous telangiectasias and arteriovenous malformations (AVMs) often presenting as epistaxis in childhood. Patients commonly experience recurrent epistaxis, gastrointestinal bleeding, and iron deficiency. Telangiectasias can be frequently seen on the nasal mucosa, oral mucosa, and lips of adults. Cerebral, hepatic, and pulmonary AVMs

may also occur in HHT patients, and screening for these sites is recommended.
- ○ Collagen-vascular disorders
  - *Ehlers-Danlos syndrome*: A group of inherited disorders of weakened connective tissue. Affects one in 5000 and features loose joints, stretchy skin, abnormal scarring, and brittle vessels.
  - *Osteogenesis imperfecta*: A phenotype associated with multiple gene mutations affecting type I collagen seen in one in 20,000 live births. Features blue sclera, brittle bones, and multiple fractures, as well as mucosal bleeding.

- **Coagulopathy**
  - ○ Iatrogenic
    - *Medications*
      - ○ Aspirin (ASA): Irreversibly inhibits platelet function
      - ○ Nonsteroidal antiinflammatory drugs (NSAIDs): Reversibly inhibit platelet function
      - ○ Clopidrogrel or ticlopidine: Platelet aggregation inhibitor
      - ○ Warfarin: Inhibits synthesis of vitamin K–dependent coagulation factors (II, VII, IX, X, proteins C and S)
    - *Blood loss*: Prolonged or rapid bleeding can consume enough coagulation factors and platelets to inhibit clotting.
  - ○ Congenital
    - Congenital factor disorders
      - ○ *Hemophilia A*: X-linked recessive factor VIII deficiency affecting one in five to 10,000 males
      - ○ *Hemophilia B*: X-linked recessive factor IX deficiency affecting one in 35 to 30,000 males
      - ○ *Factor XI deficiency*: Common in Ashkenazi Jews, unpredictably presents with variable amounts of bleeding
    - Congenital platelet dysfunction
      - ○ *Von Willebrand disease*: A mostly inherited disorder with multiple subtypes affecting 1% of the population. The absence of factors (commonly von Willebrand factor) required for platelet function causes increased bleeding times with normal platelet counts.
      - ○ *Bernard-Soulier syndrome*: A glycoprotein defect that leads to a functional and quantitative platelet defect
      - ○ *Glanzmann thromblasthenia*: A glycoprotein defect causing dysfunctional platelet aggregation
      - ○ Storage pool diseases
        - *Chédiak-Higashi syndrome*
        - *Wiskott-Aldrich syndrome*
        - *Thrombocytopenia with absent radii syndrome*
        - *Hermansky-Pudlak syndrome*

- ○ **Acquired**
  - — *Liver disease*: Many proteins involved in clotting are produced in the liver and can be reduced in severe liver disease from a variety of causes. Spider telangiectasias, jaundice, and nail changes are common. PT will be elevated.
  - — *Renal failure*: Uremia is associated with platelet dysfunction.
  - — *Malnutrition*
    - ○ Vitamin A, D, E, or K deficiency
    - ○ Scurvy (vitamin C deficiency)
  - — *Polycythemia vera*: Elevated hematocrit can be associated with epistaxis and gastrointestinal bleeding.
  - — *Thrombocytopenia*
    - ○ *Immune (idiopathic) thrombocytopenic purpura (ITP)*: May present in children or adults with estimates of symptomatic presentation around 20 per million. More women are affected and tends to follow infections in children. Defined as platelets < 50,000/μL. Petechiae are asymptomatic and not palpable, a distinction from vasculitis and drug reactions.
    - ○ *Drug reactions*
      - — Beta-lactam antibiotics
      - — Anticonvulsants
      - — Steroid-induced purpura
    - ○ *Consumptive*
      - — *Bleeding*
        - • *Kasabach-Merritt syndrome*: Thrombocytopenia associated with large hemangiomas
    - ○ Hematologic malignancies
      - — *Lymphoma*
      - — *Multiple myeloma*
      - — *Leukemia*
      - — *Myeloproliferative and myelodysplastic syndromes*

Table 29.1 Differential Diagnosis of Epistaxis by Age and Location

Age	Location	Differential Diagnosis
Infant	Anterior	Trauma or abuse Congenital coagulopathy Congenital vascular disease Tumor or malignancy
	Posterior	Tumor or malignancy Congenital coagulopathy Congenital vascular disease Trauma or abuse

Table 29.1 (*Continued*) Differential Diagnosis of Epistaxis by Age and Location

Age	Location	Differential Diagnosis
Young child	Anterior	Congenital coagulopathy Foreign body *Staphylococcus aureus* colonization Trauma
	Posterior	Congenital coagulopathy Tumor or malignancy Foreign body Adenoid hypertrophy
Child	Anterior	Foreign body *S. aureus* colonization Von Willebrand disease Hereditary hemorrhagic telangiectasia Congenital coagulopathy
	Posterior	Congenital coagulopathy Neoplasm Foreign body
Teenager, young adult	Anterior	Trauma Deviated septum Drug abuse Pyogenic granuloma Hereditary hemorrhagic telangiectasia *S. aureus* colonization Deviated septum Nasal sprays
	Posterior	Juvenile angiofibroma Lymphoma
Adult < 50 years	Anterior	Trauma Deviated septum Drug abuse Nasal sprays Pyogenic granulomas
	Posterior	Medication–coagulopathy Tumor or malignancy
Adult > 50 years	Anterior	Deviated septum Nasal oxygen Medication–coagulopathy Nasal sprays Acquired coagulopathy
	Posterior	Atherosclerotic vascular disease Medication–coagulopathy Acquired coagulopathy Tumor or malignancy

Suggested Reading

Chiu TW, McGarry GW. Prospective clinical study of bleeding sites in idiopathic adult posterior epistaxis. Otolaryngol Head Neck Surg 2007;137:390–393

Massick D, Tobin EJ. Epistaxis. In: Cummings CW, Flint PW, Haughey BH, et al, eds. Otolaryngology: Head and Neck Surgery. 4th ed. Philadelphia: Mosby; 2005:941–962

Whymark AD, Crampsey DP, Fraser L, Moore P, Williams C, Kubba H. Childhood epistaxis and nasal colonization with *Staphylococcus aureus*. Otolaryngol Head Neck Surg 2008;138:307–310

30 Nasal or Sinus Mass

K. Christopher McMains

When presented with the prospect of evaluating a patient whose chief complaint is "nasal mass," a wide variety of considerations come into play, each affecting the differential diagnosis and driving evaluation. Because many masses within the nasal cavity and sinuses are initially discovered incidentally during workup for other issues, or cause fairly nonspecific symptoms such as nasal airway obstruction, epistaxis, and hyposmia, many masses are identified late within their course. Facial distortion, nerve dysfunction, or evidence of bony destruction suggests more aggressive disease and is important to elicit for this reason. Once a nasal mass has been identified, the differential diagnosis is vast. Possibilities include anatomical variant (such as enlarged turbinate), congenital or developmental defect, result of traumatic injury, inflammatory/infectious mass, obstructive mass, and benign or malignant neoplasm. Often, thorough history and anterior rhinoscopic exam are sufficient to guide diagnosis. Rigid or flexible endoscopy can serve as a useful adjunct for posteriorly and superiorly based masses and in establishing the relationship between the mass and other structures. Radiographic investigation with computed tomography (CT), magnetic resonance imaging (MRI), or both may be of benefit in certain cases. This chapter is dedicated to the overall issues pertinent to the differential diagnosis of nasal masses.

◆ Presentation

- History: Key factors to consider:
  - Nasal airway obstruction (see Chapter 27)
    - Time course of obstruction
      - Life-long versus progressive: Life-long presence suggests congenital or chronic etiology; progression of severity can represent exacerbation of a chronic condition or progressive growth of a nasal mass.
      - Gradual versus abrupt: Gradual change can be the progression of a chronic condition such as inflammatory polyps or the slow progression of benign neoplastic disease; an abrupt change of traumatic origin can usually be traced to a specific event; abrupt change without history of trauma is worrisome for malignant neoplastic disease.
    - Unilateral versus bilateral
  - Epistaxis (see Chapter 29)
  - Hyposmia/anosmia (see Chapter 31)

- ○ Facial distortion: Although facial distortion is occasionally due to benign disease, in the majority of cases, this results from an aggressive neoplastic process.
- ○ Nerve dysfunction: Malignant neoplastic disease must be excluded if this is identified and not otherwise explained.
- ○ Serous middle ear effusion: Nasal masses that extend into the nasopharynx can physically obstruct eustachian tube outflow; unilateral middle ear effusion mandates investigation of the nasopharynx to rule out neoplasm.

- Physical examination
- Radiological evaluation

- ○ CT: A scan should be completed before biopsy unless a clear plane can be seen between attachment of the nasal mass and the skull base.
- ○ MRI: Enhancement can be affected by biopsy.

◆ Differential Diagnosis of Intranasal Mass

- **Normal anatomy** mimicking a mass: Enlarged or inflamed inferior turbinates can be mistaken for nasal masses; these are usually obvious to the specialist and will shrink with topical decongestion.
- **Anatomical variant**

  — Nasal septum

  - ○ *Maxillary crest*: A maxillary crest gives the appearance of a prominence when quadrangular cartilage is completely off of the crest and protruding into one side.
  - ○ *Deviated nasal septum*: Septal spurs or fractured cartilage can protrude unnaturally into the nasal cavity, giving the illusion of a nasal mass.

  - ○ *Concha bullosa*: Extensive pneumatization of the middle turbinate can expand this structure and appear as a well-mucosalized, unilateral mass posterior and superior to the inferior turbinate.
  - ○ *Duplicate middle turbinate*: This is a relatively rare anatomical variant resulting from atypical embryological progression from the ethmoturbinals to the turbinates.

- **Congenital/developmental**

  - ○ *Glioma*: Ectopic rest of glial tissue. Some can be visible outside the nasal vault, whereas others are located completely within the nasal cavity in the vicinity of the foramen cecum; usually well mucosalized, these do not expand with crying, although they may have a dural stalk.
  - ○ *Meningocele*: Extensions of the meninges outside of the cranial vault. Without a history of trauma, meningoceles are often located in the area of the foramen cecum; these lesions do not contain neuronal or glial tissue and are usually well mucosalized; they may expand with crying.

- ○ *Encephalocele*: Similar characteristics as meningoceles, but contain neuronal tissue within the meningeal sac.
- ○ *Mucocele*: Occurs as a result of entrapped, but productive, respiratory epithelium that continues to produce mucus and can deform or erode bony structures; usually covered with healthy mucosa.
- ○ *Dermoid*: Results from ectopic rests of ectodermal tissue; often associated with a draining tract and repeated infections; draining tracts can exit in the midline or in the medial canthal region.

- **Inflammatory/infectious**

- ○ *Rhinoscleroma*: Infectious disease resulting from *Klebsiella rhinoscleromatis*. this is usually nasal, though it may involve the nasopharynx and larynx. The process may be suppurative, granulomatous (often at the mucocutaneous junction), or cicatricial in appearance, depending on the stage of disease. Lesions may extend to distort the external nasal pyramid. Mikulicz cells are organism-containing vacuolated histiocytes characteristic of rhinoscleroma.
- ○ *Sarcoidosis*: Granulomatous autoimmune disease associated with hilar lymphadenopathy; noncaseating granulomas on pathology; more common in females and African Americans; may be associated with cranial and peripheral neuropathies; commonly involves painful mucosal and submucosal granulomata with associated crusting.
- ○ *Wegener granulomatosis*: Autoimmune disease involving necrotizing granulomatous vasculitis; associated with lower airway disease and glomerular disease; nonspecific symptoms are common, though an ill-described "deep pain" of the nose below the bony/cartilaginous junction can be the presenting symptom.
- ○ *Syphilitic gumma*: Results from untreated infection with *Treponema pallidum*; may result in an intranasal plaque, extranasal plaque, erosive septal lesion, submucosal gummas, saddle nose deformity, or more severe architectural deformity of the nose.
- ○ *Blastomycosis*: Results from infection with *Blastomyces dermatitides*; nasal involvement may be verrucous, granulomatous, or erosive and is far less common than pulmonary and laryngeal forms; associated with residents of the Ohio and Mississippi river valleys as well as immunocompromised individuals.
- ○ *Pyogenic granuloma*: Misnomer referring to a type of hemangioma; may cause nasal airway obstruction, epistaxis, or purulence.
- ○ *Nasal polyp*

- **Foreign body**

- ○ *Iatrogenic*: Usually following surgery or office procedures; can be reactive or inert materials; often accompanied by fetid odor, purulence, and nasal obstruction.
- ○ *Patient-placed*: Most common among pediatric and developmentally disabled populations; often not visible using anterior rhinoscopy alone; note: disc batteries can have similar erosive effects in the nose as in the esophagus and require immediate removal.

- *Rhinolith*: Forms when an intranasal foreign body acts as a nidus upon which salts from inspissated mucus precipitate; symptoms include purulent secretions, recurrent infections, fetid odor, and nasal obstruction; can appear as bone-density on CT.

- **Neoplasm**
  - **Benign**
    - *Juvenile nasopharyngeal angiofibroma*: Occurs in the nasopharynx. Symptoms include nasal airway obstruction (unilateral or bilateral), epistaxis, and hyposmia; usually visible as a red or white mass entering the nasal cavity posteriorly under the middle turbinate; always seen in males, usually in adolescence; CT most commonly demonstrates widening of the pterygopalatine fossa on axial cuts; MRI is useful to identify the extent of the lesion.
    - *Inverted papilloma*: Most often present with nasal obstruction and may lead to epistaxis, proptosis, epiphora, anosmia, or facial numbness; usually there is a single mucosal attachment, although there may be multifocal attachments in recurrent disease; associated with human papilloma virus (HPV) in some cases; evidence of dysplasia and malignant degeneration in a minority of cases.
    - *Hemangiopericytoma*: Most commonly presents with epistaxis, often causes nasal obstruction; well-circumscribed; arise from pericytes surrounding capillaries and venuoles; intermediate behavior, with metastases in some cases.
    - *Fibrous dysplasia*: Can cause slowly progressive disfigurement; can be monostotic, polyostotic, or with systemic associations in *McCune-Albright syndrome;* rapid enlargement suggests malignant transformation; ground-glass appearance of bone on imaging.
    - *Schwannoma*: Presents with nasal obstruction or found incidentally; rarely isolated intranasal schwannoma, often associated with schwannomas of other regions.
    - *Meningioma*: Uncommon extracranially; can be confused with mucocele; on imaging, bony wall bows toward the cranial cavity; can involve the olfactory groove, sphenoid, or clivus; association with traumatic skull fractures.
  - **Malignant**
    - *Squamous cell carcinoma*: Commonly presents with nonspecific symptoms (nasal congestion, discharge, epistaxis) resulting in delay of diagnosis. Dental complaints, facial contour distortion, and diplopia can occur.
    - *Minor salivary gland carcinoma (adenoid cystic carcinoma, mucoepidermoid carcinoma, adenocarcinoma)*: Will present as a submucosal mass, usually with bleeding or crusting, or with other local symptoms except obstruction.
    - *Sinonasal undifferentiated carcinoma (SNUC)*
    - *Esthesioneuroblastoma*: Commonly presents with nonspecific symptoms such as epistaxis, obstruction, or hyposmia; initially unilateral,

but can deform or extend through the septum; can be well mucosalized or ulcerated; located high in the nasal vault.

— *Mucosal melanoma*: Usually presents with unilateral nasal congestion/
obstruction and/or epistaxis; usually occurs lower in the nasal cavity.
Often they are amelanotic and may appear submucosal with apparently
smooth mucosa overlying; color ranges from white to dark brown.

— *Lymphoma*: Often presents with nasal obstruction, crusting, periorbital
edema, rapid expansion of the mass with distortion of the nasal pyramid, and destruction of surrounding structures; NK/T cell lymphomas
are a significant percentage of these lesions. Extranodal B cell lymphomas are common in human immunodeficiency virus (HIV) infection.

— *Sarcoma*: Very rare, submucosal mass

— *Metastasis*: Very rare, can present as mucosal or submucosal mass.

◆ Differential Diagnosis of Paranasal Sinus Mass

● Anatomical variant

- ○ *Mucus retention cyst*: Usually found incidentally on imaging or on evaluation for sinonasal complaints; symptoms can be falsely attributed to
presence of these lesions; cysts occasionally progress in size sufficiently
to obstruct the maxillary outflow.

- ○ *Aberrant carotid (lateral sphenoid)*: Also incidentally found in most cases;
bone overlying this vessel may be dehiscent; should never biopsy.

● Congenital/Developmental lesions: Presentation of these lesions origi-
nating in the paranasal sinuses does not differ significantly from those of
primarily endonasal origin.

- ○ *Glioma*
- ○ *Meningocele*
- ○ *Encephalocele*
- ○ *Mucocele*
- ○ *Vascular aneurysm*: Can be found incidentally; if symptomatic, epistaxis
is almost always the presenting symptom; can be found in the context
of current sinus infection or previous trauma; evaluation with MRA or
formal angiogram indicated.

● Traumatic

- ○ *Foreign body*

- — Bullet/missile: Presents with pain/pressure, discharge, recurrent infections, or sensation of "something moving" in the sinuses; usually with
clear history of trauma.

- — Environmental contaminant: Usually occurs in the context of head and
neck trauma in an outdoor setting with multiple facial fractures; recurrent infections or fistula formation is common.

- — Retained surgical packing: Causes malodorous discharge, recurrent infections, dysosmia, and embarrassment to the surgeon; careful history regarding time of onset.
- — Retained oil-based ointment: Can form a lipogranuloma; presents with nasal obstruction or with distorted nasal anatomy.

- ○ *Displaced bone*: Can cause sinus outflow obstruction with recurrent infections, become devascularized sequestra, serving as a nidus of infection, or be asymptomatic; can be posttraumatic or iatrogenic.
- ○ *Tooth root*: Most often occurs in the context of difficult tooth extraction with retained root tip; nidus for recurrent maxillary sinusitis; may present with maxillary pain/pressure, purulent discharge, dental pain, or fistula formation.
- ○ *Orbital fat prolapse*: May present with enophthalmos, nasal obstruction, or diplopia, or may obstruct maxillary ostium causing sinusitis; motion seen with applied pressure to the globe; may be posttraumatic or iatrogenic.
- ○ *Vascular aneurysm/pseudoaneurysm*: Can also be posttraumatic.

- ● **Physiological**: For each of the following causes, aberrant mucociliary flow results in crusting, nasal airway obstruction (either primarily or secondarily to polyp formation), and hyposmia/dysosmia with potential for recurrent infections.

- ○ *Cystic fibrosis*
- ○ *Ciliary dyskinesias*
- ○ *Postsurgical crusting*

- ● **Inflammatory or infectious**

- ○ *Fungal ball (mycetoma)*: Noninvasive collection of fungal elements usually trapped within a unilateral maxillary sinus (though can be present in other sinuses) causing intense local immune response; usually present in nonatopic, immunocompetent patients; can present with maxillary pressure, tooth pain, unilateral nasal obstruction secondary to polyp formation around the ostiomeatal complex.
- ○ *Sinonasal polyp, including antrochoanal polyps*

- ● **Neoplasm**

  - ○ **Benign**

    - — *Osseous/fibro-osseous*

      - ○ *Osteoma*: Benign, slow-growing tumors that can present in any one of the sinuses, though more common in the frontals and ethmoids; can present incidental to other evaluation, or due to postobstructive sinusitis caused by the enlarging bony mass; association with *Gardner syndrome*.
      - ○ *Ossifying fibroma*: Also known as central cementoossifying fibroma, arise from the periodontal ligament; more commonly found in mandibular sites than in maxillary sites; presents with slowly progres-

sive distortion of maxillary contour; juvenile subtype demonstrates more aggressive behavior.
   ○ *Fibrous dysplasia*

— *Odontogenic*

   ○ *Ameloblastoma*: Benign tumor of the dental epithelium; presents as painless swelling of the affected region; more common in mandibular sites; multilocular subtype is most frequently seen; described as "soap-bubble" appearance on radiography.
   ○ *Odontogenic cyst*: Several types exist, almost uniformly presenting as solitary swellings along the gingival mucosa, rarely painful; occasional transformation to squamous cell carcinoma; multiple odontogenic keratocysts presenting simultaneously is associated with *basal-cell nevus syndrome.*

— *Inverted papilloma*
— *Minor salivary gland neoplasm*: Usually an extension from minor salivary glands along the superior oral cavity, although there are minor salivary glands in the paranasal sinus mucosa as well. Most common benign neoplasms are *pleomorphic adenoma, monomorphic adenoma,* and *oncocytoma,* but benign pathology is rare in minor salivary neoplasms.
— *Neuromas*

   ○ **Malignant**

— Epithelial neoplasms

   ○ *Squamous cell carcinoma*: The most common epithelial lesion of the paranasal sinuses; relationship to the Ohngren line informs severity of disease. The Ohngren line extends from the medial canthus to the angle of the mandible; lesions above the line are generally more aggressive and invade earlier, whereas lesions below the line are considered less aggressive. Most commonly these are rapidly progressive and can be painful, with a foul smell of necrotic tissue.
   ○ *Adenocarcinoma*: Second most common nasal neoplasm of the sinuses; usually presents high within the nasal vault; associated with occupational exposures (especially wood dust).

— *Lymphoma*
— Minor salivary gland neoplasms: Eighty percent are malignant, and the most common histologies are *adenoid cystic carcinoma, mucoepidermoid carcinoma,* and *adenocarcinoma.*
— *Sarcoma*: Several types can affect this region (*osteosarcoma, chondrosarcoma, rhabdomyosarcoma*); they usually present as a rapidly growing lesion, can distort facial contour and discolor skin; osteosarcoma can have classic "sunburst" or "sunray" appearance on radiography; rhabdomyosarcoma is the most common paranasal sinus sarcoma in childhood.
— *Mucosal melanoma*: These are less common in the paranasal sinuses than in the nasal cavity, but they share similar features.

◆ Differential Diagnosis of a Nasopharynx Mass

- **Normal anatomy**: Adenoid tissue without disease; common in children
- **Anatomical variant**
  - *Adenoid hypertrophy* without disease: More common in adults with allergy
  - *Posterior pharyngeal scarring* from previous adenoidectomy
  - *Tornwaldt cyst*: Midline, mucosalized, fluid-filled cavity lying superior to the adenoid pad; embryological remnant of the notochord; usually asymptomatic and discovered incidentally. It can become infected leading to local symptoms of pain and postnasal drainage.

- **Inflammatory/Infectious**
  - *Infectious mononucleosis*
  - *Adenoiditis*

    — *Viral*

      - *Respiratory virus*
      - *Epstein-Barr virus*

    — *Bacterial*

  - *Adenoid hypertrophy*

    — *HIV infection*
    — *Lymphoproliferative disorders*

  - *Actinomycosis*
  - *Fibrosing inflammatory pseudotumor*: Associated with cranial nerve deficits and histologically mixed infiltrates without evidence of malignancy.

- **Neoplasms**
  - *Lymphoma*: Also associated with HIV infection; suspect with massive adenoid pad in an adult; attempt at complete removal can result in significant blood loss.
  - *Nasopharyngeal carcinoma*

Table 30.1 Causes of Nasal Mass, by Symptom

Symptom	Etiology
Nasal obstruction	Any nasal mass
Nasal discharge	Dermoid Rhinoscleroma Wegener granulomatosis Pyogenic granuloma Chronic invasive fungal disease Foreign body Rhinolith Inverting papilloma Cystic fibrosis Ciliary dyskinesias Postsurgical crusting Malignancies
Hyposmia/anosmia	Any mass obstructing airflow Esthesioneuroblastoma
Epistaxis	Granulomatous diseases Pyogenic granuloma Juvenile Nasopharyngeal Angiofibroma Inverting papilloma Hemangiopericytoma Aberrant carotid Aneurysm/pseudoaneurysm Malignancies
Pain	Sarcoidosis Wegener granulomatosis
Facial distortion	Syphilis Fibrous dysplasia Ossifying fibroma Odontogenic cysts Ameloblastoma Malignancies
Nerve dysfunction	Sarcoidosis Inverting papilloma Schwannomas Fibrosing inflammatory pseudotumor Malignancies

Table 30.2 Common Associations and Eponyms in Nasal and Sinus Masses

Condition	Association/"Buzzword"
Meningocele/encephalocele	Expands with crying
Dermoid	Fistulous tract
Rhinoscleroma	*Klebsiella rhinoscleromatis* Mikulicz cells
Sarcoidosis	Noncaseating granulomas
Wegener disease	Pulmonary and renal disease
Blastomycosis	Ohio and Mississippi River Valleys Immunocompromise
Unilateral nasal polyposis	Allergic fungal sinusitis Antrochoanal polyp Inverting papilloma Malignancy
Inverting papilloma	HPV infection
Juvenile nasopharyngeal angiofibroma	Adolescent males
Fibrous dysplasia	McCune-Albright syndrome
Petroleum products	Lipogranuloma
Osteoma	Gardener disease
Ameloblastoma	"Soap bubble" on radiography
Squamous cell carcinoma	Ohngren line
Adenocarcinoma	Wood dust
Osteosarcoma	"Sunburst"/"sunray" on x-ray
Mononucleosis	Atypical lymphocytosis
Nasopharyngeal carcinoma	Epstein-Barr virus
Nasopharyngeal lymphoma	HIV infection
Multiple odontogenic keratocysts	Basal cell nevus syndrome

Abbreviations: HPV, human papillovirus; HIV, human immuno-deficiency virus.

Suggested Reading

Ghaffar S, Salahuddin I. Olfactory neuroblastoma: a case report and review of the literature. Ear Nose Throat J 2005;84(3):150–152 Review

Hedlund G. Congenital frontonasal masses: developmental anatomy, malformations, and MR imaging. Pediatr Radiol 2006;36:647–662, quiz 726–727 Review

Randall DA. The nose and paranasal sinuses. In: Lee K, ed. Essential Otolaryngology. 8th ed. McGraw-Hill; 2003:747–790

31 Anosmia and Olfactory Disturbance

Mark A. Zacharek

Olfaction can be affected by many different disease processes. Olfactory disorders may be organized into categories:

- Anosmia is the loss of the ability to smell.
- Hyposmia is a diminished ability to smell.
- Parosmia is an alteration in an olfactory cue resulting in a specific smell perceived differently.
- Phantosmia is a perception of a smell when there is no external olfactory stimulation.
- Presbyosmia pertains to the smell impairment associated with age. The loss of smell is commonly the true cause of taste disturbance complaints.

◆ Review of Anatomy

The olfactory neuroepithelium is a complex network of primary and secondary neurons that make up the most ancient of the senses in humans as well as other species. This basic sensory input is more developed in other mammalian species but is critical to vertebrates and invertebrates alike.

- The primary olfactory neuroepithelium is a pseudostratified columnar epithelium lying upon the cribriform plate. Olfactory neuroepithelium is made up of several different components.

  - Olfactory receptor cells lie on the cribriform plate as well as on the superior septum and middle and superior turbinates.
  - Nerve bundles of the bipolar receptor cell then course through foramina in the cribriform plate and form the olfactory bulb, then branch out and form synaptic connections with dendrites of secondary neurons. The bipolar cells are the likely transit route by which viral and other inflammatory processes progress into the central nervous system (**Fig. 31.1**).
  - A secondary cell or sustentacular cell lies with the bipolar cells in the olfactory neuroepithelium and helps to regulate mucus production and odorant physiology.
  - Additional cells include microvillar cells, supporting cells of the secretory Bowman glands, and dark horizontal and globose basal cells, which are the primordial cells from which all the others arise (**Fig. 31.2**).

- Olfactory neuroepithelium possesses a regenerative capacity. The degree of regeneration of olfactory neuroepithelium is dependent on the severity of the inciting event.

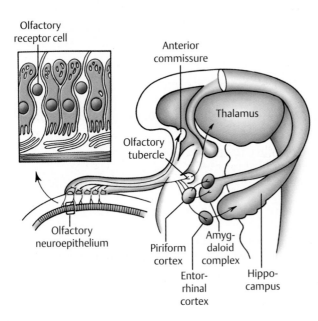

Olfactory receptor cell

Anterior commissure

Thalamus

Olfactory tubercle

Olfactory neuroepithelium

Piriform cortex

Amyg-daloid complex

Entor-rhinal cortex

Hippo-campus

Fig. 31.1 Nerve bundles of the bipolar receptor cell course through foramina in the cribriform plate and form the olfactory bulb. They then branch out and form synaptic connections with dendrites of secondary neurons. The bipolar cells are the likely transit route by which viral and other inflammatory processes progress into the central nervous system.

- The **basal globose cells** serve as the pluripotential cells, which regenerate the supporting and sensory bipolar cells. If the environmental insult is slight, then regeneration may occur. If the damage is severe, respiratory-like epithelium infiltrates the area of damage.
- This regeneration may take many years as realized in cohorts of smokers who stop their habit and realize an improvement in their sense of smell over several years.

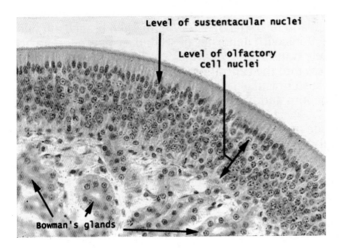

Level of sustentacular nuclei

Level of olfactory cell nuclei

Bowman's glands

Fig. 31.2 Olfactory neuro-epithelium—histology.

◆ Clinical Factors to Consider when Differentiating Causes of Small Disturbance

● The **onset** of disturbed smell is important to differentiating the cause.
  ○ A **gradual onset** is most often associated with the aging process; about 50% of patients 65 to 80 years of age have diminished olfactory function. The gradual loss is associated with additive environmental exposures, viral and bacterial damage, closure and stenosis of the cribriform foramina through which the sensory bipolar cells travel, as well as associations with dementia and neurodegenerative conditions associated with aging.
  ○ **Sudden loss** of smell is more associated with either viral inflammatory damage of the olfactory neuroepithelium or shear injury of the axonal nerve fibers at the level of the cribriform plate occurring with closed head injury.
● **Unilateral** versus **bilateral**
● **Associated symptoms**, such as memory loss, allergic rhinitis, headache, and seizure disorder

◆ Diagnostic Testing

● **Smell identification tests**
  ○ **UPSIT** (University of Pennsylvania Smell Identification Test, Sensonics, Inc., Haddon Heights, NJ). Unilateral testing can be aided by obstructing the nontest nares with a piece of tape such that cross stimulation via the nasopharynx (retronasal stimulation) does not occur. The UPSIT is a psychophysical test that is well validated and has excellent reliability compared with other testing instruments. Four booklets containing 10 odorants each are embedded on a scratch and sniff strip. Patients are asked to choose from one of four responses for each side of the nose. This test can distinguish from malingering because a 10 out of 40 response is statistically the chance performance. Lower scores suggest malingering. The UPSIT is scored on norms based on age and sex.
● **Electrophysiological tests** are available, including **odor event-related potentials (OERPs),** which involve the electroencephalographic (EEG) measurement of brain activity with surface scalp electrodes while the patient is administered odorants.
  ○ The **electroolfactogram (EOG)** involves electrode application onto the surface of the olfactory neuroepithelium, which measures generator potentials of the sensory neuronal activity. This testing is experimental and not widely available.
● **Radiographic testing**
  ○ Computed tomography
  ○ Magnetic resonance imaging

◆ Useful Clinical Classification

- **Conductive** versus **sensorineural** impairments of olfaction. Olfactory disturbance may occur from a multitude of causes. A helpful classification schema involves organizing disease processes based on **conductive/obstructive** processes versus malfunction at the level of the neuroepithelium.
  - **Conductive/obstructive**: Primary disruption or injury to the olfactory system may occur by affecting the transporting system of odorants to the olfactory sensory organ. These include sinonasal disease, chronic rhinosinusitis (CRS), nasal tumor, or mass.
  - The **sensorineural** impairment of olfaction occurs from direct damage to the neuroepithelium by virus, bacterial infection, trauma, or exposure to industrial toxins.
  - Combined **conductive** and **sensorineural** processes can occur in the same patient. This classification schema is helpful to allow for counseling of patients. In general, conductive causes of olfactory disturbance are more easily treatable than those associated with sensorineural damage. Sensorineural causes, however, are more common.

◆ Differential Diagnosis of Conductive Causes of Anosmia

- **Inflammatory disease**: Very common
  - *Allergic and nonallergic rhinitis*: Nasal mucosal edema and an increase in mucous secretion causes obstruction of odorants reaching the olfactory neuroepithelium.
  - *Nonallergic triggers*: Including barometric and temperature changes result in mucosal inflammation and may affect smell as well.
- **Infectious** etiology
  - *Viral rhinosinusitis*: Inflammatory infections of the nose commonly due to the Rhinovirus family. Several other viruses including adenovirus may damage the neuroepithelium with either partial or complete disruption resulting in sensorineural deficit. If no neurological damage occurs, the edema and resultant effect on smell are limited by the duration of the viral illness. Viral infection can also cause **sensorineural anosmia.**
  - *Bacterial rhinosinusitis*: Cause in acute inflammatory infiltration in the sinonasal cavity with resultant nasal obstruction and transient olfactory dysfunction.
- **Neoplasms**: Usually associated with nasal obstruction or epistaxis. See Chapter 30 for extensive differential diagnosis of neoplasms.
  - *Esthesioneuroblastoma* is the most common neoplasm presenting with anosmia as the only symptom.

- **Fixed obstruction**. Anatomical variants can result in obstructive symptoms but are less likely to affect odorant transmission to the roof of the nose as described for the foregoing processes. Examples include the following:
  - *Paradoxical turbinates*
  - *Nasal septal deformity/septal spurs*
  - *Turbinate hypertrophy*
  - *Atrophic rhinitis*
  - *Nasal-bypassing surgery,* such as *laryngectomy* or *tracheotomy*
- **Trauma**
  - *Iatrogenic conductive defect,* from septoplasty, rhinoplasty, iatrogenic synechia, and so on.

◆ Differential Diagnosis of Sensorineural Causes of Anosmia (Table 31.1)

- *Aging process*: The association of aging with the progression of loss of smell is well established. Approximately 1% of the population younger than 65 years has significant smell dysfunction compared with greater than 50% of those individuals between 65 and 80 years of age. In those individuals greater than 80 years old, 75% have a significant decrease in their sense of smell.
- *Viral rhinitis* and resultant damage to the olfactory neuroepithelium at the roof of the nose is the second most common cause of permanent smell disturbance. The culprit virus can be one of many different families of viruses: primarily what occurs is the reduction of the number of olfactory receptors. The severity of damage to the basal cell layer determines whether regeneration occurs. Usually, the residual olfactory neuroepithelium is abnormal in histologic appearance.
  - *Human immunodeficiency virus (HIV)* infection can also affect olfactory function.
- **Trauma**
  - *Shear injury from head trauma* is another common cause of smell disturbance. Studies vary in the incidence of anosmia after head trauma, from 5 to 19%. Olfactory loss in childhood head trauma occurs less frequently. The location of injury, loss of consciousness, and Glasgow Coma Scale are factors affecting the severity of olfaction injury: lower Glasgow Coma Scale scores and head injuries associated with anterior skull base fractures, dural tears and cerebrospinal fluid leaks, and bilateral frontal lobe injuries are more associated with smell disturbance. The force or blow to the occipital or frontal regions of the head is more likely to damage olfaction than a blow to the temporal or parietal region.
  - *Iatrogenic injury* from nasal surgery (septoplasty, rhinoplasty turbinate resection, sinus surgery) more commonly causes conductive anosmia,

but if force is transmitted to the cribriform plate, then sensorineural anosmia can result.

- **Intracranial neoplasms** of the olfactory bulb
  - *Meningioma*
  - *Frontal lobe glioblastoma multiforme*
  - *Astrocytomas*
  - *Metastatic lesions*
- **Neurological causes** of olfactory dysfunction must also be considered in the geriatric population.
  - Olfactory loss may be the first symptom of *Alzheimer or Parkinson disease.*
    - *Alzheimer disease*: Neurofibrillary tangles associated with Alzheimer disease are deposited in the highest concentrations in regions of the brain responsible for processing olfactory bulb sensorineural input.
    - *Parkinson disease*: Can result in significant olfactory dysfunction, although the mechanism is poorly understood.
  - *Multiple sclerosis*: Can be associated with olfactory disturbance.
  - *Temporal lobe seizures*: Can cause transient anosmia; usually caused by Ramsay Hunt syndrome, trauma, or primary seizure disorders. Patients can have hyperosmic symptoms in the postictal period.
- **Metabolic causes**
  - *Alcohol abuse*
  - *Chronic renal insufficiency*
  - *End-stage liver disease with cirrhosis*
  - *Vitamin and mineral deficiency (zinc, copper, vitamins A, B6, B12)*
- **Medications**
  - Several *antimicrobials* including *macrolides, penicillins, tetracyclines*
  - *Zinc sulfate irrigations* have recently been associated with altered sense of smell; *zinc sulfate* may damage the neuroepithelium in susceptible patients.
  - *Methotrexate*
  - Rarely, *nasal steroid sprays*
- **Endocrine disorders**
  - *Addison disease*
  - *Cushing disease and Cushing syndrome*
  - *Diabetes mellitus*
  - *Acromegaly*
  - *Hypothyroidism*
  - The effects of *pregnancy* and the elevated level of follicle-stimulating hormone (FSH) and luteinizing hormone (LH) are thought to effect a hyperosmic sense in some women.
  - *Kallmann syndrome* is due to maldevelopment of the olfactory bulbs characterized by hyposmia or anosmia and associated hypothalamic lesions

resulting in gonadal dysfunction. This is an X-linked mutation resulting in a reduction of hypothalamic gonadotropin-releasing hormone. Both autosomal recessive and dominant forms of the condition exist and can have variable expression in females as well.

- **Psychiatric** causes of olfactory dysfunction must be considered in some patients.
  - *Malingering* may be a result of a patient's underlying intent to pursue legal action. The malingering patient can be distinguished from the truly olfactory dysfunctioning patient by the administration of the UPSIT. Malingerers will score very low (less than 10 out of 40 responses correct). Because the test is a forced choice test, patients who are malingering will avoid choosing the proper answer.
  - *Depressive disorders* are also associated with anosmia and hyposmia.
  - *Schizophrenia*

Table 31.1 Differential Diagnosis of Anosmia

Conductive Etiology	Sensorineural Etiology
Inflammatory causes Allergic and nonallergic rhinitis	*Aging process*
Infectious Viral rhinosinusitis Bacterial rhinosinusitis	*Infectious* Viral rhinitis with olfactory damage
Neoplasm Benign Inverting papilloma Malignant Esthesioneuroblastoma Squamous cell carcinoma Lymphoma Salivary carcinoma Sinonasal undifferentiated carcinoma	*Trauma* Frontal or occipital blow with shearing of nerves at cribriform Iatrogenic injury to cribriform from surgery
Fixed nasal obstruction Paradoxical turbinates Nasal-septal deformity Turbinate hypertrophy Rhinoplasty Sinus surgery Iatrogenic synechiae Atrophic rhinitis	*Intracranial neoplasm* Meningioma Glioblastoma Astrocytoma Metastasis

(continued on page 166)

Table 31.1 *(Continued)* Differential Diagnosis of Anosmia

Conductive Etiology	Sensorineural Etiology
Decreased nasal airflow Laryngectomy Tracheostomy	*Neurologic* Alzheimer disease Parkinson disease Multiple sclerosis Temporal lobe seizure
Trauma Fracture causing airway obstruction	*Metabolic* EtOH Chronic renal failure Chronic liver failure Vitamin and mineral deficiency
	Medications Antimicrobials Zinc sulfate irrigation Methotrexate Nasal steroid sprays *Endocrine* Addison disease Cushing disease Diabetes Acromegaly Hypothyroidism Kallmann syndrome
	Psychiatric Malingering Depression Schizophrenia

Abbrevation: EtOH, ethyl alcohol.

Suggested Reading

Bailey BJ, Johnson JT, Newlands SD, eds. Head and Neck Surgery–Otolaryngology. Vol 1. 4th ed. Philadelphia: Lippincott Williams & Wilkins; 2006

Cummings CW, Flint PW, Harker LA, et al, eds. Otolaryngology Head and Neck Surgery, Vol. 2. 4th ed. Philadelphia: Elsevier Mosby; 2005

Doty RL. Handbook of Olfaction and Gestation. 2nd ed. New York: Marcel Dekker; 2003

Fong KJ, Zacharek MA. Olfaction and aging. In: Calhoun KH, Eibling DE, eds. Geriatric Otolaryngology. New York: Taylor & Francis Group; 2006:173–180

32 Foul Odor

Mark A. Zacharek

The perception of an abnormal odor in the patient's nose can suggest many different pathologies.

◆ Pertinent History

- **Duration**
  - Short periods are suggestive of acute infection or inflammation.
  - Longer periods are suggestive of an obstructing mass or chronic infectious process.
- **Associated complaints**
  - Pain
  - Loose dentition
  - Numbness: Suggests tumor infiltration
    - — Superior alveolar nerve
    - — Infraorbital nerve
  - Nasal airway obstruction
- **Previous trauma**
- **Previous nasal or sinus surgery**

◆ Physical Examination

- Attention to the facial symmetry of the patient is important. Observed mass effect on the septum or nasal vestibule, particularly when unilateral, raises suspicion for a tumor or congenital or odontogenic process.
- Unilateral serous effusion may suggest eustachian tube obstruction or nasopharyngeal mass.
- Cranial nerve exam
- Anterior rhinoscopy
- Nasal endoscopic (flexible or rigid) examination

◆ Radiology

- **Computed tomographic (CT) scan** with contrast
- **Magnetic resonance imaging (MRI) scan** with contrast

◆ Etiologies of Foul Smell in Nose

- An actual smell in nose
  - From nose or sinus
  - From nasopharynx
  - Halitosis, from base of tongue, with retronasal smell sense
- False sensation of smell in nose
  - Disorder of olfactory epithelium
  - Central neurological etiology
  - Psychiatric disorder
  - Malingering

◆ Differential Diagnosis of Specific Sites of Foul Odor from the Nose

- **Nasal or sinus source**
  - **Infectious**
    - *Bacterial rhinitis or rhinosinusitis* can cause foul smell, directly from purulence
    - *Nontuberculous mycobacteria infection*
    - *Chronic granulomatous fungal infection*
    - *Actinomycosis*
  - **Foreign body**
    - *Rhinolith*
    - *Surgical packing*
    - *Other foreign body*
  - **Odontogenic** etiologies: Infection associated with periodontal pathology, such as *periapical cyst, nasopalatine duct cyst,* primary jaw tumor such as *ameloblastoma.*

○ **Neoplasm** of the nasal or sinus cavity (see Chapter 30). Foul smell can be due to nose or sinus obstruction with bacterial overgrowth, tumor necrosis, or tumor colonization or superinfection.

○ **Atrophic rhinitis:** The "empty nose syndrome" can occur as a result of excessive surgical resection of turbinates bilaterally and stripping of nasal mucosa. It gives rise to nasal crusting and drying and affects olfaction. Also known as rhinitis sicca, the disease results from either bacterial infection with *Klebsiella ozaenae* or *Corynebacterium diphtheriae* (atoxic form). The bacteria cause ciliary dysfunction in the sinus and nasal cavity with resultant foul-smelling crusts and sloughing off of large portions of mucosa with loss of normal pseudostratified respiratory epithelium that undergoes metaplasia to areas of keratinized squamous epithelium. The infectious form of atrophic rhinitis is more common in developing nations and in individuals with poor hygiene. The atrophic form is invariably caused by excessive surgery, or nasal trauma or manipulation, such as from drug abuse.

○ **Nasal septal perforation:** Buildup of crust and debris can cause foul odor.

● **Nasopharynx source**

  ○ **Infectious**

  — *Adenoiditis*
  — *Tornwaldt cyst* can become secondarily infected resulting in nasal obstructive symptoms and foul discharge from the nose.

  ○ **Neoplasm** (see Chapter 30): The most common neoplasms are:

  — *Nasopharyngeal carcinoma*
  — *Lymphoma*

● **Neurological source:** When a distorted sense of smell is perceived (ie, something pleasant smells unpleasant to the affected patient), it is referred to as parosmia. When the patient perceives a smell that is not actually present, it is referred to as phantosmia; phantosmias are usually unpleasant, such as rotten eggs, dying tissue, or other fetid smells.

  ○ *Olfactory epithelial damage:* Usually causes parosmia. Most common etiologies from viral injury, toxic inhalation, or trauma. The parosmia usually only occurs during the initial postinjury phase and resolves or can be permanent.

  ○ *Central neurological etiology:* Can cause parosmia or phantosmia.

  — *Brain tumor*
  — *Temporal lobe epilepsy*
  — *Cerebrovascular disease*

● **Psychiatric disorders:** Can cause parosmia and phantosmia and is particularly seen in somatization disorders.

Table 32.1 Sources of Foul Smell from the Nose

Source	Infection	Foreign Body	Neoplasm
Nasal cavity	Viral or bacterial infection Tuberculosis Fungal Odontogenic abscess Atrophic rhinitis Postsurgical Primary infection	Extracorporeal tissue Nasal crusting Rhinolith Retained surgical packing	Benign or malignant
Paranasal Sinus	Acute and chronic rhinosinusitis Odontogenic abscess Atypical mycobacterial infection Fungal infection	Extracorporeal tissue Rhinolith Retained surgical packing	Benign or malignant
Nasopharynx	Adenoiditis Infected Tornwaldt cyst	Nasopharyngeal Rhinolith	Benign or malignant
Neurological or psychiatric			

Suggested Reading

Bailey BJ, Johnson JT, Newlands SD, eds. Head and Neck Surgery–Otolaryngology. Vol 1. 4th ed. Philadelphia: Lippincott Williams & Wilkins; 2006

Cummings CW, Flint PW, Harker LA, et al, eds. Otolaryngology Head and Neck Surgery. Vol 2. 4th ed. Philadelphia: Elsevier Mosby; 2005

Doty RL. Handbook of Olfaction and Gestation. 2nd ed. New York: Marcel Dekker; 2003

V Differential Diagnosis in Pediatric Rhinology and Sinus Disease

Section Editors: *Max M. April and Robert F. Ward*

33 Nasal Obstruction in Children

Dale Amanda Tylor and Seth M. Pransky

◆ Background

- Nasal obstruction is an extremely common complaint in the pediatric population, which can significantly impact the child's quality of life.
- Significant confusion and misuse surrounding pediatric "sinusitis" versus nasal issues exists in the lay press and among medical colleagues.
- Neonates are obligate nasal breathers for the first several months of life, and nasal obstruction in this instance can be life threatening.
- The etiology of pediatric nasal obstruction can be categorized into the classifications of infectious/inflammatory, congenital, iatrogenic/traumatic, immunologic/other, and neoplastic.
- The evaluation and management of pediatric sinonasal complaints are approached differently than in adults for several reasons including the following:
  - Decreased ability to provide a reliable history
  - Different underlying disease processes, often related to growth, development, and exposure to infectious organisms
  - Less cooperative with diagnostic procedures
  - Possible decreased compliance with treatments (such as nasal saline irrigations)

This chapter covers **nasal obstruction** in children. Other presenting symptoms of sinonasal disease include rhinorrhea, epistaxis, mass, and anosmia, and those are covered in detail—including pediatric diagnosis—in Chapters 28 through 32.

◆ Infectious/Inflammatory Etiologies

By far, these are the most common causes of nasal airway obstruction in the pediatric population.

- *Rhinitis, rhinosinusitis, adenoiditis*: Viral infection (much more commonly than bacterial infection) resulting in inflammation of one or more areas of the uppermost aspect of the respiratory tract. Children develop six to eight upper respiratory infections (URIs) per year, and 0.5 to 5.0% of these URIs will be complicated with acute sinusitis.

- *Allergic rhinitis*: Episodic, seasonal, or perennial nasal obstruction, often associated with complaints of sneezing, pruritic eyes or nose, or lacrimation. Allergy testing may or may not reveal the allergen; consider *nonallergic rhinosinusitis with eosinophilia syndrome* (NARES) if testing is negative.
- *Adenoid hypertrophy*: Extremely common, often with associated mouth breathing and snoring, with characteristic facies (open mouth, long and narrow face, short upper lip)
- *Nasal polyposis*: In children usually associated with *asthma, cystic fibrosis,* or allergic rhinitis.
- *Antrochoanal polyp*: Originates in the maxillary sinus and can grow to very large sizes, even extending into the nasopharynx or oropharynx.
- *Neonatal rhinitis*: Can be related to nasal trauma in the neonatal period (vigorous suctioning), viral URIs, milk/soy allergies, extraesophageal reflux, or an idiopathic etiology.
- *Chronic rhinitis of childhood*, or "daycare nose": Typically, occurs in children less than 6 years of age, with ongoing mucopurulent rhinorrhea and nasal airway obstruction.
- *Gastroesophageal reflux or extraesophageal reflux*: Commonly identified in children and may be "silent" apart from nasal complaints.
- *Vasomotor rhinitis*: Excessive cholinergic response related to head position, food intake, temperature changes, or environmental irritants, leading to turbinate hypertrophy and nasal congestion; rare in children.

◆ Congenital Etiologies

- *Choanal stenosis* or *choanal atresia*: More often bony than membranous, other congenital anomalies are present in up to 50% of cases. Classic finding in bilateral disease is "cyclical cyanosis" with cyanotic episodes associated with feeding; crying bypasses the obstruction. Unilateral disease may not present until later childhood, with unilateral obstruction and rhinorrhea.
- *Piriform aperture stenosis*: Can be associated with *holoprosencephaly* (and single maxillary mega-incisor), endocrine abnormalities, and other maxillary dental anomalies.
- *Nasal malformations*: Facial dysostosis, clefts, partial to complete absence of nasal structures
- *Tornwaldt cyst*: In nasopharynx just superior to adenoid; is an embryological remnant of the notochord and tends to present in older children and adults.
- Midline nasal masses
  - *Dermoid cyst*: Presents at birth, generally in the midline. A sinus tract is frequently present, often with associated hair or sebaceous material.
  - *Encephalocele*: Sixty percent external nose, 30% intranasal, 10% mixed
  - *Glioma*: Typically intranasal and can resemble a nasal polyp.
  - *Teratoma*: Can present anywhere, but nasopharynx is a common location; very rarely can undergo malignant transformation.

◆ Iatrogenic/Traumatic Etiologies

- *Foreign body*: Often in the setting of unilateral purulent rhinorrhea. If a button battery is suspected, emergent removal should be performed because of the risk of septal perforation.
- *Trauma*: Blunt or penetrating. Can occur at birth, with severe *septal deviation* requiring closed reduction in the first week of life. Nasal fractures are associated with *septal hematomas* in children more frequently than in adults. Septal hematoma can lead to septal cartilage devitalization and subsequent septal perforation and/or saddle nose deformity if not managed expeditiously with surgical drainage. Synechiae or septal perforations can also develop with penetrating trauma.
- *Nasopharyngeal stenosis*: Rare complication associated with use of laser or aggressive nasal cautery during adenoid surgery or palatal procedures, with scarring of the tonsil pillars and soft palate to the posterior pharyngeal wall.
- *Surgical repair of velopharyngeal insufficiency*: Pharyngeal flap, posterior pharyngeal wall augmentation, and velopharyngeal sphincteroplasty can all result in nasal airway obstruction.
- *Rhinitis medicamentosa*: Prolonged use of topical nasal decongestants leads to a rebound nasal mucosal dilation. This is very rare in the pediatric population.

◆ Immunologic/Other Etiologies

- *Cystic fibrosis*: Presenting symptoms may include nasal obstruction or recurrent sinusitis; nasal polyposis is often identified. CT scans commonly reveal extensive sinus disease even in fairly asymptomatic patients.
- *Immune deficiencies*: Can be present in up to 0.5% of the population. *Common variable immunodeficiency* (CVID), *immunoglobulin G (IgG) subclass deficiency*, and *selective antibody immune deficiencies*, in descending order, are most prevalent in the pediatric population.
- *Ciliary dyskinesia*: Can be a primary diagnosis or can be associated with a syndrome including recurrent respiratory infections, sinusitis, otitis media, male infertility, and situs inversus (*Kartagener syndrome*); very rare.

◆ Neoplastic Etiologies

- Benign masses
  - *Hemangioma*: Most common benign tumor of neonates; often involves the septum.

- ○ *Pyogenic granuloma*: Often posttraumatic in nature, associated with epistaxis and nasal obstruction.
- ○ *Juvenile nasopharyngeal angiofibroma*: Typically, occurs in adolescent males, presenting with epistaxis, nasal obstruction, and rhinorrhea.
- ○ Other very rare benign neoplasms
  - — *Craniopharyngioma*
  - — *Chordoma*
  - — *Lipoma*
  - — *Chondroma*
  - — *Hemangiopericytoma*
  - — *Schwannoma*
  - — *Neurofibroma*
  - — *Rhabdomyoma*
  - — *Pleomorphic adenoma*

- Malignant masses
  - ○ *Lymphoma*: Usually Hodgkin or non-Hodgkin lymphoma
  - ○ *Rhabdomyosarcoma*: Most common malignant head and neck soft tissue neoplasms in children
  - ○ *Esthesioneuroblastoma*: Mainly in teenagers and young adults
  - ○ *Nasopharyngeal carcinoma*: Very rare in young children but can present in teenage years; 70% have neck metastases at presentation.
  - ○ Other very rare masses
    - — *Squamous cell carcinoma*
    - — *Adenocarcinoma*
    - — *Neuroendocrine or neuroectodermal tumors*
      - ○ *Small cell carcinoma, Ewing sarcoma*
    - — *Soft tissue tumors*
      - ○ *Fibrosarcoma, neurofibrosarcoma, malignant fibrous histiocytoma*
    - — Germ cell tumor: *Yolk sac tumor*

Table 33.1 The 5 A's of Assessment of the Most Common Causes of Sinusitis/Nasal Obstruction in Children

Allergy	Allergy symptoms present in over 50% of children with nasal obstruction. All children warrant assessment of allergies if symptomatic.
Adenoids	Can be assessed with rhinoscopic exam, fiberoptic nasopharyngoscopy, or lateral neck x-ray. Adenoids are a bacterial reservoir and the surface can harbor a biofilm. In children with adenoid hypertrophy who undergo adenoidectomy, a majority have significantly improved nasal obstructive symptoms.
Acid	Many children with chronic sinusitis can be found to have gastroesophageal reflux disease on pH probe studies, and treatment of the reflux can resolve sinus symptoms in some of these patients.
Anatomy	Look for septal deviation, turbinate abnormalities, sinus disease, and anatomical abnormality. Plain x-rays of the sinuses are not typically useful, and computed tomographic scan is preferred.
All other	Cystic fibrosis workup, immune deficiency workup, or ciliary motility assessment can be performed if the history or clinical course is suspicious.

Suggested Reading

Benoit MM, Bhattacharyya N, Faquin W, Cunningham M. Cancer of the nasal cavity in the pediatric population. Pediatrics 2008;121:e141–e145

Lusk R. Pediatric chronic rhinosinusitis. Curr Opin Otolaryngol Head Neck Surg 2006; 14:393–396

Myer CM III, Cotton RT. Nasal obstruction in the pediatric patient. Pediatrics 1983;72:766–777

Smart BA. Pediatric rhinosinusitis and its relationship to asthma and allergic rhinitis. Pediatr Asthma Aller 2005;18:88–98

VI Differential Diagnosis in the Oral Cavity (Adult and Pediatric)

Section Editor: *Jason G. Newman*

34 Oral Pain

Mark H. Terris

The symptom of oral pain, although nonspecific, can be an indicator of localized or systemic dysfunction. Oral pain can be associated with a myriad of disorders and diseases. Thorough history taking and evaluation of the oral cavity during the otolaryngological examination can often aid the clinician in establishing a definitive diagnosis. Many times, however, laboratory testing is required to confirm the clinical suspicion.

In evaluating the etiologies of oral pain, it is convenient to consider the various conditions by the areas or systems affected, which is the approach taken in this chapter. Oral pain can be a result of diseases affecting the tongue (glossitis), lips (cheilitis), or any other region of oral mucosa (stomatitis). Dental disorders can be an alternative source of oral pain. Similarly, it may be secondary to a salivary gland, pharyngeal, neurological, or psychological disorder. Individual descriptions of the disorders are beyond the scope of this text.

The differential diagnosis of etiologies affecting the lips, tongue, or oral cavity mucosa causing pain is vast. Certain infectious causes of oral pain may result in fever or leukocytosis. Systemic diseases with oral manifestations will often have symptoms and signs of disease outside the oral cavity that can be elicited with a thorough history, physical examination, and laboratory testing. Although many of the conditions following here are benign, the cause of oral pain secondary to precancerous or malignant lesions must always be considered. Suspicious lesions should always be considered neoplastic until otherwise determined. Biopsy with histopathological analysis is often necessary. Most infectious lesions listed here will have other findings, such as ulceration, blistering, or mucosal change, which are covered in detail in Chapter 36.

◆ Infectious Disease

● Viral

- *Herpetic gingivostomatitis*
- *Varicella*
- *Herpangina (Coxsackie A or B)*
- *Hand, foot, and mouth disease (Coxsackie A)*
- *Human papilloma virus*
- *Human immunodeficiency virus (HIV)*

● Bacterial

- *Staphylococcus/Streptococcus*
- *Tuberculosis*

- ○ *Syphilis*
- ○ *Diphtheria*
- ○ *Gonorrhea*
- ○ *Rhinoscleroma*
- ○ *Leprosy*

- **Fungal**

  - ○ *Candidiasis*
  - ○ *Actinomycosis*
  - ○ *Blastomycosis*
  - ○ *Histoplasmosis*
  - ○ *Sporotrichiosis*

◆ Inflammatory Disease

- *Aphthous ulcers*
- *Lichen planus*: Lichen planus (LP) is a cell-mediated immune response that causes pruritic, papular eruptions. Lesions are most commonly found on the tongue and the buccal mucosa; they are characterized by white or gray streaks forming a linear or reticular pattern on a violaceous background.
- *Behçet syndrome*: This rare syndrome is characterized by ocular inflammation and recurrent aphthous ulcers of the oral mucosa and the genitalia.
- *Eagle syndrome*: Oral pain, usually oropharyngeal, and unilateral, is secondary to inflammation around a calcified stylohyoid ligament.
- *Xerostomia*: Is more notable for the dry mouth but can cause oral pain. Causes include the following:

  - ○ *Obligatory mouth breathing*
  - ○ *Medications*
  - ○ *Collagen vascular disorders*, such as *scleroderma* and *Sjögren syndrome*
  - ○ *Radiation therapy*

◆ Bullous Disease

In the pemphigus disease group, the blisters are broken easily; therefore, they are rarely observed clinically. Instead, erosions and superficial ulcers are more likely observed. In the pemphigoid disease group, because the blisters are situated deeply, they are more likely to be observed intact clinically.

- *Pemphigus vulgaris*
- *Bullous pemphigoid*
- *Epidermolysis bullosa*
- *Erythema multiforme*

◆ Noninfectious Granulomatous Disease

- *Sarcoidosis*: Patients may present with a malar butterfly rash and oral or cutaneous lesions consisting of elevated erythematous plaques, hypopigmented edges, and alopecia. Pulmonary involvement may cause a concurrent cough, and patients often also have lymphadenopathy.
- *Langerhans cell histiocytosis (histiocytosis X)* and *eosinophilic granuloma*: The clinical presentation is varied, with patients presenting with acute mastoiditis, middle ear granulation tissue, tympanic membrane perforations, proptosis, diabetes insipidus, or facial nerve paralysis.
- *Wegener granulomatosis*: The disease is characterized by a triad of airway necrotizing granulomas, systemic vasculitis, and focal glomerulonephritis. In addition to oral ulcerations, patients may have septal perforations, saddle nose deformities, sinusitis, otitis media, cough, or hemoptysis.
- *"Idiopathic midline destructive disease"*: This disease category probably no longer exists because most former cases are now known to be *Wegener granulomatosis, lymphomatoid granulomatosis (polymorphic reticulosis),* or *low-grade lymphoma.* Disease is localized to the head and the neck, and it may present with pansinusitis and ulceration of the nasal floor and septal ulcerations.
- *Melkersson-Rosenthal syndrome*: Lip swelling, fissured or plicated tongue, and facial palsy may be observed.

◆ Metabolic Disorders

- *Irondeficiency anemia (Plummer-Vinson syndrome aka Paterson-Brown-Kelly syndrome)*: Anemia, brittle nails, confusion, constipation, depression, and dizziness may occur with glossitis.
- *Vitamin B deficiency*: Patients may have anemia, mood disturbances, dizziness, intestinal disturbances, headaches, loss of vibration sensation, numbness, or spinal cord degeneration.
- *Pellagra*: Patients often have a triad of diarrhea, dermatitis, and dementia.
- *Vitamin A deficiency*: Acne, dry hair, insomnia, hyperkeratosis (thickening and roughness of skin), and night blindness may be noted.
- *Diabetes mellitus*

◆ Precancerous Lesion/Neoplasm

See Chapter 37.

◆ Allergy

- *Food allergy*
- *Food sensitivity*

◆ Trauma

- *Scalds*
- *Caustic injury*
- *Foreign body*
- *Blunt*
- *Penetrating*

◆ Idiopathic

- *Burning mouth syndrome*

◆ Dental and Periodontal Disease

The disorders presented here are common, affecting at least 20% of the adult population. Poorly fitting dentures or sharp teeth can irritate the oral mucosa producing pain, especially if secondary infections develop. Patients with gingival or periodontal disease will often present with painful, bleeding gums, resorption of the gingival margin, or bacterial plaques.

- *Acute necrotizing ulcerative gingivitis (Vincent angina)*
- *Periodontitis*
- *Osteitis and osteomyelitis*
- *Dentures/poor dentition*

◆ Neurogenic

Consideration and detection of neurogenic causes of oral pain most often requires a comprehensive neurological examination. Proper cranial nerve, cerebellar, and peripheral motor and sensory nerve examination can most often detect the following causes of oral pain.

- *Organic brain disease (cerebral atrophic syndrome)*
- *Glossopharyngeal neuralgia, intermedius neuralgia, lingual neuralgia*: Attacks are brief and occur intermittently, but they cause excruciating pain. Attacks may be triggered by a particular action, such as chewing, swallowing, talking, coughing, or sneezing.
- *Progressive paralysis and tabes dorsalis*: Tabes dorsalis occurs in tertiary syphilis and is a slowly progressive degenerative disease involving the posterior columns (ie, demyelination) and posterior roots (ie, inflammatory change with fibrosis) of the spinal cord. Thus the neurological presentation is one of ongoing loss of pain sensation, loss of peripheral reflexes, impairment of vibration and position senses, and progressive ataxia.

◆ Psychogenic

Eliciting specific characteristics of oral pain, including onset, severity, frequency, aggravating/alleviating factors, can help determine psychogenic etiologies. Additionally, obtaining a thorough social history may shed light on any psychosocial causes of oral pain.

◆ Salivary Gland Disease

See Chapter 39.

Suggested Reading

Campana JP, Meyers AD. The surgical management of oral cancer. Otolaryngol Clin North Am 2006;39:331–348

Gonsalves WC, Chi AC, Neville BW. Common oral lesions, I: Superficial mucosal lesions. Am Fam Physician 2007;75:501–507

Gonsalves WC, Chi AC, Neville BW. Common oral lesions, II: Masses and neoplasia. Am Fam Physician 2007;75:509–512

Jabaley ME, Clement RL, Bryant WM. Recognizing oral lesions. Am Fam Physician 1976;13:604

McDowell JD. An overview of epidemiology and common risk factors for oral squamous cell carcinoma. Otolaryngol Clin North Am 2006;39:277–294

Neville BW, Day TA. Oral cancer and precancerous lesions. CA Cancer J Clin 2002;52:195–215

Touger-Decker R, Mobley CC; American Dietetic Association. Position of the American Dietetic Association: oral health and nutrition. J Am Diet Assoc 2007;107:1418–1428

35 Oral Inflammation

Michael Medina and Miriam Lango

Stomatitis and mucositis may cause diffuse mouth discomfort. By definition, stomatitis refers to any inflammatory reaction affecting the oral mucosa, with or without ulceration, that may be caused or intensified by local factors. Mucositis refers to inflammation affecting the gastrointestinal (GI) system anywhere from the mouth to anus, most commonly in response to chemotherapeutic agents or ionizing radiation. Frequently, the terms *stomatitis* and *mucositis* are used interchangeably. There may be predominant involvement of the tongue (glossitis) or gums (gingivitis). Individuals with diminished immunity due to malignancy, human immunodeficiency virus (HIV), malnutrition, pregnancy, or infancy are subject to severe and potentially life-threatening stomatitis. The most common causes of stomatitis in this population are listed in **Table 35.1**.

◆ Stomatitis in Immunodeficient Individuals

- *Candidiasis*: The white plaques of pseudomembranous candidiasis are usually asymptomatic, although burning or a foul taste in the mouth may be reported. Individuals with erythematous or atrophic candidiasis may complain of a "scalded mouth." Diffuse loss of filiform papillae yields a reddened "bald" tongue. In immunodeficient patients it may be refractory to usual measures. Hyperplastic candidiasis and chronic multifocal candidiasis are also encountered in this population.
- *Aphthous stomatitis*: Frequent, extensive outbreaks that may lead to severe infection.
- *Viral infections*: Including *Herpes simplex virus, Varicella-zoster virus,* and *Epstein-Barr virus*
- *Vitamin deficiency*

  - *Vitamin B deficiency (niacin, B6, B12)*: Can cause stomatitis and glossitis even in patients without symptomatic anemia or macrocytosis. There may be associated angular cheilitis. A red beefy tongue is characteristic. Infants and children demonstrate developmental and growth delays. Pregnant or lactating women, alcoholics, and patients with malignancies or malabsorption are also at high risk.
  - *Iron-deficiency anemia, Plummer-Vinson syndrome,* and *folate deficiency anemia*: presents with glossitis and recurrent aphthous ulcers
  - *Vitamin C deficiency*: Causes generalized gingival swelling with spontaneous hemorrhage, ulceration, tooth mobility (*scorbutic gingivitis*) associated with widespread petechial hemorrhages and ecchymoses.

Table 35.1 Common Causes of Stomatitis/Mucositis

Immunodeficient patient	**Any age**	Candidiasis Aphthous stomatitis Viral Necrotizing ulcerative gingivitis/noma Drug/radiation treatment Leukemia/plasma cell gingival hyperplasia Graft versus host disease
Immunocompetent patient	**Children/young adults**	Viral Kawasaki disease Drug reaction Contact stomatitis Trauma Poisoning Emesis Diarrhea (Crohn/celiac disease) Malnutrition
	Middle-aged and older adults	Aphthous stomatitis Smoking Poor oral hygiene Trauma Emesis Malnutrition Candidal stomatitis Contact stomatitis Denture stomatitis Drug reaction Lichen planus Behçet syndrome Pemphigoid Systemic lupus erythematosus Mouth breathing Orthodontic work Geographic tongue Uremia Burning mouth/burning tongue syndrome

- *Noma* (or *cancrum oris,* or *necrotizing/gangrenous stomatitis*): Occurs in individuals with immune suppression as a result of malignancy (leukemia) or HIV and is an opportunistic infection of the oral flora. Malnutrition, dehydration, poor oral hygiene, are other predisposing factors. The process frequently starts as an acute necrotizing ulcerative gingivitis. This condition primarily affects 2- to 10-year-olds, but is rare in the United States. HIV-related gingivitis and periodontitis are common.
- *Acute mucositis* secondary to *chemotherapy, radiotherapy, radioactive iodine ablation*: is common. These treatments disrupt the mucosal cell cycle causing mucosal erythema and random, focal-to-diffuse, ulcerative lesions. Methotrexate, 5-fluorouracil (5-FU), and cytarabine in particular are associated with increased stomatotoxicity. The combination of radiation with chemotherapy increases the incidence and severity of mucositis in head and neck cancer patients. Mucosal breakdown and impaired wound healing promote infection and tissue loss.
- *Graft versus host disease (GVHD)*: Following bone marrow transplantation may result in the donor's immunocompetent cells attacking host mucosa causing stomatitis. Eighty percent of patients with chronic GVHD will have oral symptoms, including burning, atrophic mucosa, ulceration, xerostomia, and other mucosal changes.
- *Plasma cell gingivitis* and *leukemic gingival hyperplasia*
- *Kaposi sarcoma* in HIV patients

◆ Stomatitis in Immunocompetent Individuals

For those with intact immune systems, the causes of stomatitis vary by patient age. For children, viral causes are most common, although allergic contact stomatitis, drug reactions, malnutrition, poisoning, and associated GI symptoms should be kept in mind. In older adults, denture use, poor oral hygiene, smoking, medication use, and associated cutaneous lesions need to be assessed.

- **Fevers** and the presence of **mucosal vesiculoerosive lesions** suggest an infectious etiology, more frequently seen in young children and immunocompromised patients.

  - *Viral*

    - *Acute herpetic gingivostomatitis (HSV1)*
    - *Hand, foot, and mouth disease (Coxsackievirus)*
    - *Herpangina (Coxsackievirus)*
    - *Kawasaki disease*: Young children with conjunctivitis, erythematous mucus membranes, and "strawberry tongue." Arthralgias, skin rashes, and cardiac abnormalities may be present. Asian males under 5 years of age are at greatest risk.

  - *Candidal stomatitis*: May develop after antibiotic use, but is also encountered in HIV patients, leukemic patients, and infants. Pseudomembranous candidiasis is most common after antibiotic use. Erythematous and mucocutaneous candidiasis may also be seen.

- ○ *Drug-related anaphylactic stomatitis*: May be associated with generalized anaphylaxis but may also present as isolated findings. Mucosal erythema with or without numerous aphthous-like ulcerations may be present. Numerous drugs can cause such reactions, but penicillins and sulfa drugs are most common. *Barbiturates, dapsone, salicylates, sulfonamides,* and *tetracycline* have also been associated with fixed mucosal eruptions, reappearing 30 minutes to 8 hours after drug administration.

- ● *Allergic contact stomatitis*: Arises in response to oral flavorings (eg, cinnamon), preservatives, and dental materials (metals, acrylates, resins, impression compounds). Sensitivity to mouthwashes, toothpaste, alcohol, spicy foods, and tobacco has been implicated. Allergic contact stomatitis can be acute or chronic. Burning pain is the main symptom. The affected mucosa may be erythematous or normal. Desquamation or hyperkeratotic changes can be seen.

- ● *Aphthous stomatitis*: Recurrent superficial ulcers, etiology is still unclear but genetic and immunologic causes are currently most accepted. Painful mucosal macules undergo superficial ulceration, measure 3 to 10 mm, resolve in 14 days, and are almost exclusively on nonkeratinized mucosa. Larger, more persistent lesions may occur and are more common in immunocompromised patients. Patients with *Behçet syndrome* and *Crohn disease* may have similar intraoral findings.

- ● *Poisoning*: May cause stomatitis associated with cognitive changes, neuropsychiatric symptoms, or language delay. Acute toxicity may be associated with abdominal pain, nausea and vomiting, pharyngitis, and gingivitis. Signs and symptoms may be nonspecific, especially with chronic, low-dose exposures.

  - ○ *Mercury toxicity*: Neurological symptoms and GI symptoms may be present. Metallic taste, ulcerative stomatitis, enlargement of the salivary glands, gingiva, and tongue are reported. The gingiva may have a bluish or grayish discoloration. Destruction of alveolar bone leads to early tooth loss. In children, chronic mercury exposure leads to acrodynia (Swift disease).

  - ○ *Lead toxicity (Plumbism)*: May present with ulcerative stomatitis and a gingival lead line, a bluish line along the gingival sulcus, representing a lead sulfide precipitate. Gray areas may also be noted on the buccal mucosa and tongue. Other associated symptoms may include tongue tremor, advanced periodontal disease, excessive salivation, and metallic taste in the mouth.

  - ○ *Bismuth toxicity*: Like lead toxicity, frequently leads to the development of a blue-gray line along the gingival margin. There may be diffuse discoloration of the oral mucosa, skin, and conjunctiva. Ulcerative stomatitis and ptyalism may be seen.

- ● Stomatitis and *malnutrition/vitamin deficiency*: See above.
- ● Stomatitis with **diarrhea and weight loss**

  - ○ Although abdominal cramping and pain, diarrhea, fevers, weight loss, and a constellation of oral cavity findings in a teenager suggest *Crohn disease*, oral lesions precede GI lesions in as many as 30% of cases. Patients develop diffuse nodular swelling of the oral and perioral tissues, cobble-stoning of the oral mucosa, aphthous-like oral ulcerations, and occasionally metallic dysgeusia. Patients with *celiac disease* may also present at this age, with GI symptoms and stomatitis due to B-vitamin deficiency.

  ○ *Emesis-related mucosal reactions*

  — *Emesis* can cause a sore throat, throat swelling, dysphagia, and odynophagia. Gastroesophageal reflux disease can cause a chronic sore throat.
  — Individuals with *bulimia*: Most frequently young women, may develop gingivitis, erosion of dental enamel causing dental sensitivity, parotid gland enlargement, and characteristic cuts over the back of the fingers.
  — *Gastric bypass* patients: Subject to vomiting after overeating and/or may develop B-vitamin deficiencies.

- Intraoral mucosal inflammation associated with **cutaneous lesions**

  ○ *Lichen planus*: A common chronic dermatologic disease that often affects the oral mucosa. Middle-aged adults develop purple pruritic papules, usually affecting the extremities. Intraoral involvement may include the buccal mucosa, tongue, or gingiva. *Lichenoid drug reactions* may also occur. Arsenic, bismuth, gold, quinidine, propranolol, and naproxen have been implicated. Patients with suspicious erosive lesions should be biopsied to rule out cancer.
  ○ *Cicatricial pemphigoid*: Most patients exhibit areas of erythema and diffuse irregular ulceration. Involvement of other sites (conjunctival, nasal cavity, esophagus, larynx) is less common but associated with scar formation and stricture at these sites.
  ○ *Behçet syndrome*: Middle-aged men (thirties) develop aphthous-like ulcerations involving the soft palate and oropharynx. Frequently six or more ulcerations may be present at once. Oral involvement precedes cutaneous and genital lesions, and uveitis, in 25 to 75% of cases.
  ○ *Systemic lupus erythematosus*: Malar or discoid rash, arthritis, and oral ulcers support this diagnosis. Up to 40% of patients with lupus have mucosal changes in the palate, buccal mucosa, and gingivae. Variable ulceration, redness, and hyperkeratosis are present. Patients with *discoid lupus* may also have oral lesions.

- *Geographic tongue* or *Erythema migrans*: Is characterized by multiple well-demarcated zones of erythema over the tip and lateral borders of the anterior tongue with a whitish border. Lesions come and go. Most patients are asymptomatic, although some report sensitivity to spicy foods or a burning type of discomfort.
- *Melkersson-Rosenthal syndrome*: A fissured tongue associated with periodic nodular swelling of the lips or face. This disease has a hereditary basis.
- *Denture stomatitis*: Characterized by erythema localizing to the denture-bearing mucosa of the maxillary alveolus. Affected individuals admit to wearing the denture continuously, and sometimes also develop chronic atrophic candidiasis. Most individuals are asymptomatic.

- *Poor oral hygiene*: May lead to the development of gingivitis and stomatitis. Diabetes, mouth breathing, smoking, and poor nutrition may contribute. Patients develop swollen, erythematous gingiva. Breach of the mucosa may lead to secondary infection by the oral flora. There may be an accumulation of dental plaque and dental calculi. In predisposed individuals, *acute necrotizing ulcerative gingivitis (trench mouth)* may develop.
- *Smoking-related stomatitis*
  - Pipe or cigar smoking, reverse smoking, may cause stomatitis. White keratotic changes over the palate are common. Changes due to reverse smoking are usually precancerous.

- *Trauma* (cheek biting, ill-fitting dentures): Can cause mucosal injury, which may be secondarily infected. Chronic ingestion of very hot beverages can also cause changes over the palate similar to those found with smoking-related stomatitis.
- *Mouth breathing*
- *Orthodontic treatment*
- *Uremic stomatitis*: Has been described in particular in individuals in acute renal failure. There is an abrupt onset of white plaques or crusts on the buccal mucosa, tongue, and floor of mouth, associated with burning pain. Urea may be broken down by the oral flora into ammonia, which damages oral mucosa. Dialysis helps.
- *Burning mouth syndrome* (*Stomatopyrosis*) and *burning tongue syndrome* (*Glossopyrosis*) are diagnoses of exclusion. May be associated with abnormal taste (usually bitter and/or metallic). Some postmenopausal women with mouth discomfort benefit from hormone replacements. Risks must be weighed against possible benefits.

Suggested Reading

Eisen D. The clinical features, malignant potential, and systemic associations of oral lichen planus: a study of 723 patients. J Am Acad Dermatol 2002;46:207–214

Eisenberg E. Diagnosis and treatment of recurrent aphthous stomatitis. Oral Maxillofac Surg Clin North Am 2003;15:111–122

Epstein JB. Mucositis in the cancer patient and immunosuppressed host. Infect Dis Clin North Am 2007;21:503–522, vii

Field EA, Speechley JA, Rugman FR, Varga E, Tyldesley WR. Oral signs and symptoms in patients with undiagnosed vitamin B12 deficiency. J Oral Pathol Med 1995;24:468–470

LeSueur BW, Yiannias JA. Contact stomatitis. Dermatol Clin 2003;21:105–114, vii

Neville BW, Damm DD, Allen CM, et al. Oral and Maxillofacial Pathology. Philadelphia: WB Saunders; 1995

Schubert MM, Correa ME. Oral graft-versus-host disease. Dent Clin North Am 2008;52:79–109, viii–ix

Zunt SL. Vesiculobullous disease of the oral cavity. Dermatol Clin 1996;14:291–302

36 Mucosal Ulceration or Lesion

Bryan C. Ego-Osuala and Duane Sewell

Diagnosis of lesions in the oral cavity can usually be made clinically, with biopsy reserved for suspected malignant lesions. A proper history and physical exam, however, are essential. To distinguish between the various causes of ulcers and lesions, several aspects of the history must be elucidated. History of lesion/ulcer: onset, duration, progression, pain, bleeding, changes in appearance. Other factors: trauma (eg, from poorly fitting dentures), risk factors for malignancy (EtOH and tobacco use), autoimmune disease, history of previous lesion, taste or sensory disturbances, hoarseness, sore throat, trismus, fever, or malaise.

◆ Lesions That Present as *Ulcers*

- *Pemphigus vulgaris*: Autoimmune disease. Can affect mucosa of oral cavity, nasal cavity, pharynx and larynx. Typically seen in older adults in the fifth decade and above. It is a chronic illness, and typically presents as erosions, blisters, and ulcerations. The blisters tend to be short lived, and as old blisters rupture and collapse, new ones form. These ruptured lesions ulcerate and cause pain.
- *Cicatricial pemphigoid* or *mucous membrane pemphigoid*: Also an autoimmune disease. Can affect the oral cavity, nasal cavity, pharynx, and larynx. These usually present as patchy distribution of erythematous vesicles and bullae, usually beneath a collapsed bulla as an ulcer. The lesions have a predilection for the palate and gingiva. It is less commonly seen on the buccal mucosa.
- *Bullous pemphigoid*: Chronic autoimmune skin disease involving the formation of blisters below the surface of the skin and antibodies against the type XVII collagen component of hemidesmosomes. It can also involve the mucous membranes in the head and neck, but only rarely.
- *Herpes simplex virus*: This will be covered in the inflammation section but these very shallow painful ulcers present as small vesicles on the oral mucosa that are short lived and quickly become ulcers with a surrounding erythematous ring.
- *Aphthous stomatitis (canker sores)*: Usually seen on the labial, buccal, ventral tongue, floor of mouth, lateral tongue, soft palate, and tonsillar pillars. According to studies, this is prevalent in people of high socioeconomic status, nonsmokers, and members of professional groups. They can be very painful, but they typically last 7 to 10 days. They heal without scarring.
- *Erythema multiforme (EM)*: This is a self-limiting mucocutaneous hypersensitivity reaction characterized by cutaneous or oral cavity ulcerations. Usually involves the mucosa in a symmetrical distribution. On close examination, you will see target or iris lesions that are usually irregular in size.

- *Eosinophilic granuloma (traumatic granuloma)*: This condition usually presents as painful ulcers that develop along the lateral and ventral tongue, although sometimes on the dorsum of the tongue as well. They usually range in size from 1 to 2 cm; the periphery is sharply marginated, firm, and indurated.
- *Malignancy*: Any nonhealing ulceration could potentially represent carcinoma and should be biopsied or referred to an otolaryngologist for biopsy and definitive diagnosis. The most common cancer in the oral cavity is *squamous cell carcinoma*. Risk factors include smoking and drinking alcohol.

◆ Lesions That Present as *Changes of Mucosa Color*

- *Leukoplakia (white plaque)*: Appears white, usually benign (less than 10% will be malignant or show severe dysplasia). Leukoplakia is a hyperkeratotic lesion that may or may not be associated with dysplastic change on histologic examination.
- *Erythroplakia (red plaque)*: Appears red. The chance of malignancy is higher than with leukoplakia; sometimes seen in association with leukoplakia. Approximately half will show carcinoma or dysplasia on biopsy.
- *Nodular leukoplakia (mixed white and red plaques)*: Same chance of malignancy as erythroplakia. Sometimes seen in association with invasive cancer in the oral cavity, usually squamous cell carcinoma (SCCA).
- *Hairy leukoplakia*: Usually seen along the lateral tongue margins bilaterally, and ranges from subtle white keratotic vertical streaks to thick corrugated and sometimes shaggy alterations. The Epstein-Barr virus is considered an etiologic agent for this lesion.
- *Lichen planus (LP)*: Typically presents as white striaform lesions that occur bilaterally, it can also be symmetric in distribution. Usually asymptomatic in the above form. LP can also present as an erosive/ulcerative lesion; these will usually be painful. LP is a disease of immunologic origin that is T cell mediated. The erosive form may progress to SCCA.
- *Candidiasis*: This entity will be covered further in the inflammation section; however, it does present as a white pseudomembrane that can usually be scraped off with a tongue depressor. Patients with this might also have odynophagia secondary to pain.
- *Anemia*: Globally pale mucosa
- *Bismuth and/or arsenic intoxication*: Black or brown discoloration
- *Lead intoxication*: Blue-gray gingival discoloration, also known as Burton lines
- *Polycythemia vera, hepatic insufficiency*: Global erythema of mucosa
- *Peutz-Jeghers syndrome (gastrointestinal hamartomatous polyps)*: Perioral melanotic macules
- *Fordyce disease (overgrown ectopic sebaceous glands)*: Small yellow spots. This is a very rare disease that occurs mostly on the skin. It is a chronic pruritic papular eruption that localizes to areas where apocrine glands are found.
- *Hyperplastic filiform papillae/black hairy tongue*: This is caused when the papilla do not fall off as they normally do. As the length of the papilla in-

creases, debris collects and bacteria grow, producing the characteristic dark appearance. This may be associated with antibiotic use.

- *Osler-Weber-Rendu disease*: Multiple mucosal telangiectasias. Frequent nosebleeds are often present, though bleeds could occur in the oral cavity as well. Look for port wine stain. This is a genetic disease with autosomal dominant inheritance pattern.
- *Addison disease*: Diffuse hyperpigmentation of the oral mucosa. Look for skin changes such as areas of hyperpigmentation, or dark tanning, covering exposed and nonexposed parts of the body. This darkening of the skin is most evident on scars; skin folds; pressure points such as the elbows, knees, knuckles, and toes; lips; and mucous membranes.
- *Hemochromatosis*: Bronze pigmentation
- *Xanthomatous disease*: Yellow/gray pigmentation
- *Kaposi sarcoma (HIV+)*: Violaceous macules. On exam one would note patches of abnormal tissue on the skin, in the oral mucosa, nose, and throat, or in other organs. The patches are usually red or purple and are made up of cancerous cells and blood cells. The red and purple patches often cause no symptoms; sometimes, however, they may be painful.
- *Amalgam tattoo*: Usually in people who have had dental work. Usually occurs from inadvertent implantation of dental amalgam into the adjacent gingiva or mucosa.
- *Melanoma*: May be flat, heterogeneously pigmented, irregular in shape. Most oral cavity melanoma will occur on the soft palate, some will occur on the gingiva.

◆ Lesions That Present as *Masses*

- *Torus*: These are developmental anomalies that grow out of the bone. They usually present in the second decade of life and continue to grow throughout life. On the mandible; torus mandibularis: found in the anterior mandible. On the palate, torus palatinus—found in the midline.
- *Lingual thyroid*: Bulge seen on the dorsum of the tongue in the area of the foramen cecum. Represents the lack of descent of thyroid tissue during development. Some of these patients will have hypothyroidism.
- *Fibroma*: Common in the oral cavity, it represents an inflammatory and fibrous hyperplastic response to chronic irritation.
- *Lipoma*: Uncommon, seen in patients after the third decade of life. Presents as a soft, slowly enlarging, mucosa-covered, smooth painless mass. Can be found in the buccal, lingual, and floor areas of the mouth.
- Malignancy: Tumors in the oral cavity could also represent malignancy. In general, pain, weight loss, bleeding, and sometimes night sweats will accompany a malignancy. They are generally indurated on palpation. They need to be biopsied to determine the diagnosis.
- Benign neoplasm: These include vascular tumors such as *hemangiomas*, which tend to have a quiescent phase and a rapid growth phase. *Vascular malformations (venous and lymphatic types)* do not have a proliferative

growth phase like hemangiomas. *Lymphangiomas* are found commonly in the tongue and floor of mouth.

◆ Lesions Due to *Trauma*

● *Laceration*

Suggested Reading

Carpenter CCJ, Griggs RC, Loscalzo J. Cecil's Essential of Medicine. Philadelphia: WB Saunders; 2001

Cummings CW. Otolaryngology–Head and Neck Surgery. Vol 2. 4th ed. Philadelphia: Mosby; 2005

Lalwani AK. Current Diagnosis and Treatment in Otolaryngology–Head and Neck Surgery. 2nd ed. New York: McGraw-Hill; 2008

Lee KJ. Essential Otolaryngology–Head and Neck Surgery. 8th ed. New York: McGraw-Hill; 2003

37 Mass in the Oral Cavity

David M. Cognetti and Robert L. Ferris

The oral cavity extends from the vermilion border of the lips anteriorly to the junction of the hard and soft palates and the circumvallate papillae of the tongue posteriorly. A wide variety of masses, both benign and malignant, can present in the oral cavity. Masses can arise from any of the various tissue types present in the oral cavity, including the mucosa, salivary glands, teeth, and bone. Most benign lesions are asymptomatic and present as slow-growing painless masses. Malignant lesions are more commonly associated with pain and ulceration, which can lead to difficulty eating and weight loss. More than 90% of malignant lesions of the oral cavity are squamous cell carcinomas, which are linked to tobacco and alcohol use. Therefore, assessment of these risk factors is important when evaluating a patient with an oral cavity mass. Infection with human papilloma virus (HPV) has been associated with oropharyngeal cancer and to a lesser degree with oral cavity cancer. This section reviews both benign and malignant oral cavity masses categorized by anatomical subsite. Each diagnosis is discussed according to the **site of most common occurrence**, with the exception of squamous cell carcinoma, which is detailed by subsite.

◆ Lip

- *Mucus retention cysts*: Due to an obstructed salivary duct, which leads to epithelial proliferation. As a result, they have an epithelial lining. They are submucosal, slow growing, fluctuant, and painless.
- *Mucus escape reaction, or mucocele*: Due to extravasation of mucus secondary to traumatic severance/interruption of a salivary gland duct. These are cystlike and painless and differ from *mucus retention cysts* in that they lack an epithelial lining. The lower lip is the most common site, followed by the buccal mucosa.
- *Squamous cell carcinoma*: Accounts for > 90% of cancers of the lips, of which > 90% occur on the lower lip. The most important risk factor for lip cancer is sun exposure, which likely explains the much higher rate of lower lip involvement. Although *basal cell carcinomas* are frequently described to involve the upper lip, these tumors likely arise from the cutaneous portion of the lip and are not true oral cavity lesions.
- *Minor salivary gland tumors*: See Palate section.

◆ Tongue

- *Granular cell tumor*: Small, benign, painless, submucosal mass thought to arise from Schwann cells. Tongue is the most common site. These tumors can be confused with squamous cell carcinoma on microscopic examination due to pseudoepitheliomatous hyperplasia.
- *Papilloma*: Benign squamous proliferation due to human papilloma virus (HPV). Different serotypes (HPV 6 and 11) account for benign papillomas than for HPV-related squamous cell carcinoma (HPV 16). Presents as a pedunculated mass with fingerlike projections. Usually painless and nonulcerated but may have a white surface change due to keratinization.
- *Squamous cell carcinoma*: Commonly occurs on the lateral border of the oral tongue (**Fig. 37.1**). Typically presents as a painless, nonhealing ulcer in the middle portion of the lateral tongue. Pain, referred otalgia, and dysarthria can develop with advanced lesions. Squamous cell carcinoma very rarely occurs in the midportion of the dorsum of the oral tongue. Diagnosis of squamous cell carcinoma in this location should raise suspicion of misdiagnosis and warrants a second histologic opinion.
- *Leukoplakia*: Clinical description for white plaque that cannot be rubbed off. Diagnosis of exclusion with up to 10% malignant transformation rate.
- *Erythroplakia*: Clinical description for a red mucosal plaque that cannot be explained by another clinical or pathological condition. Typically friable and has a much higher malignant transformation rate than *leukoplakia*.
- *Irritation fibroma*: Firm lesion, on lateral border of oral tongue (**Fig. 37.2**)
- *Verrucous carcinoma* (see Buccal Mucosa section)
- *Pyogenic granuloma* (see Alveolar Ridge section)

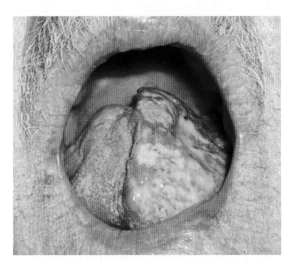

Fig. 37.1 Squamous cell carcinoma of the left lateral tongue.

Fig. 37.2   Irritation fibroma of the lateral tongue.

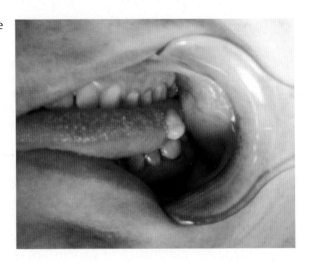

◆ Floor of Mouth

- *Wharton duct*: Main salivary duct of the submandibular gland. The papilla opens in the anterior floor of the mouth, and the duct may be mistaken for a mass.
- *Ranula*: Mucocele occurring in the floor of the mouth in association with the sublingual gland. Named for its resemblance to the undersurface of a frog. *Plunging ranula* refers to a ranula that extends below the mylohyoid muscle into the neck.
- *Sialolithiasis*: Large stones in the Wharton or Stensen ducts may be palpable in the floor of the mouth or buccal region. Usually associated with sialadenitis of the associated salivary gland.
- *Dermoid cyst*: Occurs in the floor of the mouth and is secondary to entrapment of the midline epithelium during closure of the mandibular and hyoid branchial arches. It is an *epidermoid cyst* (**Figs. 37.3, 37.4**) when the lining consists of only epithelium, whereas a *dermoid* contains skin adnexa, such as hair follicles, sweat, and sebaceous glands. Typically presents in young adults and is painless. May result in dysphagia and dysarthria as well as obstructive sleep apnea from posterior displacement of the tongue.
- *Torus mandibularis*: Bony growth on the lingual surface of the anterior mandible. Almost always occurs bilaterally. Large tori may interfere with direct laryngoscopy.
- *Squamous cell carcinoma*: Similar to squamous cell carcinoma of the oral tongue in regard to frequency and symptoms. Usually asymptomatic when discovered early but can lead to pain, ulceration, and bleeding as the disease progresses. Due to the proximity of the Wharton duct, the hypoglossal nerve, and the lingual nerve, larger floor of mouth squamous cell cancers can lead to submandibular duct obstruction, decreased tongue mobility, and numbness.

- See also *leukoplakia* (see Tongue section), *erythroplakia* (Tongue section), *verrucous carcinoma* (Buccal Mucosa section).

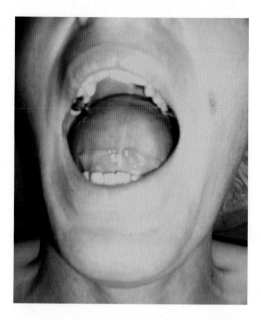

Fig. 37.3 Large epidermoid cyst of the floor of the mouth with posterior displacement of the tongue.

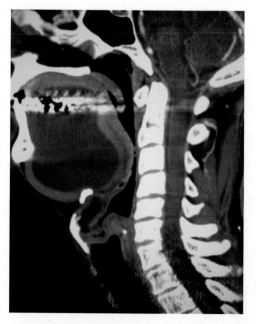

Fig. 37.4 Sagittal computed tomographic scan demonstrating upper airway compromise caused by a floor of mouth cyst and displacement of tongue musculature.

◆ Buccal Mucosa

- *Stensen duct*: Main salivary duct of the parotid gland. Papilla opens in the buccal mucosal opposite the second maxillary molar and may be mistaken for a mass.
- *Irritation fibroma*: Nodular and nonulcerative lesion reactive to trauma or irritant. It most frequently occurs on the buccal mucosa along plane of occlusion of the teeth.
- *Verrucous carcinoma*: Wartlike, extremely well-differentiated squamous cell neoplasm that lacks metastatic potential. Slow growing and can become quite large. Associated with tobacco use, especially smokeless forms. Typically involves the buccal mucosa. When it exists in a hybrid form with conventional squamous cell carcinoma, metastatic potential is present due to the conventional part.
- *Squamous cell carcinoma*: Frequently presents as a nonhealing ulcer. Extensive lesions (**Fig. 37.5**) can extend into surrounding musculature as well as the parotid gland, which can lead to pain, trismus, and even facial paralysis.
- See also *leukoplakia* (Tongue section), *erythroplakia* (Tongue section), *verrucous carcinoma* (Buccal mucosa), *minor salivary gland tumors* (Palate section).

◆ Palate

- *Torus palatinus*: Bony growth on the hard palate. Typically occurs in the midline. It is common and occurs more frequently than mandibular torus. Ulceration can occasionally form due to repeated trauma or denture irritation.

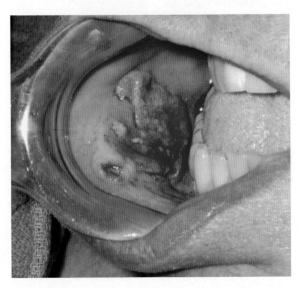

Fig. 37.5 Squamous cell carcinoma of the right buccal mucosa.

- *Necrotizing sialometaplasia*: Benign, ulcerative condition affecting the minor salivary glands that can be mistaken clinically and histologically for carcinoma. Usually occurs at the junction of hard and soft palates and is typically painless. The clinical course includes spontaneous regression.
- *Nasopalatine duct (incisive canal) cyst*: most common nonodontogenic cyst. Presents as a slowly enlarging mass in the midline of the anterior hard palate. Typically occurs in the fifth or sixth decade.
- *Non-Hodgkin lymphoma*: Can rarely present in the oral cavity as a painless mass. Typically polypoid in appearance and can be ulcerated in up to one third of cases. Palate and gingiva are most common sites. Risk is higher in the human immunodeficiency virus (HIV) population.
- *Kaposi sarcoma*: Presents as red, purple, blue, or brown papular lesions on the hard palate or gingiva. Typically asymptomatic but may become painful or ulcerated. It is caused by human herpesvirus 8 (HHV8) and is common among immunosuppressed acquired immunodeficiency syndrome or transplant patients.
- *Melanoma*: May arise from any mucosal surface. Hard palate and maxillary gingiva are the most common sites in the oral cavity. It typically presents as a pigmented macule, but can be unpigmented. Ulceration is common.
- *Minor Salivary Gland Tumors*: Present as a submucosal, firm, painless mass that rarely ulcerates.

  - *Pleomorphic adenoma*: Benign salivary gland tumor that can arise from minor salivary glands in the oral cavity. Within the oral cavity, the palate is the most common site, followed by lip and buccal mucosa.
  - *Mucoepidermoid carcinoma*: Malignant salivary gland tumor that can arise in the oral cavity from a minor salivary gland. Can be low or high grade; high-grade mucoepidermoid carcinoma is distinguished from squamous cell carcinoma by the presence of mucin staining.
  - *Adenoid cystic carcinoma*: Most common type of malignant salivary gland tumor to arise in the minor salivary glands. Three histologic subtypes exist: cribriform, tubular, and solid. Perineural spread is common. Characterized by an indolent course with a high rate of delayed distant metastases.
  - *Polymorphous low-grade adenocarcinoma*: Presents as a painless mass that can be longstanding. Usually presents in the sixth or seventh decade and is more common in women. Typically well circumscribed and nonaggressive.

- *Squamous cell carcinoma*: Painless mucosal lesion that is usually ulcerated. It occurs rarely on the hard palate in comparison with other subsites. Care must be taken to avoid misdiagnosis of one of the minor salivary lesions as a squamous cell carcinoma.

◆ Alveolar Ridge

- *Gingival*

  - *Pyogenic granuloma*: Pedunculated, reactive lesion occurring on the gingival mucosa of children, young adults, and pregnant women. Ulceration and bleeding can occur. Its vascular nature has led to the more histologically appropriate name *lobular capillary hemangioma*. Also referred to as *pregnancy epulis* when it occurs in gravid women and likely has a hormonal association.

- ○ *Epulis fissuratum*: Benign mucosal hyperplasia reactionary to denture flange. May be ulcerated. Also known as *denture epulis*.
- ○ *Peripheral giant cell granuloma (giant cell epulis)*: Protruding and reactive lesion of the gingival mucosa. Clinically similar to *pyogenic granuloma*, but histologically distinct. Typically nonulcerative and more bluish in color than pyogenic granulomas. *Central giant cell granulomas* occur within the mandible or maxilla.
- ○ *Peripheral ossifying fibroma*: Another reactive gingival lesion common in young adults. Typically nodular and ulcerated and may be sessile or pedunculated. Some may arise from a long-standing *pyogenic granuloma*.
- ○ *Squamous cell carcinoma*: Usually occurs on the lower alveolar ridge in an edentulous area (**Fig. 37.6**). Patients often complain of ill-fitting dentures or loose teeth, pain, bleeding, and difficulty chewing related to a nonhealing, ulcerated lesion. Mandibular invasion is common and can present with numbness related to inferior alveolar nerve involvement.
- ○ See also *leukoplakia* (Tongue section), *erythroplakia* (Tongue section), *non-Hodgkin lymphoma* (Palate section), *Kaposi sarcoma* (Palate section), *melanoma* (Palate section).

◆ Odontogenic

- ○ *Periapical (radicular) cyst*: Most common cyst of the jaws. Develops at the apex of a nonvital tooth. Typically is asymptomatic and generally does not produce bone expansion.

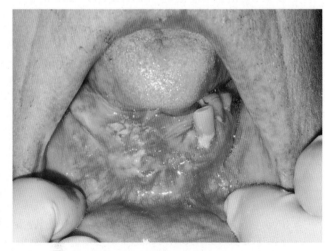

Fig. 37.6 Squamous cell carcinoma of the alveolar ridge with associated leukoplakia of the anterior floor of the mouth.

○ *Dentigerous cyst*: Second most common cyst of the jaws. Developmental cyst that occurs during the second and third decades in association with an unerupted tooth. Mandibular third molars and maxillary canine teeth are common sites. It is usually asymptomatic, but cortical bone expansion is possible.

○ *Odontogenic keratocyst*: Aggressive developmental cyst that arises from the dental lamina. Most occur in the mandible in the region of the third molar and can present with buccal expansion. May be multiple and associated with basal cell–nevus syndrome.

○ *Ameloblastoma*: Most common odontogenic tumor. Most occur in the mandible. Presents most commonly in fourth and fifth decades and characterized by painless, gradual expansion of bone. Benign, but locally aggressive. Malignant transformation can rarely occur.

○ *Dental abscess*: May present as a fluctuant and painful mass involving the gingiva. Typically warm and erythematous and associated with dental caries and poor oral hygiene. Most commonly involves the lower third molar or other posterior mandibular teeth.

Suggested Reading

Mills SE, Gaffey MJ, Frierson HF. Atlas of Tumor Pathology: Tumors of the Upper Aerodigestive Tract and Ear. Washington, DC: Armed Forces Institute of Pathology; 2000

Myers EN, Ferris RL. Salivary Gland Disorders. Berlin, Heidelberg, New York: Springer; 2007

Myers EN, Simental AA. Cancer of the oral cavity. In: Myers EN, Suen JY, Myers JN, Hanna EY, eds. Cancer of the Head and Neck. Philadelphia: Saunders; 2003

Regezi JA, Sciubba JJ, Jordan RCK. Oral Pathology: Clinical Pathologic Correlations. St. Louis: Mosby; 2008

38 Neurological Dysfunction (Including Taste and Dysarthria)

Niels Kokot and Ara A. Chalian

The oral cavity is responsible for both the chemosensory functions of taste and sensation, as well as the motor functions of speech and swallowing. Neurological dysfunction leads to problems with taste disturbance, dysarthria, and dysphagia (see Chapter 48 for causes of dysphagia).

◆ Taste Disturbance

Disorders of taste must be distinguished from disorders of olfaction. There are four genuine taste qualities: salty, sweet, sour, and bitter. Recently a fifth taste quality, "umani," the taste of glutamate, aspartate, and certain ribonucleotides, has been described. The overall taste perception is dependent on not only the true taste sensation but also the smell, texture, and temperature. In addition, taste is dependent on saliva, which is required to dissolve the tastants so they may be detected by the taste receptors. During mastication, odorants are released from food and detected in the olfactory cleft through retronasal olfaction via the nasopharynx. The combination of smell and taste contributes to flavor, which is often mistakenly called taste. The smell or aroma of food and drink is the most important contributor to flavor.

Taste buds are located in the fungiform, foliate, and circumvallate papillae, but not the filiform papillae. Fungiform papillae are located at the tip and lateral edge of the anterior two thirds of the tongue, whereas foliate papillae are located at the posterolateral tongue. Circumvallate papillae are arranged in a V shape at the junction of the anterior two thirds and posterior one third of the tongue. Filiform papillae are located throughout the tongue. Despite the historical perception that there is a topographic mapping of taste sensation on the tongue, this is incorrect. All five taste sensations are perceived by each taste receptor, although it may be more sensitive to one type of stimulus. Taste to the oral tongue (chorda tympani) and the palate (greater superficial petrosal) is mediated by CN VII, whereas CN IX mediates taste to the tongue base, the vallecula, and the pharynx. Taste buds on the laryngeal surface of the epiglottis are innervated by CN X, but their role in everyday taste perception is unknown. All taste afferents converge in the nucleus solitarius in the medulla. Higher neural pathways are less well understood.

Taste disturbances can be categorized as taste loss, taste intensification, or taste phantoms. Taste loss may either be complete (ageusia) or partial (hypogeusia). Taste intensifications, or hypergeusias, are much less common than taste losses. Phantoms, or dysgeusias/parageusias, are tastes experienced in the absence of overt stimulation.

Common causes of taste disturbance include the following (**Table 38.1**):

- *Primary smell disorder*: Eighty percent of taste disorders are actually primary smell disorders. The three most common causes of smell disturbances are *obstructive nasal and sinus disease, upper respiratory infection*, and *head trauma*. The history and physical, as well as the subsequent workup, should be directed toward these causes.
- *Upper respiratory infection*: Probably the second most common cause of taste alteration, independent of olfactory loss. It is hypothesized that this is due to damage to the chorda tympani nerve through the path from the eustachian tube to the middle ear.
- *Poor oral health*: Oral infections, including *candidiasis, herpes simplex, periodontitis*, and *sialadenitis* can all lead to taste alteration. This may be due to overgrowth or colonization of the taste pore, or due to foul chemicals released as a result of the infection. Tooth loss, replacement with a removable prosthesis, and a subsequent decline in masticatory function may result from poor oral hygiene. The decreased mastication leads to decreased release of tastants from the food, preventing access to the taste buds. Furthermore, mastication leads to release of odorants from the food, allowing for retronasal olfaction that contributes to the sensation of flavor.
- *Chorda tympani injury*: Can occur secondary to ear surgery, or infections such as chronic otitis media, Bell palsy, Ramsay Hunt syndrome, or Lyme disease. Patients typically complain of a metallic taste rather than a taste loss. Dysgeusia is frequently temporary due to bilateral innervation.
- *Medications*: Over 250 medications affect the chemical senses. Although the exact mechanism by which various drugs alter taste sensation may be unknown, common effects of medications include *xerostomia*, secretion of the drug into saliva causing an adverse taste sensation or interference with the taste conduction pathway, or alteration of cell turnover.

  - *ACE-inhibitors*: Captopril is among the most commonly noted medications associated with taste disturbance. Frequent complaints include hypogeusia and a strongly metallic, bitter, or sweet taste.
  - *Anticholinergics*: These medications cause excessive drying of saliva. Decreased saliva prevents tastants from dissolving, leading to hypogeusia and dysgeusia. Xerostomia may also cause the taste buds to close, preventing access of the tastants. Other medications that cause drying of saliva include *antidepressants* and *antihistamines*.
  - *Other*: *Antibacterial mouthwash, aspirin, antiparkinson drugs, acetazolamide, lithium, lipid-lowering drugs, antibiotics, antineoplastic drugs*, and *penicillamine*

- *Age*: Taste perception, like olfactory function, becomes somewhat impaired with normal aging, although the effects of aging on taste are less pronounced. Elderly tend to complain of tastes being less intense. In addition to diminished taste perception found with aging, the elderly population is susceptible to many other factors that alter taste. Age-related disease states, surgery, poor dentition, multiple medications, or cumulative exposure to toxins are all contributing factors.

Less common causes of taste disturbance include the following:

- *Nutritional deficiencies*: Vitamin deficiencies (eg, B_3 or B_{12}) or trace metal deficiencies (eg, zinc, copper), whether isolated or due to generalized malnutrition, can result in taste disturbances.
- Medical disorders
    - *Renal failure*: Renal disease has been associated with both taste loss and taste phantoms (metallic, bitter). This improves with dialysis.
    - *Diabetes mellitus*: Patients exhibit a specific deficit to glucose as well as a generalized taste neuropathy. In addition, dehydration due to polydipsia can lead to taste disturbance due to decreased saliva.
- *Head and neck cancer*: Squamous cell carcinomas of the floor of oral cavity, oropharynx, and hypopharynx may cause taste disturbance by damaging peripheral nerve branches of CN VII or IX, or as a result of injury to the nerves from ablative surgery. In addition, CN IX can be damaged by tumors of the carotid sheath or jugular foramen. CPA tumors can cause taste disturbance from injury to CN VII.
- *Post-surgical*: As noted previously, damage to CN VII or CN IX may result from middle ear surgery or ablative cancer surgery. Other operations have also been associated with postoperative taste dysfunction. Notably, third molar extractions or submandibular gland excision can damage the lingual nerve, whereas tonsillectomy has been associated with glossopharyngeal nerve injury. The majority of these injuries are self-limited.
- *Radiation therapy*: External beam radiation leads to xerostomia and concomitant hypogeusia and dysgeusia. Radiation can also cause hypogeusia by direct damage to taste receptors or decreased turnover of taste receptors.

Table 38.1 Causes of Taste Disturbance

Common Causes	Less Common Causes	Uncommon Causes
Primary smell disorder	Nutritional deficiencies	Gustatory aura
Upper respiratory infection	Renal disease	Psychiatric conditions
Poor oral health	Diabetes mellitus	Endocrine disorders
Medications	Head and neck cancer	Head trauma
Chorda tympani injury	Radiation therapy	Toxins
Age		

Uncommon causes of taste disturbance include the following:

- *Gustatory aura*: Taste disturbance can occur as a part of a gustatory aura in association with *epilepsy* or *migraine*.
- *Psychiatric conditions*: *Depression, anorexia nervosa,* and *bulimia* have all been associated with taste disturbances.
- *Neurologic conditions*: *Stroke, multiple sclerosis*, or any neurological or neoplastic lesion along the taste pathway can cause taste disturbance.

- *Endocrine disorders*: *Hypothyroidism, panhypopituitarism, adrenocortical insufficiency*, and *pregnancy* have all been associated with taste disturbances.
- *Inflammatory disease*: *Sjögren syndrome* can lead to xerostomia and resultant taste disturbance.
- *Head trauma*: The incidence of taste loss in head trauma is reported to be 0.4 to 0.5%.
- *Toxic chemical exposure*: Benzene, benzol, butyl acetate, carbon disulfide, chlorine, ethyl acetate, formaldehyde, hydrogen selenide, paint solvents, sulfuric acid, trichloroethylene, chromium, lead, and copper can all cause taste changes.
- *Burning mouth syndrome*: This syndrome of idiopathic oral cavity pain is seen most commonly in postmenopausal women and has frequently been associated with dry mouth and altered taste, including dysgeusias or changes in taste intensity.

Evaluation of the patient with taste disturbances should be directed by a thorough history and physical exam directed toward the common causes as outlined earlier. Objective gustatory or olfactory testing is largely limited to research or academic settings. Taste testing involves threshold and suprathreshold perceived intensities. Taste detection thresholds measure the concentration for the absolute threshold of taste sensation, whereas taste recognition threshold measures the lowest concentration at which a tastant is identified correctly. Typical stimuli to test the individual taste qualities include sodium chloride, sucrose, quinine hydrochloride or quinine sulfate, and citric acid (salty, sweet, bitter, sour). Imaging is directed based on suspicion of a potential lesion. Computed tomographic (CT) scanning is most effective for suspected sinonasal causes or temporal bone causes of gustatory dysfunction. Magnetic resonance imaging (MRI), on the other hand, is more effective for soft tissue detail and is the test of choice for defining the facial nerve and intracranial causes of chemosensory dysfunction. Unfortunately, in most cases, even if the cause of the taste disorder is known, there are few effective therapies.

◆ Dysarthria

The act of speaking involves a highly coordinated sequence of actions of the respiratory musculature, larynx, pharynx, palate, tongue, and lips. Innervation is via the vagal, hypoglossal, facial, and phrenic nerves, the nuclei of which are by both motor cortices through the corticobulbar tracts. As with all movements, control of the muscles involved in speech is subject to extrapyramidal influences from the cerebellum and basal ganglia.

Phonation, the production of vocal sounds, is a function of the larynx. Sounds are then modulated as they pass through the nasopharynx and mouth, which act as resonators. Articulation consists of contractions of the pharynx, palate, tongue, and lips, which alter the vocal sounds. Hoarseness and dysphonia (discussed in Chapter 43) refer to altered phonation, whereas dysarthria consists of defective articulation. Vowels are of laryngeal origin, whereas most consonants are formed during articulation. The consonants *m, b,* and *p* are labial, *l* and *t* are lingual, and *nk* and *ng* are guttural (pharynx and soft palate). Test phrases or rapid repetition of lingual, labial, and guttural consonants can bring out the particular abnormality (eg, *la-la-la, me-me-me, k-k-k*).

Defects in **articulation** can be divided into several types (**Table 38.2**):

- **Flaccid dysarthria:** Also known as *neuromuscular, lower motor neuron dysarthria,* or *atrophic bulbar paralysis,* this is due to weakness or paralysis of the articulatory muscles as a result of diseases affecting motor nuclei or lower motor neurons. In advanced forms the tongue will be atrophic with fasciculations, whereas the lips are lax and tremulous. This leads to difficulty with labial and lingual consonants, and bilateral palatal paralysis can cause hypernasality.

  ○ *Progressive bulbar palsy*: A form of motor neuron disease, causes bilateral palate paralysis leading to hypernasality. In the past diphtheria and poliomyelitis were common causes of this disease.
  ○ *Myasthenia gravis*: Affects the neuromuscular junction and can cause varying degrees of palatal and labial paralysis.
  ○ *Lyme disease*: Leads to bilateral paralysis of the lips and interferes with enunciation of labial consonants.

- **Spastic dysarthria**: Diseases that affect bilateral upper motor neurons or neurodegenerative diseases result in the syndrome of *spastic bulbar,* or *pseudobulbar, palsy*. This is typically due to vascular, demyelinative, or motor system disease.

  ○ *Stroke*: Patients may have had a clinically inevident vascular lesion at some time affecting the corticobulbar fibers of one side. Then when another stroke occurs on the contralateral side, the patient immediately becomes dysarthric, with paresis of the tongue and facial muscles. This condition involves no atrophy or fasciculations of the paralyzed muscles. Facial reflexes usually become exaggerated, the palatal reflexes are retained or increased, and emotional control may be impaired.
  ○ *Anterior opercular syndrome*: Damage to the cerebral cortex and subcortical white matter in the dominant frontal operculum leads to dysarthria as a result of voluntary paralysis of masticatory, facial, pharyngeal, and lingual muscles. Autonomic and emotional control is not impaired.

- **Rigid dysarthria**: *Extrapyramidal diseases* are associated with rigidity in muscle.

  ○ *Parkinson disease*: The dysarthria associated with Parkinson disease is characterized by rapid mumbling and cluttered utterance and slurring of words and syllables with trailing off in volume at the ends of sentences. The words are spoken hastily and run together. Dysarthria associated with Parkinson disease has also been termed **hypokinetic.**
  ○ *Chorea and myoclonus*: Speech associated with these disorders is loud, harsh, improperly stressed or accented, and poorly coordinated with breathing. It has also been called **hyperkinetic** speech. These diseases also cause abrupt interruptions of the words by superimposition of involuntary movements of bulbar muscles, also described as "hiccup" speech.

○ *Cerebral palsy*

- **Ataxic dysarthia:** This condition is characteristic of acute and chronic cerebellar lesions. The primary abnormalities are slowness of speech, slurring, and monotony. Another characteristic is scanning speech, or unnatural separation of the syllables of words. Speech and breathing may be uncoordinated, leading to whispered speech at times and explosive speech at others. Ataxic dysarthria is observed in conditions such as *multiple sclerosis*, various degenerative diseases involving the cerebellum or its peduncles, or as a sequel of *anoxic encephalopathy* and rarely of *heat stroke.*
- **Mixed dysarthrias:** Some diseases are associated with speech disturbances that combine elements of more than one category of dysarthria.

  ○ *Multiple sclerosis*: This disease is a demyelinating disease of the central nervous system producing a variety of motor, sensory, and cognitive impairments. It is most commonly associated with a mixed **spastic** and **ataxic** dysarthria. Scanning speech is the classic disturbance.
  ○ *Amyotrophic lateral sclerosis*: ALS is a rapidly progressive condition involving motor neurons of the brain and spinal cord. This produces a mixed **spastic** and **flaccid** dysarthria. These patients have tongue muscle wasting with fasciculations, also described as a "bag of worms."
  ○ *Traumatic brain injury*

- *Neoplastic*: *Brain tumors* can cause dysarthria depending on their location. In addition, neoplasms of the floor of mouth, tongue, and pharynx can cause dysarthria as a result of decreased mobility. Finally, skull base neoplasms such as *chordoma, nasopharyngeal carcinoma, paraganglioma*, and various *metastases* that cause paralysis of CN IX, X, XII, can lead to dysarthria.
- *Isolated CN XII injury*: Paralysis of CN XII without other cranial neuropathies is uncommon but can occur due to a variety of reasons. Vascular disease such as brainstem vascular loops or carotid artery aneurysms can lead to hypoglossal paralysis. Common surgeries that can lead to CN XII injury include carotid endarterectomy and submandibular gland excision, as well as ablative head and neck cancer operations. Uncommonly hypoglossal paralysis can occur as a result of infectious or inflammatory processes such as viral infection similar to Bell palsy, Lyme disease, rheumatoid arthritis, and Wegener granulomatosis. Finally, CN XII paralysis can occur as a result of radiation neuronitis from treatment of head and neck cancer.

Table 38.2 Causes of Dysarthria

Flaccid	Spastic	Rigid	Ataxic	Mixed
Progressive bulbar palsy	Pseudobulbar palsy	Parkinson disease	Cerebellar lesions	Multiple sclerosis
Myasthenia gravis	Stroke	Chorea		Amyotrophic lateral sclerosis
Guillain-Barré syndrome	Anterior opercular syndrome	Myoclonus		Traumatic brain injury
Lyme disease		Cerebral palsy		Neoplasm

Dysarthria is rarely the only presenting sign or symptom of many of the foregoing diseases. Evaluation of these patients should focus on a detailed neurological exam. If the physical exam does not clearly indicate the cause of dysarthria, analysis of the patient's speech will determine the type of dysarthria. Test phrases or rapid repetition of lingual, labial, and guttural consonants can bring out the particular abnormality (eg, *la-la-la, me-me-me, k-k-k*). If a particular lesion is suspected, imaging with MRI or CT scan may be helpful. In general, patients receive benefit from speech therapy with a speech and language pathologist.

Suggested Reading

Bromley SM. Smell and taste disorders: a primary care approach. Am Fam Physician 2000;61:427–436, 438

Reiter ER, DiNardo LJ, Costanzo RM. Effects of head injury on olfaction and taste. Otolaryngol Clin North Am 2004;37:1167–1184

Roper AH, Brown RH. Adams and Victor's Principles of Neurology. 8th ed. New York: McGraw-Hill; 2005

39 Salivary Disturbance (Xerostomia, Sialorrhea) and Halitosis

Chia Haddad and Devraj Basu

Salivary glands are distributed throughout the head and neck and can be divided into major and minor glands. The major salivary glands include the paired parotid, submandibular, and sublingual glands. The minor salivary glands consist of over 500 much smaller submucosal structures distributed throughout the upper aerodigestive tract.

Disorders of the salivary glands can manifest with a variety of symptoms. Rapid onset of pain, diffuse enlargement, and tenderness of major salivary glands, either unilateral or bilateral, is typically associated with acute infectious processes. These conditions may be accompanied by systemic symptoms such as fever and fatigue. However, a painful, swollen gland may also be seen with a variety of other conditions. An isolated, persistent salivary gland mass is more suggestive of neoplasm and often presents without other symptoms. When this is associated with pain or facial paralysis, it is strongly suggestive of malignancy. Sialadenosis is a noninflammatory, nonneoplastic enlargement of a salivary gland that is generally asymptomatic. Xerostomia is dry mouth due to a lack of saliva production. Sialorrhea or ptyalism is the excessive production or impaired swallowing of saliva, often leading to drooling. Halitosis is oral malodor (bad breath), a small subset of which is secondary to salivary gland disturbance.

◆ Presenting Symptom

Painful Swelling of a Major Salivary Gland

- Viral infection

  - *Mumps* (systemic paramyxovirus): Remains an important cause of diffuse painful parotid enlargement despite a precipitous decline in cases since the introduction of vaccination in 1964. The virus has an incubation time of 2 to 3 weeks, after which diffuse pain and swelling can occur in one or both parotid glands. Often there will be a prodrome of fever, malaise, and myalgia. Major associated complications include sudden sensorineural hearing loss, meningitis, encephalitis, orchitis/oophoritis, and pancreatitis. Chronic obstructive sialadenitis may also develop as a sequela of the acute infection.
  - *Cytomegalovirus, coxsackievirus, echovirus, and influenza A*: Can all cause similar syndromes that include salivary gland swelling mimicking mumps

- Bacterial infection

  - *Acute suppurative sialadenitis*: Most commonly involves the parotid gland but also frequently affects the submandibular gland. It can be bilateral in up to 20% of cases. Patients will present with pain, tenderness, and swelling, and may also complain of increased pain with eating. Often purulence can be expressed from the duct orifice with gland massage and milking the duct, and appearance of pus with this maneuver is considered diagnostic. *Staphylococcus aureus* is the most common pathogen, although other bacteria such as *Streptococcus pneumoniae, Escherichia coli,* and *Haemophilus influenzae* can be etiologies. Salivary stasis is thought to be the major predisposing factor. Stasis can be caused by obstruction secondary to a salivary stone or stricture, medications that decrease saliva production, or dehydration. It often appears in a postoperative setting and in elderly, debilitated patients. Infections can be complicated by abscess formation, which requires aspiration or open surgical drainage.
  - *Chronic sialadenitis*: Can be a sequela of recurrent acute infection, other inflammatory disease, partial plugging of salivary ducts with calculi, and/or ductal stricture. These changes result in decreased secretion and overall stasis. Chronic sialadenitis is most common in the parotid gland. Patients typically describe a mildly painful recurrent swelling that is worsened by eating, and they may also complain of xerostomia. Occasionally, another treatable anatomical cause may exist, such as an extractable stone or an isolated stricture that may be dilated.
  - *Cat scratch disease*: A self-limited disease caused by *Bartonella henselae.* Although this disease does not directly involve the salivary glands, it can present as acute painful swelling of intraparotid lymph nodes, though typically producing an ill-defined mass rather than diffuse gland enlargement. Some cases may mimic the symptoms of a malignant parotid neoplasm (see later discussion).
  - *Primary salivary tuberculosis*: Very rare. The disease is most often unilateral and involves the parotid gland.

- *Sialolithiasis* (salivary calculi): Eighty percent of stones occur within the submandibular gland, with most of the remainder in the parotid gland. Patients will complain of recurrent pain and swelling of the involved gland, especially while eating. A calculus may be palpable within the duct, and most stones are identifiable on computed tomography. Secondary acute bacterial sialadenitis may develop as the presenting symptom. Other complications include ductal ectasia and/or stricture, predisposing to recurrent or chronic sialadenitis.
- Noninfectious granulomatous disease

  - *Sarcoidosis*: Can manifest as diffuse salivary gland enlargement in up to 33% of cases. *Uveoparotid fever* is a syndromic manifestation of sarcoid characterized by the association of uveitis, parotid enlargement, and facial paralysis.

Mass within a Salivary Gland

- Benign neoplasms: These represent 75 to 80% of all parotid neoplasms, 50% of submandibular neoplasms, and < 40% of sublingual and minor salivary gland neoplasms. These lesions typically present with painless, gradual enlargement over time without facial nerve paralysis.

  - *Pleomorphic adenoma* (benign mixed tumor): Accounts for 65% of salivary gland tumors.
  - *Warthin tumor* (papillary cystadenoma lymphomatosum): The second most common benign salivary neoplasm. These are more common in men and almost exclusively seen in smokers. Ten percent are bilateral.
  - *Oncocytoma, monomorphic adenoma, intraductal papilloma, lipoma,* and *hemangioma*: Other less common benign neoplasms included in the differential

- Malignant neoplasms: These make up 20% of parotid neoplasms, with higher incidence in the submandibular, sublingual, and minor salivary glands. Primary salivary malignancies may present very similarly to benign neoplasms but can also present with rapid enlargement, pain, facial paralysis, cystic necrosis, and involvement of the overlying skin.

  - *Mucoepidermoid carcinoma*: The most common malignancy in the parotid gland; subcategorized as low, intermediate, and high grade based on multiple histologic criteria.
  - *Adenoid cystic carcinoma*: The most common malignancy of the submandibular and minor salivary glands
  - *Acinic cell carcinoma, carcinoma ex-pleomorphic adenoma, adenocarcinoma, squamous cell carcinoma, sarcoma,* and *lymphoma*: Other less common malignant tumors of the salivary glands

- *Metastatic cancers*: Also presenting as a parotid mass, intraparotid lymph nodes can be a site of regional metastasis for head and neck malignancies, and, very rarely, a site of distant metastasis from other cancers.
- Cystic nonneoplastic lesions: Cystic lesions within the major salivary glands are most common in the parotid and can be divided into congenital and acquired cysts.

  - Benign congenital cysts include *lymphatic malformation, salivary cyst,* and *dermoid cyst. First branchial cleft cysts* can also occur in close association with the parotid gland, with a tract to the ear canal that is in intimate relation to the facial nerve. The association of a draining cutaneous pit also suggests a diagnosis of type I branchial cleft anomaly.
  - *Acquired cysts* may develop in the setting of traumatic injury (eg, hematoma from blunt trauma or sialocele after penetrating injury), or bacterial parotitis.
  - *Lymphoepithelial cysts* are designated simply on the basis of significant lymphoid tissue in the cyst wall. These lesions commonly arise in human immunodeficiency virus (HIV) infection, and can be a presenting sign. These

can be multiple within the gland and bilateral. An associated solid mass should raise particular concern for parotid lymphoma in an HIV+ patient.
- *Ranulas*: Salivary pseudocysts arising in association with the sublingual gland or, occasionally, the submandibular gland. They present as bluish cystic lesions in the floor of the mouth and arise from escaped mucus from an injured excretory duct or ductal obstruction. Cervical or "plunging" ranulas include a component that extends through the mylohyoid muscle into the upper neck to produce a cystic mass in the submandibular triangle.

Sialadenosis (Nonneoplastic, Noninflammatory Enlargement of a Salivary Gland)

- A long list of systemic and metabolic conditions may be associated with sialadenosis, which is itself a benign entity. *Malnutrition* in conditions such as *anorexia nervosa, bulimia* (caused by both malnutrition and the hypersalivation stimulated by induced vomiting), *kwashiorkor, pellagra,* and *beriberi* lead to acinar hypertrophy. Bilateral parotid enlargement will also eventually occur in approximately half of the patients with *cirrhosis*. Other diseases that affect protein absorption may also cause sialadenosis: *Chagas disease, celiac sprue, esophageal cancer, uremia,* and *chronic pancreatitis.*
- *Obesity* alone can cause a bilateral asymptomatic enlargement of the parotid glands due to fat hypertrophy.

Xerostomia (Dry Mouth)

- *Medications* are the most common cause of xerostomia. Antihypertension agents, diuretics, antianxiety agents, antidepressants, antihistamines, anticholinergics, decongestants, and pain killers are the most common pharmacological culprits.
- *Dehydration*
- *Aging* itself leads to deceased saliva production, resulting in part from gradual replacement of secretory glandular components in the major glands by fatty tissue.
- *Radiation* to the head and neck causes chronic and often intractable xerostomia, particularly in patients receiving high total doses to both parotid glands.
- *Congenital aplasia* of the major salivary glands is a rare, poorly characterized condition that results in xerostomia and multiple dental caries. It may occur as an isolated defect or in the context of other congenital anomalies, and hereditary cases usually show autosomal dominant transmission.
- Systemic diseases that can secondarily affect the salivary function are numerous and include *diabetes, Parkinson disease, rheumatoid arthritis, systemic lupus erythematosus, scleroderma, sarcoidosis, amyloidosis, cystic fibrosis, thyroid dysfunction,* and multiple *neurological diseases. Sjögren syndrome* is the most common disease causing xerostomia and is an autoimmune syndrome characterized by lymphocyte-mediated destruction of exocrine glands, predominantly in postmenopausal women. Some cases are also characterized by any of several extraglandular manifestations that

overlap various rheumatologic illnesses, such as arthritis, nephritis, Raynaud phenomenon, myalgia, vasculitis, and the like. Typical symptoms include xerostomia from major salivary gland (particularly parotid) involvement and keratoconjunctivitis sicca (dry eye) from lacrimal gland involvement. Recurrent/chronic sialadenitis often ensues, often with enlargement of the major salivary and lacrimal glands. Development of a parotid mass, however, should raise concern for malignancy and in particular parotid lymphoma, which has a high incidence in this population.

Sialorrhea (Drooling)

Sialorrhea arises from either excess saliva production (hypersecretion) or impaired swallowing of saliva.

- Hypersecretion can be seen with *teething, parasympathomimetic* or *sympatholytic drugs, rabies*, and *irritants* such as capsaicin.
- Impaired swallowing

  - Infectious/inflammatory/neoplastic causes are invariably accompanied by other more prominent symptoms of the disease process. These entities include severe *pharyngitis, tonsillitis, epiglottitis, peritonsillar abscess, parapharyngeal/retropharyngeal abscess, submandibular abscess/Ludwig angina, allergic angioedema,* and *pharyngeal* or *esophageal masses.*
  - *Neurological impairment* can cause sialorrhea from peripheral denervation or loss of central motor coordination. Adult cases arise from *severe brain injury* of any etiology, advanced *neurodegenerative disease,* or multiple *cranial nerve dysfunction* of any other cause.

Halitosis (Oral Malodor)

- The chemistry of halitosis is complex. Anaerobic bacterial organisms usually play a prominent role in breaking down aminoacids into volatile, foul-smelling, sulfur-containing compounds. The causes of halitosis are best considered by anatomical site.

  - Oral: Multiple subsites and processes in the oral cavity and oropharynx can contribute to halitosis.

    - Tongue: The most common site for oral halitosis is the *tongue.* The posterior tongue is relatively dry and poorly cleansed, predisposing it to bacterial overgrowth. Accumulated food particles, dead epithelium, crypts in lingual tonsil tissue, and postnasal secretions can sustain this overgrowth.
    - Gingiva: *Periodontal disease* can also lead to overgrowth of anaerobes and resultant halitosis.
    - Tonsils: Within palatine tonsillar crypts, debris aggregates into *tonsilloliths,* which become malodorous as they are exposed to the oral cavity. Although a variety of cleansing strategies exist, the occasional patient may benefit from tonsillectomy for intractable halitosis from this source.

— *Xerostomia*: Can contribute to halitosis. This effect is likely related to poor oral clearance, alterations in microbial flora, and exacerbation of periodontal disease.

— *Oral malignancies*: Particularly larger tumors with significant necrotic components, can produce prominent and distinctive halitosis, though rarely a presenting symptom in such cases.

○ Nasal

— *Sinusitis*: Can lead to excessive mucus production, bacterial overgrowth, and postnasal drip as contributing factors.

— *Nasal foreign bodies*: In children may present with halitosis along with a unilateral foul smelling rhinorrhea.

○ Pulmonary

— *Pulmonary infections*: Can also contribute to halitosis.

○ Esophageal/gastric: In the setting of severe *gastroesophageal reflux*, putrid substances may rise from the stomach leading to halitosis. Similarly esophageal or gastric carcinomas may contribute to halitosis.

● Systemic disease: *Fetor hepaticus* is a late sign of liver failure where certain volatile compounds normally cleared in the liver are shunted to the systemic circulation and reach the lungs. *Renal failure*, poorly controlled *diabetes*, and other forms of *metabolic dysfunction* can all lead to halitosis. The breath of a type I diabetic in *ketoacidosis* can have a distinctive odor of acetone.

● *Halitophobia*: A psychiatric condition consisting of a highly exaggerated concern about halitosis and falls on the spectrum of social anxiety disorders. This entity is also called *delusional halitosis* and is a subcategory of *olfactory reference syndrome*, which describes pathological preoccupation with any body odor.

Suggested Reading

ADA Council on Scientific Affairs. Oral malodor. J Am Dent Assoc 2003;134:209–214

Carlson GW. The salivary glands: embryology, anatomy, and surgical applications. Surg Clin North Am 2000;80:261–273, xii

Guggenheimer J, Moore PA. Xerostomia: etiology, recognition and treatment. J Am Dent Assoc 2003;134:61–69, quiz 118–119

Rice DH. Noninflammatory, non-neoplastic disorders of the salivary glands. Otolaryngol Clin North Am 1999;32:835–843

Shah JP, Ihde JK. Salivary gland tumors. Curr Probl Surg 1990;27:775–883

VII Differential Diagnosis in the Larynx, Pharynx, Trachea, and Esophagus (Adult and Pediatric)

Section Editor: *Jason G. Newman*

40 Sore Throat

Jason Leibowitz and Jason G. Newman

- Throat pain is a ubiquitous symptom. It may be acute or chronic, constant or intermittent, and mild to severe. The time course of the pain is a critical factor in establishing the diagnosis because **acute** pain tends to be associated with infectious etiologies or trauma, whereas **chronic** pain may be associated with chronic inflammation or neoplasm. Key points of the history include the following:
    - Time course of symptoms
    - Otalgia (unilateral otalgia in the absence of ear disease may indicate an underlying malignancy)
    - Dysphagia or odynophagia
    - Stridor or other respiratory symptoms (may indicate an underlying airway obstruction)
    - Reflux or heartburn-related symptoms
    - Neck mass
    - Hemoptysis
    - Inflammatory symptoms such as fever and malaise
    - Constitutional symptoms such as weight loss or night sweats
    - Patient risk factors (tobacco, alcohol, sick contacts, trauma, or foreign body ingestion)

A full head and neck exam is essential. Careful attention should be paid to the ears, mucosal membranes of the upper aerodigestive tract, and neck.

◆ Infectious Causes of Throat Pain

Infectious causes of throat pain include the following:

- **Pharynx**
    - *Viral pharyngitis*: Most common infectious etiology. Sore throat associated with malaise, low-grade fever, and upper respiratory infection (URI) symptoms. Commonly caused by adenovirus and rhinovirus. Other causes of acute viral pharyngitis include the following:
        - *Herpes simplex virus*: Sore throat may be seen in both primary infection and reactivation with associated vesicular or ulcerative lesions.
        - *Measles*: Sore throat, coryza, and conjunctivitis. Intraoral Koplik spots (erythematous spots on buccal mucosa) are pathognomonic.
        - *Infectious mononucleosis*: Epstein-Barr virus (EBV). Symptoms include severe sore throat with odynophagia, dysphagia, high fevers, posterior cervical lymphadenopathy, rashes, exudative tonsillitis, and hepatosplenomegaly.

- *HIV*: Initial infection presents with acute retroviral syndrome (similar to EBV) with myalgias, photophobia, joint pain and rash.
  ○ *Bacterial pharyngitis*: Acute onset, significant throat pain with otalgia, dysphagia, odynophagia, cervical adenitis, and high fevers. May see tonsillar and posterior pharyngeal erythema with exudates on physical exam. Most common bacterial cause is group A β-hemolytic streptococcus. Other bacterial causes include the following:

    - *Staphylococcus*: Mucopurulent drainage and localized pustules on the tonsils
    - *Diphtheroid*: Usually seen in children > 6 years old who are not immunized. Exam reveals gray-black membrane firmly adherent to the underlying pharyngeal mucosa, with extension to the larynx or nasopharynx. Symptoms include sore throat and airway obstruction.
    - *Pertussis*: Acute onset of sore throat in children associated with a whooping cough.
    - *Gonorrhea*: Sexually active patient with sore throat, tonsillar hypertrophy, and cervical adenitis
    - *Syphilis*: May appear as a painless papule that ulcerates in the primary stage in the tonsils, or as a pharyngitis/tonsillitis in later stages (painless superficial erosions with raised erythematous margins in the pharynx).

  ○ *Acute tonsillitis*: Hypertrophied tonsils with purulent exudates. May be associated with trismus, dysphagia, and odynophagia. May progress to peritonsillar or neck abscess.
  ○ *Chronic tonsillitis*: Hypertrophied cryptic tonsils with chronic sore throat, recurrent tonsillitis/pharyngitis, halitosis, malaise, and cervical adenopathy
  ○ *Peritonsillar abscess*: "Hot potato" voice, trismus, soft palate edema/erythema with uvular deviation, drooling, inability to tolerate secretions, and otalgia.
  ○ *Cervical adenitis*: Viral or bacterial lymphadenitis of the neck usually preceded by URI or pharyngitis. May progress to neck abscess (fluctuant mass with high spiking fevers).
  ○ *PFAPA (periodic fever, aphthous stomatitis, pharyngitis,* and *cervical adenitis)*: Syndrome of periodic fever, aphthous stomatitis, pharyngitis and cervical adenitis. Symptoms last ~5 days and occur in a cyclical manner (once every 28 days). Cause is unknown.
  ○ *Fungal pharyngitis*: Rare and is seen in immunocompromised patients, in poorly controlled diabetics, or with long-term antibiotic use.

● **Larynx and trachea**

  ○ *Croup*: Symptoms include insidious sore throat associated with stridor (inspiratory or biphasic) and barking cough, commonly seen in children.
  ○ *Acute epiglottitis*: Rarely seen since widespread H influenza B vaccine. Symptoms include acute onset of sore throat, high fever, drooling, dysphagia, airway obstruction, and tripoding. A cherry red, edematous epiglottis is seen on exam.

○ *Supraglottitis*: Associated with high fever, muffled voice, drooling, and inspiratory stridor with supraglottic edema and erythema seen on examination. Symptoms may progress quickly to acute airway obstruction.
○ *Bacterial tracheitis*: Diagnosed by thick purulent secretions in the airway. May require intubation for pulmonary toilet.
○ *Acute infectious laryngitis*: Associated symptoms include voice changes (hoarseness/raspy voice), postnasal drip, low-grade fevers, cough, malaise, and URI. Viral causes most common, but may be bacterial or fungal (tuberculosis, syphilitic, scleroma, leprosy).

● **Esophagus infection.** Esophageal infection may also cause sore throat. Common causes are *Candida* and herpesvirus.

◆ Inflammation

Inflammation may be a cause of sore throat by involving the upper aerodigestive tract. Causes include the following:

● *Laryngitis*: Associated with dysphonia, globus sensation, and chronic cough. Causes include the following:

○ *Infectious* (see earlier)
○ *Traumatic*

— *Vocal abuse*: May cause throat pain associated with dysphonia and hoarseness
— *Thermal injury*: Steam, smoke, hot liquids/foods
— *Overuse trauma*: Including vocal fold ulcers or contact granulomas, vocal cord nodules, or polyps. *Chronic cough* can be an etiology of overuse trauma.
— *Instrumentation*: Surgery, laryngoscopy, intubation, nasogastric tube
— *Radiation*: Atrophic changes due to radiation and reduced salivation
— *Retained foreign body*

○ Systemic inflammatory disorders: *Wegener granulomatosis, rheumatoid arthritis, amyloidosis, relapsing polychondritis, systemic lupus erythematosis,* and *sarcoidosis*
○ Integumental disorders: *Stevens-Johnson syndrome, pemphigus, bullous pemphigoid,* and *epidermolysis bullosa* may present with sore throat due to pharyngeal involvement as well as typical skin and mucosal changes (painful vesiculobullous lesions with ulceration, crusting, and bleeding).
○ *Allergic laryngitis*: Chronic and recurrent dysphonia; associated with typical allergic picture of nasal polyps, boggy nasal mucosa, and allergic shiners.
○ *Granulomatous disease*: A rare cause of sore throat. The clinical picture is that of a presumed infectious etiology that does not respond to empirical antibiotic treatment. Infectious and noninfectious etiologies include the following:

— *Mycobacteria*
— *Leprosy*

— *Parasites*

— *Crohn disease*: Primarily affects small and large intestine with 9% pharyngeal involvement.

○ *Toxin exposure* (eg, tobacco)

- *Laryngopharyngeal reflux*: Symptoms include hoarseness (typically worse in the morning), regurgitation, heartburn, chronic cough, globus sensation, and chronic throat clearing. May have choking spells at night. Indirect laryngoscopy reveals supraglottic edema with interarytenoid erythema.
- **Esophageal inflammation** causing sore throat will usually also present with significant swallowing disorders and odynophagia. Etiologies include the following:

  ○ *Esophagitis*: Etiologies include reflux (most common), infectious, drug-related, and radiation.
  ○ *Diffuse esophageal spasm*: Associated with odynophagia, dysphagia, and chest pain.
  ○ *Esophageal webs*
  ○ *Esophageal diverticula*
  ○ *Esophageal trauma*
  ○ *Esophageal foreign body*

◆ Neoplasms

Neoplasms may be benign or malignant. Unilateral otalgia in the absence of ear pathology is an ominous sign. Long-term tobacco and alcohol use are major risk factors. Airway evaluation is critical to assess adequacy of the airway. Metastatic tumors (eg, breast or renal) or systemic tumors (eg, lymphoma) are rare causes.

◆ Thyroid Disorders

Acute thyroid inflammation as well as large masses or goiters may cause pain referred to the throat. Other symptoms include thyroid mass or enlargement, hoarseness, swallowing difficulties, neck mass, and symptoms of hyper- or hypothyroidism.

◆ Other Causes of Throat Pain

- *Glossopharyngeal neuralgia*: Severe lancinating pain from the posterior pharynx to the ear, neck, and head that is short lived (lasts seconds). The pain can be triggered by swallowing, chewing, or coughing.

- *Eagle syndrome*: Pain along the course of the stylohyoid ligament. It is associated with a chronic sore throat, difficulty swallowing or globus sensation.
- *Drugs*: Rarely, drug reactions may cause sore throat. For example, inhaled steroids may cause laryngitis associated with dysphagia, odynophagia, globus sensation, dysphonia, and diffuse inflammation (seen on laryngoscopy).

Suggested Reading

Bailey BJ, Johnson JT. Head and Neck Surgery–Otolaryngology. Philadelphia: Lippincott Williams & Wilkins; 2006

Cummings CW. Otolaryngology–Head and Neck Surgery. Philadelphia: Mosby; 2005

Lucente FE, Gady HE. Essentials of Otolaryngology. Philadelphia: Lippincott Williams & Wilkins; 2004

41 Throat Ulcer or Lesion

Melonie A. Nance and Christine G. Gourin

The surface of the upper aerodigestive tract is lined with smooth, pink, moist mucosa containing minor salivary glands and lymphoid tissue. Interruptions in this smooth surface layer may result from an ulcer or a lesion of the oropharynx, pharynx, larynx, or trachea. An *ulcer* (or ulcerative lesion) is a concave area of tissue erosion. Natural progression can lead to a variety of outcomes from spontaneous healing to spreading tissue necrosis. Ulcers found on the laryngeal/pharyngeal mucosal surface are often painful and may be described by the patient as a "raw" area. **Lesion** is a general term that describes a circumscribed area of tissue irregularity, which may represent an area of discoloration, rough texture convexity, or raised tissue. Lesions may have areas of ulceration from concurrent trauma or necrosis, further confounding the distinction between the two terms.

Duration, location, and size, along with history, often provide definitive clues to etiology. It is important to determine whether the ulcer or lesion exists alone or if it is a sign of systemic pathology such as an inflammatory or infectious disorder, or extends beyond the surface epithelium as in the case of an ulcerative mass. Associated symptoms such as pain, increased sensitivity, rapid growth, exudative drainage, or bleeding are important clinical indicators in determining the pathological cause. These causes can be divided into three categories: **inflammatory**, **traumatic**, and **neoplastic**. Although supportive care can alleviate mild general symptoms, definitive treatment is ultimately determined by the specific etiology.

All lesions/ulcers in this area should be followed carefully by a physician. Without clear signs of spontaneous healing or clinical resolution, a biopsy should be considered early in the course of disease. Once the histopathologic diagnosis is established, definitive medical or surgical therapy can be selected with confidence.

◆ Inflammatory Causes

Inflammatory ulcers can be caused by local or systemic infection of bacteria, fungi, or viruses. They often present with erythema and can be covered with exudate. They are usually painful and have a short onset of symptoms. Knowledge of the patient's medical history can help to elucidate the patient's degree of immunocompromise. Social history, including sexual history, can point to important factors in terms of behavioral risk of orally transmitted sexually transmitted diseases (STDs), as well as immunocompromise from human immunodeficiency virus (HIV).

- **Infection**
  - ○ **Systemic granulomatous fungal infections**
    - — *Histoplasmosis*
    - — *Blastoplasmosis*
    - — *Coccidioidomycosis*
    - — *Cryptococcosis*
    - — *Candidiasis* is more frequently found in the oral cavity and oropharynx; however, it can also be found in the pharynx and esophagus.
  - ○ *Syphilis*: Primary disease presents as a painless ulcer, whereas secondary disease presents with multiple gray mucous membrane ulcerations.
  - ○ *Herpes*
  - ○ *Respiratory papillomatosis*
  - ○ *Leprosy*
- **Inflammatory noninfectious** lesions can look similar to infectious ulcers or lesions. These are associated with an autoimmune or systemic disease that is not caused by an infectious organism. For some patients these lesions may be the initial presenting symptom, so no associated medical history will be known. Laboratory investigations can be very helpful; however, biopsy is usually required for definitive diagnosis.
  - ○ **Autoimmune inflammation**
    - — *Rheumatoid arthritis*
    - — *Lupus (systemic lupus erythematosus [SLE])*
    - — *Crohn disease*
  - ○ **Granulomatous inflammation**
    - — *Sarcoidosis*
    - — *Wegener granulomatosis*
  - ○ *Amyloidosis*
  - ○ *Pemphigus vulgaris*
  - ○ *Mucous membrane (cicatricial) pemphigoid*
  - ○ *Behçet syndrome*: A rare vasculitis that can present with painful aphthous ulcers that frequently recur. Because this is a systemic disease, ulcers may exist in genital, skin, and ocular ulcers, arthritis, and central nervous system (CNS) involvement may occur.
  - ○ *Lichen planus*: Has an unclear etiology but is associated with immune or allergic reactions. Clinically this appears as small, pale, bumps that form a lacy network. Symptoms can include pain, tenderness, burning, itching, or dryness.
  - ○ *Aphthous ulcer*: Aphthous ulcers, also called *canker sores*, present as small, shallow, pale ulcers with a halo of surrounding erythema. They may be multiple and recurrent and are often quite painful and usually spontaneously resolve.
  - ○ *Pseudoepitheliomatous hyperplasia*: An inflammatory process involving the superficial proliferation of tongues of epithelial cells into deeper tissues along with inflammatory cell infiltrate. It can be painful and often looks

grossly suspicious for malignant neoplasm. Pseudoepitheliomatous hyperplasia is associated with lesions such as *granular cell tumor, respiratory papillomatosis, pyogenic granuloma, tuberculosis, syphilis,* and *blastomycosis.*

◆ Traumatic Causes

Traumatic ulcerations or lesions described following here are of the chronic variety. Minor lacerations or abrasions to normal mucosa should heal within a few days. If healing is prolonged (> 2 weeks) or complicated, an underlying cause should be investigated.

- **Contact**
  - *Contact ulcer* of the true vocal fold is along the spectrum of *vocal fold granuloma.* The lesion is an erythematous localized area of inflammation, most often at the vocal process of the true cord. The lesion originates from chronic inflammation and irritation of the perichondrium of the arytenoid cartilage. Eventually the area can become raised and become an inflammatory mass. These are commonly seen with a history of intubation or laryngeal reflux.
  - *Vocal fold hemorrhage*: This is a localized red or brown lesion on the surface of the true vocal fold that is most often a result of vocal overuse.

- **Chemical**
  - *Acid reflux laryngopharyngitis*: Acid reflux in the pharynx/larynx can cause irritation and erythema, usually localized to the posterior glottis or cricopharyngeal mucosa. Minimally visible irritation can cause vocal disturbances and increase susceptibility to vocal fold lesions.
  - *Caustic ingestion*: Tissue damage and severity are determined by the amount, pH, and concentration of the substance ingested. Compounds with basic pH (> 7) cause liquefaction necrosis, early disintegration of mucosa with deep penetration into tissues. Acidic compounds cause coagulation necrosis, forming a coagulum on the mucosal surface and limiting deeper absorption and injury.

◆ Neoplastic Causes

Neoplastic lesions are caused by abnormal growth of tissue, usually leading to a localized mass, and can be benign or malignant. If this is suspected, biopsy is recommended for histopathologic diagnosis.

- **Benign/premalignant**
  - *Pseudoepitheliomatous hyperplasia* is associated with benign lesions such as *granular cell tumors, papilloma, pyogenic granuloma, tuberculosis, syphilis,* and *blastomycosis.*

○ *Leukoplakia* is a white colored lesion of the mucosa. It is often described as having a leathery surface.
○ *Erythroplakia* is a red-colored, well-circumscribed lesion of the mucosa. Texture can vary from smooth and velvety to irregular and granular on the surface.
○ *Carcinoma in situ*

● **Malignant lesions** can appear as small, seemingly minor lesions or as large invasive tumors. Clinically they appear similar to inflammatory lesions with redness and pain. Often ulceration can be quite deep and aggressive. It is important to remember that biopsy of all nonhealing ulcers/lesions is absolutely necessary. A wide variety of tumor types may arise in the upper aerodigestive tract; however, the majority belong to just a few histologic types.

○ *Squamous cell carcinoma* is the most common malignancy found in the pharynx/larynx. Small or shallow lesions may appear to be leukoplakia. Often these lesions appear ulcerated or friable and may bleed.
○ *Spindle cell carcinoma*
○ *Sarcoma*
○ *Lymphoepithelial carcinoma*
○ **Minor salivary gland carcinoma** can exist anywhere in the upper aerodigestive tract due to the high concentration of minor salivary glands. As suggested earlier, mucosal ulcers or nonhealing lesions should be biopsied to establish an early diagnosis.

— *Mucoepidermoid carcinoma*
— *Adenoid cystic carcinoma*
— *Adenocarcinoma*

Suggested Reading

Alper CM, Myers EN, Eibling DE. Decision Making in Ear, Nose, and Throat Disorders. Philadelphia: WB Saunders; 2001

Bailey B, Johnson JT, Newlands SD, Calhoun KH. Head and Neck Surgery–Otolaryngology. 4th ed. Head and Neck Surgery, Vol 2. Philadelphia: Lippincott Williams & Wilkins; 2006

Cummings CW, Haugey BH, Thomas JR, Harker LA, Flint PW. Cummings Otolaryngology–Head and Neck Surgery, Vol 2, 4 vols. 4th ed. St Louis: Mosby; 2004

Laskaris G. Color Atlas of Oral Diseases. 3rd ed. New York: Thieme; 2006

42 Throat Mass

Ronda E. Alexander, Nazaneen N. Grant, and Andrew Blitzer

The finding of a mass in the upper aerodigestive tract is often discovered as a part of an investigation of a symptomatic complaint. These may include dysphonia, aphonia, dysphagia, dyspnea, hemoptysis, and odynophagia. This symptom directs the physician's investigation to the site of the lesion. A mass may be congenital, infectious, inflammatory, neoplastic, or traumatic in nature, and there may be some overlap. Also, any lesion can cause bleeding if it is sufficiently traumatized. Historical points to consider include symptom duration, the presence of exacerbating or ameliorating factors, tobacco exposure, as well as recent travel and occupational risks. We divide the differential diagnosis of "mass" into groups according to the **primary** associated symptom; obviously some masses will cause multiple symptoms.

◆ Primary Associated Symptom

Dysphagia

Dysphagia: To solids worse than liquids is indicative of a mass lesion within the upper digestive tract. The mass may be either intrinsic to the esophagus or an internal deformation caused by an external compression. Dysphagia may occur with or without odynophagia (painful swallowing).

- **Intrinsic mass**
  - *Foreign body granuloma*: An irregularity overlying an ingested object; the mucosa may be intact or ulcerated.
  - *Actinomycosis*: May be associated with immumocompromise, although not always.
  - Epithelial malignancy (*squamous cell carcinoma*): May appear as an ulcerated elevation or as an irregularly elevated area of mucosa.
  - Glandular malignancy (ie, *adenocarcinoma*): Usually in the distal portion of the esophagus and associated with chronic changes related to gastroesophageal reflux
  - *Sarcoma*: Remember that striated muscle predominates in the proximal one third of the esophagus.
  - *Neurofibromatosis type I*: Plexiform neurofibroma may cause mechanical obstruction but it may also progress to pseudochalasia and liquid dysphagia.
  - *Leiomyoma*: A smooth, submucosal mass in the distal two thirds of the esophagus
  - *Amyloid deposit*: A smooth submucosal mass

○ *Hemangioma*: Although these usually present during childhood, they may remain silent depending on size.
○ *Lymphatic malformation*: Either infiltrative or externally compressive

● **External lesions impinging on the aerodigestive tract**

○ *Thoracic and mediastinal lymphadenopathy*: Multiple etiologies

— Infectious, bacterial, or mycobacterial
— Neoplastic, usually from pulmonary primary neoplasm
— Autoimmune processes, most commonly *sarcoidosis*

○ Thoracic vascular anomalies: *Anomalous arterial* or *venous origin, aortic anomalies, aneurysms*
○ *Paraganglioma*: Carotid body tumor, glomus vagale
○ *Thyroid and parathyroid neoplasia*: Benign or malignant
○ *Ectopic thyroid*: Often described in the tongue base, the mass effect of this tissue may impair lingual mobility and the passage of food bolus from the oral cavity to the pharynx.
○ *Thyroglossal duct cyst* and patent tract remnants: If high in the neck, these may compress/displace aspects of the pharynx.
○ *Thymoma*
○ *Neck space abscess*: *Retropharyngeal, prevertebral spaces*

Dyspnea

Dyspnea: Can result from lesions at any point along the upper respiratory tract. The type of associated stridor is suggestive of the location of pathology. Inspiratory stridor is associated with obstruction in the upper airway (proximal to the glottis), whereas expiratory phase stridor is more indicative of issues within the lower respiratory tract (distal trachea and lungs). Biphasic stridor (inspiratory and expiratory) indicates pathology at the level of the glottis or trachea. These patients may have been treated inappropriately for reactive airway disease or chronic obstructive pulmonary disease (COPD) and, thus, may present with advanced lesions.

● *Squamous cell carcinoma*
● **Glandular neoplasm**

○ *Adenoid cystic carcinoma* (very common in this trachea)
○ *Pleomorphic adenoma*
○ *Oncocytoma*

● *Carcinoid tumor*: Often metabolically active; occurs in the tracheobronchial tree.
● *Chondroma/chondrosarcoma*: A continuum of cartilaginous neoplasia most common at the posterior lamina of the cricoid cartilage. It begins as a submucosal fullness but may progress to become an obstructing mass or result in fixation of the cricoarytenoid joint and resultant vocal fold paresis.
● *Sarcoma*: *Rhabdomyosarcoma* in youth, *malignant fibrous histiocytoma* in adults

- *Small cell tumor*: Although usually centered in the distal lung parenchyma, they may compress the trachea should they grow to sufficient size.
- *Lipoma*: Especially in the preepiglottic or paraglottic adipose tissue
- *Granular cell tumor*: A smooth, submucosal mass usually located in the larynx.
- *Paraganglioma*: Rare finding of deep fullness laterally within the larynx, which may be associated with impaired vocal fold mobility due to inadequate abduction secondary to the mass lesion.
- *Wegener granulomatosis*: Tracheal and subglottic mass or stenosis; or airway collapse (from chronic cartilaginous inflammation); or hemoptysis
- *Amyloidosis*: Submucosal deposits may present within the larynx or trachea.
- *Respiratory papillomatosis*: Presents with progressive symptoms that often recur despite initial management. Lesions are often centered around the glottis but can extend into the trachea; lesions often have a characteristic "stippled" appearance that is a macroscopic manifestation of the microscopic structure of the papilloma. This can mimic or, importantly, contain foci of squamous carcinoma. Biopsy is required to differentiate this process from the variants of squamous cell carcinoma.
- *Hemangioma*: Although commonly described in the pediatric subglottis, these may present throughout the airway.
- *Lymphatic malformation*
- *Arteriovenous malformation*
- *Laryngocele*: an air- or mucus-filled cavity formed by invagination of the endolaryngeal mucosa of the ventricle that often deforms the false vocal fold.
  - Internal laryngocele: Stays within the confines of the larynx
  - External laryngocele: Extends outside the larynx, usually through the thyrohyoid membrane.
- *Saccular cyst*: An anterior mucus-filled cavity formed from trapped mucus in the laryngeal saccule, a small area at the anterior-superior aspect of the ventricle.
- Autoimmune bullae: *Pemphigus vulgaris, bullous pemphigoid*
- *Infectious supraglottitis*: The deformation of the edematous laryngeal architecture may be mistaken for or obscure a mass, particularly within the epiglottis.

Dysphonia

Dysphonia: Results from derangements of the glottic vibratory mechanism. It may result from benign mucosal disorders or malignancy that interferes with either vocal fold motion or vibratory function. Processes that prevent proper vocal fold adduction also result in air escape, which manifests as breathy dysphonia and phonatory dyspnea. There is significant overlap with the causes of dyspnea.

- *Phonotraumatic nodules*: Found in women and preadolescent youth, at the junction of the anterior one third and posterior two thirds of the vocal folds and are often bilateral.

- *Polyps*: Degradation of the normal architecture, often after a subepithelial hemorrhage
- *Reinke edema*: A spectrum of myxomatous edema of the lamina propria of the true vocal folds usually found in patients with a history of cigarette smoking; initially presents with dysphonia but, if massive, may result in airway obstruction
- *Granuloma*: Presents on the posterior one third of the vocal fold; usually starts as posterior chondritis of the vocal process of the arytenoid; typically results from interruptions in the mucosa from intubation, excessive phonatory force perhaps from coughing, or surgery and can be exacerbated by peptic reflux
- **Cysts**
  - *Inclusion cyst*: Keratinaceous collections prevent appropriate mucosal vibration.
  - *Retention cyst*: Mucus glands may obstruct and enlarge into the structure of the vocal fold.

- *Rheumatoid nodules*: In the setting of autoimmune disease, deposits collect beneath the epithelium of the vocal folds. Often overlying edema and erythema can obscure the masses, and voice rest with or without an oral steroid taper can reveal the pathology.
- *Sarcoidosis*: May affect the supraglottis, glottis, or large airway with submucosal granulomata. Observe for the classic finding of "turban epiglottis."
- *Wegener granulomatosis*: Tracheal stenosis and/or collapse may impair the power generator of the vocal mechanism.
- *Respiratory papillomatosis*
- Epithelial malignancy: *Glottic squamous cell carcinoma* impairs mucosal vibratory function and may appear as leukoplakia, erythroplakia, or raised patches on one vocal fold.
- *Candidiasis*: On the vocal fold, this appears as a white patch and can result from local immunosuppression from systemic medications or pulmonary inhalers. The pseudomembranous form may also affect the larynx in the form of patches that can be raised or erosive.
- *Lipoma*
- *Laryngocele*
- *Saccular cyst*
- *Sarcoma*

Suggested Reading

Blitzer A, Schwartz JS, Song P, Young N. Oxford American Handbook of Otolaryngology. New York: Oxford University Press; 2008

Lalwani A. Current Diagnosis and Treatment in Otolaryngology–Head and Neck Surgery. 2nd ed. New York: McGraw-Hill Medical; 2007

43 Hoarseness and Voice Change (Breathy, Tremulous)

Robert T. Sataloff and Mary J. Hawkshaw

The symptom of hoarseness (coarse, scratchy sound) is caused by abnormalities of the vibratory margin of the vocal fold that cause turbulent airflow and acoustic perturbations. Hoarseness can be chronic or acute, persistent or intermittent. It can be associated with other symptoms, including postnasal drip, throat tickle, throat clearing, globus sensation, cough, fever, voice breaks, inability to project voice, voice fatigue, pain (throat, neck, or referred to ear), dysphagia, and weight loss. Hoarseness should be differentiated from other voice complaints that are often incorrectly described as hoarseness. The most common of these include breathiness, voice fatigue, volume disturbance, prolonged warm-up time, and tickling or choking during speech or singing.

Breathiness is caused by anything that interferes with glottal closure (*masses, paralysis, neuromuscular weakness, cricoarytenoid joint dysfunction,* and other abnormalities) and permits excessive air escape during phonation. **Voice fatigue** is the inability to continue to phonate for extended periods of time without change in voice quality. It may be caused by problems such as *voice abuse* or *misuse (muscle tension dysphonia), generalized fatigue, neurological disorders* (such as *myasthenia gravis,* or *mild vocal fold paresis with hyperfunctional compensation*). **Volume disturbance** is the inability to speak or sing loudly or to phonate softly. If not due to intrinsic limitations of the voice, the most common causes are technical errors in voice production. However, *hormonal changes, aging, superior laryngeal nerve paresis,* and other etiologies may be causal. **Prolonged warm-up time** is reported most commonly among singers. Normally, only 10 to 20 minutes are required for voice warm-up, even in the morning. The most common cause of prolonged warm-up time is *laryngopharyngeal reflux.* Tickling or choking during speech or singing may be caused by voice abuse, but it may also be a symptom of vibratory margin pathology. **Odynophonia** (pain while vocalizing) is most commonly due to *muscle tension dysphonia.* However, less common structural problems must be ruled out, including *infection, laryngopharyngeal reflux,* some *laryngeal granulomas* (although most are painless), *laryngeal joint arthritis,* and *malignancy.*

True hoarseness is most commonly caused by inflammation, edema, growths (benign and malignant), or vocal fold scarring.

Sudden onset hoarseness/voice change can be caused by infectious laryngitis, vocal fold hemorrhage, mucosal tear, and more serious problems, including neoplasm (onset of which may be sudden or gradual).

- *Infectious and inflammatory laryngitis* generally involves both vocal folds and may be associated with infection involving the entire supraglottic and/ or subglottic vocal tract (trachea and lungs). Concomitant problems can include excessive secretions, including mucopurulence, nasal obstruction, postnasal drip, throat clearing, dryness, throat tickle, and inflammation, and other mucosal changes due to irritants, including allergies, environmental fumes or particles, and acid reflux.

- *Vocal fold hemorrhage* or *mucosal tear* can be unilateral (usually) or bilateral, and both conditions can occur concomitantly. They are often associated with voice abuse and misuse (phonotrauma), acute infectious laryngitis, chronic laryngitis (especially secondary to acid reflux), allergy and sneezing, coughing, prolonged vomiting, systemic anticoagulation (including aspirin and ibuprofen), hormonal problems, blunt trauma to the anterior neck, and trauma secondary to intubation/extubation.
- Hoarseness is a hallmark sign of *laryngeal cancer*, which can be unilateral or bilateral. Concomitant problems may include irritation and edema, vocal fold paresis or mechanical fixation; paralysis, cough, hemoptysis, shortness of breath, dyspnea on exertion, throat pain, and/or referred otalgia. It is most often associated with smoking, although laryngopharyngeal reflux and papilloma infection may also be significant. Cancer usually causes **chronic** hoarseness, but it can present with sudden hoarseness when there is mucosal disruption or bleeding into the tumor.
- *Benign lesions* can be unilateral or bilateral. If bilateral, they can be the same pathology or different lesions, with one lesion often causing the contralateral lesion secondary to repeated trauma. These lesions can cause sudden hoarseness and may be associated with acute voice abuse or vocal trauma, although **gradual onset** of hoarseness is more typical. In addition to voice abuse, they are often associated with vocal fold hemorrhage or trauma. Some benign lesions can be treated successfully with voice therapy and medical management. Some will require surgical excision.

Chronic hoarseness can be constant or intermittent, and it can be associated with concomitant problems such as laryngopharyngeal reflux, allergy, hormonal problems, voice abuse/misuse, smoking, and other etiologies.

- *Inflammation* caused by inhalants and irritants (chemical and environmental, including smoking, stage special effects, and steroid inhaler use), *vocal fold scar* secondary to trauma, *voice abuse, voice misuse, benign lesions, malignant lesions,* and *viruses* such as human papilloma virus. Voice abuse/misuse is commonly associated with "abdominal support" problems, which may be technical, but which also may be caused by pulmonary dysfunction such as asthma or emphysema. Lung function should be considered and assessed as appropriate in voice patients.
- Mass lesions associated with *amyloidosis, sarcoidosis, tuberculosis, rheumatoid arthritis,* and other conditions may cause chronic hoarseness.
- Intermittent chronic hoarseness is commonly the result of *edema,* often associated with *upper respiratory infection, sneezing, coughing, extensive periods of voice overuse/abuse,* and *hormonal fluctuation.* Chronic infection from fungi may also cause intermittent hoarseness, as may smoking, irritant exposure, and the use of steroid inhalers.
- *Laryngopharyngeal reflux* causes chronic hoarseness in most patients who have the condition, but fluctuation is typical and may be associated with dietary indiscretions, increased stress, activities that increase abdominal pressure, and other factors that aggravate reflux.

- *Benign vocal fold lesions*, including polyps, cysts, and nodules may cause consistent or intermittent hoarseness. The intermittency is caused by fluctuating edema over the lesion or contralateral to the lesion at the point of contact.
- *Chronic abuse* of the voice during speaking and/or singing commonly causes hoarseness that improves at least partially during periods of relative voice rest.
- *Neurolaryngologic* problems such as *vocal fold paresis* or *myasthenia gravis* are less common causes of hoarseness, but not rare. Intermittency is typically associated with increased vocal demand, vocal effort, and stress. Hoarseness can also be associated with systemic neurological disease such as multiple sclerosis, amyotrophic lateral sclerosis, and Parkinson disease.
- *Laryngeal cancer* typically causes chronic hoarseness.

◆ Conclusion

The symptom of hoarseness requires medical evaluation in all cases other than mild-to-moderate hoarseness associated with acute laryngitis and upper respiratory infection, and which resolves within no more than about 1 to 2 weeks, even if untreated. Hoarseness that does not resolve must be evaluated promptly to rule out serious causes. Sudden hoarseness should always be evaluated immediately to determine whether vocal fold hemorrhage or mucosal tear is present because most laryngologists agree that these conditions require treatment with a brief course of absolute voice rest. Severe hoarseness even associated with an upper respiratory infection warrants physical examination for the same reason. New-onset hoarseness unassociated with an obvious etiology (such as upper respiratory infection) should lead to prompt otolaryngologic assessment.

Suggested Reading

Fried MP, Ferlito A, eds. The Larynx. San Diego: Plural Publications; 2008

Ossoff RH, Shapshay SM, Woodson GE, Netterville JL. The Larynx. Philadelphia: Lippincott, Williams and Wilkins; 2003

Rubin J, Sataloff RT, Korovin G. Diagnosis and Treatment of Voice Disorders. 3rd ed. San Diego: Plural Publishing; 2006

Sataloff RT. Professional Voice: The Science and Art of Clinical Care. 3rd ed. San Diego: Plural Publishing; 2005

Sataloff RT, Castell DO, Katz PO, Sataloff DM. Reflux Laryngitis and Related Disorders. 3rd ed. San Diego: Plural Publishing; 2006

Sataloff RT, Hawkshaw MJ, Eller R. Atlas of Laryngoscopy. 2nd ed. San Diego: Plural Publishing; 2006

Sataloff RT, Mandel S, Heman-Ackah YD, Manon-Espaillat R, Abaza M. Laryngeal Electromyography. 2nd ed. San Diego: Plural Publishing; 2006

Sulica L, Blitzer A. Vocal Fold Paralysis. New York: Springer; 2006

44 Cough or Hemoptysis

Nadia G. Mohyuddin, J. Kenneth Byrd, and Terry A. Day

Cough, derived from the Latin word *tussis*, is an expulsion of air from the lungs that is often accompanied by a characteristic sound. It is usually produced as a response to foreign matter irritating the lining of the respiratory tract, including the larynx, trachea, and distal airways. Furthermore, cough can be divided into acute, lasting less than 3 weeks, subacute, lasting 3 to 8 weeks, or chronic, lasting greater than 8 weeks.

Additionally, hemoptysis is the expectoration of blood or blood-tinged sputum from any area within the airway passages, including the nose, mouth, laryngopharynx, trachea, bronchi, alveoli, and lung parenchyma. This word itself is a derivative from the Greek words *haima*, meaning blood, and *ptyein*, meaning to spit.

◆ Pathophysiology

The involuntary cough reflex is a primitive, protective action initiated by mechanical stimulation of both myelinated and unmyelinated sensory afferent nerve fibers from the larynx and lungs, chemoreceptors in the distal airway, and stretch receptors in the lungs (**Fig. 44.1**). Additional afferent fibers from the Arnold nerve transmit signals from the external auditory canal and tympanic membrane. These afferent signals are then transmitted by the vagus nerve directly to the medulla. The efferent cascade is initiated with the inspiration of air followed by closure of the epiglottis. The vocal cords then adduct to entrap the air within the lungs. Next, the expiratory and accessory muscles simultaneously contract, resulting in increased intrathoracic pressure reaching upward of 300 mm Hg. The epiglottis and vocal cords then open widely, resulting in both a rapid release of air and production of a distinctive noise. This sudden gush of air can reach velocities as high as 75 to 100 miles per hour. The noncartilaginous portions of the bronchi and trachea collapse inward, thereby allowing the air passing through to carry with it the irritants present within the airway.

The act of coughing can also be a voluntary event based on supramedullary central cortical stimulation, resulting in an alteration of the expiratory and accessory muscles' activities. Voluntary control of the force of muscle contractility results in variation of cough intensity. This cough is not directly mediated by irritation of the respiratory tract, but rather as a conscious effort by the individual.

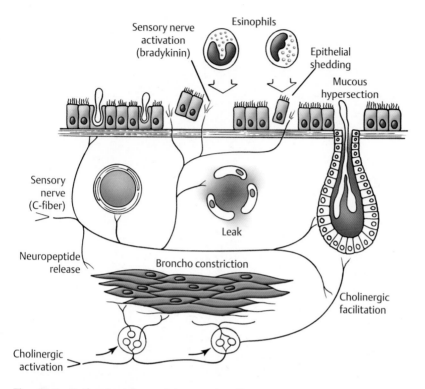

Fig. 44.1   Pathophysiology of the cough reflex in response to neurogenic inflammation in asthma.

◆ Etiology

Cough can be due to various etiologies, including self-limited benign illnesses to more significant and potentially fatal diseases. It can be dry or productive, the latter being associated with the expulsion of sputum, mucus, or exudate, suggestive of a possible underlying infection, a systemic disease, or even a malignancy. Hemoptysis can be a symptom of a much more severe and possibly life-threatening disease process that warrants immediate investigation. If the hemoptysis is of bronchogenic origin, it is often massive due to the pressures of the systemic circulation, whereas bleeding from the pulmonary circulation is less profuse. In adults, the differential diagnosis for both cough and hemoptysis is broad; however, the causes can be simplified into several general categories (**Table 44.1**).

(Text continues on page 245)

Table 44.1 Differential Diagnosis for Cough and Hemoptysis

Etiology	Description	Presentation	Diagnosis	Treatment
Vascular				
Pulmonary embolism	Blood clot in the lungs	Sudden onset dyspnea, hemoptysis, pleuritic chest pain, hypoxia	CT angiogram	Anticoagulation with heparin or Coumadin
Congestive heart failure	Decreased pumping ability of the heart	Dry hacking or wet frothy cough, worse when lying down, peripheral edema	Echocardiogram	Diuretics, ACE-I, digoxin, β blockers, cardiac transplant
Aortic aneurysm	Dilation of the aorta due to weakness in the vessel wall	Asymptomatic until aneurysm expands leading to chronic cough	CT scan, ultrasonography	Surgical repair
Mitral valve stenosis	Stiff and poorly compliant cardiac valve	Palpitations, enlargement of left atrium leads to left recurrent laryngeal nerve paralysis (*Ortner syndrome*); dry cough and hemoptysis	Echocardiography, cardiac catheterization	Valve replacement; need antibiotic prophylaxis before any surgical procedure
Arteriovenous malformation	Direct communication between an artery and a vein	Epistaxis, platypnea (dyspnea while erect relieved by lying down), chronic cough, frank hemoptysis	Angiography	Embolization, surgical resection

Table 44.1 (*Continued*) Differential Diagnosis for Cough and Hemoptysis

Etiology	Description	Presentation	Diagnosis	Treatment
Infectious/Inflammatory				
Rhinosinusitis	Inflammation of the sinonasal mucosa	Nasal congestion, postnasal drip leading to cough worse when laying flat	Nasal endoscopy, CT scan	Antiinflammatory agents, antibiotics, sinus surgery
Pharyngitis, laryngitis, sinusitis, pneumonia	Infection and inflammation due to viral, bacterial, fungal, or parasitic pathogens	Acute cough becoming chronic, mild hemoptysis, hoarseness	Physical examination, endoscopy, CXR	Antimicrobial agents, supportive care
Lung abscess	Polymicrobial cavitary lung lesion; due to aspiration in the debilitated or alcoholic patient	Chronic productive cough, foul-smelling sputum, hemoptysis	CXR	Broad-spectrum antibiotics
Tuberculosis	Inhaled bacterial pathogen *Mycobacterium tuberculosis*	Frank hemoptysis, chronic cough, caseating granulomas, cavitary lung lesions	CXR, sputum culture	Four-drug therapy: isoniazid, rifampin, ethambutol, pyrazinamide; contact precautions
Gastroesophageal reflux	Gastric contents entering the esophagus leading to mucosal damage	Throat clearing, globus sensation, nonproductive cough worse at night, hoarseness, chest pain	Endoscopy, pH probe	Lifestyle modification, H2 blockers, proton pump inhibitors, Nissen fundoplication

(Continued on page 240)

Table 44.1 (Continued) Differential Diagnosis for Cough and Hemoptysis

Etiology	Description	Presentation	Diagnosis	Treatment
Neoplasm				
Benign	Enlarged tonsils, vocal polyps or nodules, bronchogenic adenomas	Dry cough, hoarseness	Endoscopy, laryngoscopy, CXR	Conservative measures, voice rest, surgery
Malignant	Carcinomas of the aerodigestive tract	Chronic cough, gross hemoptysis, upper airway obstruction, dyspnea, weight loss	Aerodigestive endoscopy, biopsy, bronchial washings	Chemotherapy, radiation therapy, surgery
Degenerative/Deficiency				
Pulmonary fibrosis	Progressive lung scarring	Chronic dry hacking cough, restrictive breathing pattern	Pulmonary function tests, CXR	Oxygen, pulmonary rehabilitation, lung transplant
Emphysema bulla	Destruction of the alveolar walls with enlargement of the air spaces	Chronic dry cough, air trapping, hypoxia, obstructive breathing pattern	Pulmonary function tests, α-1 antitrypsin deficiency	Bronchodilators, anticholinergics, oxygen, lung transplant
Intoxication				
Smoke	Fire or tobacco exposure	Acute, chronic, dry or productive cough; paralysis of cilia resulting in impaired airway clearance	Known exposure; firefighters, smokers	Avoid exposure
Inhalants	Chemicals, perfumes, cleaning agents	Allergic reaction or exacerbate underlying condition	Known exposure, occupational activities	Avoid exposure

Table 44.1 (*Continued*) Differential Diagnosis for Cough and Hemoptysis

Etiology	Description	Presentation	Diagnosis	Treatment
Medications	ACE-I leads to elevated bradykinin and hyperreactive airways	Dry chronic cough in ~20% users	Review of medication list	Discontinue and start ARB
Congenital				
Cystic fibrosis	CFTR gene mutation	Chronic productive cough, copious secretions	Sweat-chloride and genetic testing	Gene therapy, mucolytics, antimicrobials
Bronchiectasis	Irreversible dilation of distal airways, poor respiratory clearance	Hemoptysis, chronic productive cough worse when leaning forward; situs inversus, chronic sinusitis, and ciliary dyskinesia (*Kartagener syndrome*)	High-resolution CT scan	Bronchopulmonary hygiene, antimicrobials, antiinflammatory agents
Tracheoesophageal fistula	Abnormal communication between the trachea and esophagus	Life-threatening aspiration, chronic cough, choking, cyanosis after eating	CXR, upper airway endoscopy	Surgical correction
Vascular ring	Anomalous aorta or associated vessel configuration encompassing the aerodigestive tract	High-pitched, brassy cough, tracheo- and bronchomalacia, dysphagia	Barium esophagram, echocardiogram, endoscopy	Surgical correction

(Continued on page 242)

Table 44.1 (Continued) Differential Diagnosis for Cough and Hemoptysis

Etiology	Description	Presentation	Diagnosis	Treatment
Autoimmune/Allergic				
Asthma	Hyperreactive airway leading to inflammation, narrowing, and mucus secretion	Dyspnea, wheezing; a leading cause of chronic cough; nasal polyposis and ASA sensitivity (*Samter triad*)	Pulmonary function tests	Bronchodilators, anti-inflammatory agents, β-2 agonists, oxygen, heliox
Angioedema	Leaky postcapillary venules, C1 esterase deficiency	Rapid subcutaneous, mucosal and submucosal swelling, airway obstruction	Physical examination, upper airway endoscopy	Airway protection, epinephrine, H1/H2 blockers, steroids, FFP
Goodpasture syndrome	Necrotizing lesions of kidneys and lungs	Frank hemoptysis, cough, renal failure	Tissue biopsy	Corticosteroids, cyclophosphamide, dialysis
Granulomatous diseases	*Wegener granulomatosis, vasculitis*	Nasal septal perforation, dyspnea, chronic cough, mild hemoptysis	C-ANCA (Wegener's), ACE levels (sarcoid), tissue biopsy	Immunosuppressants
Hay fever/seasonal allergies	Pollens or other airborne agents leading to airway hypersensitivity, elevated IgE	Sneezing, rhinorrhea, postnasal drip, dry, acute or chronic cough	Allergy testing, IgE levels	Avoid inciting factors, antihistamines, antiinflammatory agents
Eosinophilic bronchitis	Abundance of eosinophils and metachromatic cells	Dry chronic cough, mimics asthma	Normal spirometry	Corticosteroids

Table 44.1 (Continued) Differential Diagnosis for Cough and Hemoptysis

Etiology	Description	Presentation	Diagnosis	Treatment
Trauma				
Foreign body	Ingestion or aspiration leads to irritation	Acute cough, stridor, mild hemoptysis; if lodged in distal airway, develop chronic dry cough and wheezing	CXR, CT scan, aerodigestive endoscopy	Surgical removal
Pneumothorax and pneumomediastinum	Air in the intrapleural space or mediastinum can lead to lung collapse	Dry, acute, or chronic cough with dyspnea, chest pain, hemoptysis, subcutaneous emphysema	CXR, CT scan	Tube thoracotomy, needle decompression
Blunt/penetrating trauma	MVA, GSW, stab injury	Variable; acute dry or productive cough, blood-tinged sputum to frank hemoptysis and aerodigestive tract hemorrhage	CXR, CT scan, urgent/emergent aerodigestive tract endoscopy	Dependent on the injury type ranging from conservative to aggressive surgical intervention
Endocrine				
Thyroid	Substernal compression or vocal cord/tracheal involvement by neoplastic process	Hoarseness, dysphagia, chronic dry cough, dyspnea	Ultrasonography, noncontrasted CT scan, thyroid uptake scan	Suppressive hormone therapy, surgical removal, radioactive iodine therapy

(Continued on page 244)

Table 44.1 (*Continued*) Differential Diagnosis for Cough and Hemoptysis

Etiology	Description	Presentation	Diagnosis	Treatment
		Other		
Psychogenic	Adolescent population; stress induced	Cough which is absent in sleep and disappears when enjoyable distractions available	Diagnosis of exclusion	Counseling, behavioral therapy
Otogenic	Reflex arch from afferent fibers of Arnold's nerve from EAC	Chronic dry cough made worse with EAC manipulation	Stimulation of the EAC	Remove stimulating factor from ear canal

Abbreviations: ACE-I, angiotensin-converting enzyme inhibitor; ARB, angiotensin receptor blocker; ASA, aspirin; C-ANCA, c-anti-neutrophil cytoplasmic antibody; CFTR, cystic fibrosis transmembrane conductance regulator; CT, computed tomography; CXR, chest x-ray; EAC, external auditory canal; FFP, fresh frozen plasma; GSW, gunshot wound; MVA, motor vehicle accident.

- **Cardiovascular etiology**

  - *Pulmonary embolism (PE)*: Associated with a sudden onset of dyspnea, hemoptysis, pleuritic chest pain, and hypoxia. Hemoptysis can occur in the setting of a massive PE. Risk factors include immobility, recent surgery, obesity, malignancy, history of thromboembolism, and smoking. Clinical symptoms include tachycardia, tachypnea, hypoxia, rales or decreased breath sounds, and elevated jugular venous distension. It is second only to coronary artery disease as the most common cause of unexpected natural death in any age group.

  - *Congestive heart failure (CHF)*: Can have either a dry hacking or a wet frothy cough that may worsen when lying down or on exertion. Impaired systolic function results in a sympathetically mediated retention of salt and water, thereby leading to systemic as well as pulmonary fluid overload. The most common risk factors for CHF include heart disease, hypertension, and diabetes.

  - *Aortic aneurysm*: Patients often remain asymptomatic until the aneurysm begins to expand, at which time they may develop a chronic cough due to pressure on the respiratory tract or recurrent laryngeal nerve. This vascular pathology is associated with hypertension, autoimmune diseases, syphilis, and genetic defects in structural proteins (eg, *Marfan syndrome*).

  - *Mitral valve stenosis*: This can lead to left atrial enlargement, which can exert pressure on and possible paralysis of the left recurrent laryngeal nerve, resulting in a dry cough and hoarseness (*Ortner syndrome*). This disease process is most often seen in patients with a history of rheumatic fever, although congenital stenosis has also been reported.

  - *Arteriovenous malformation*: Can afflict various systems; however, respiratory tract involvement may lead to frequent epistaxis, platypnea (difficulty in breathing while erect often relieved by lying down), chronic cough, and massive hemoptysis.

- **Infectious/inflammatory etiology**

  - *Acute or chronic rhinosinusitis*: Results in postnasal drip, which is one of the leading causes for cough. This is exacerbated by lying flat. Bacterial infections will lead to a productive cough and discolored rhinorrhea.

  - *Pharyngitis, laryngitis, bronchitis, sinusitis,* and *pneumonia*: These processes can be due to several viral, bacterial, fungal, or parasitic pathogens; however, most are self-limiting. Patients may develop an acute cough, which can eventually become chronic, often lingering for several weeks. If the cough is severe enough, patients may experience blood-tinged sputum. Gross hemoptysis is less common.

  - *Lung abscess*: A polymicrobial infection often associated with anaerobic pathogens accompanied by chronic productive cough with foul-smelling sputum and hemoptysis. Patients can be quite debilitated, alcoholic, or immunosuppressed.

  - *Tuberculosis*: Inhaled bacterial pathogen that infects the lungs leading to frank hemoptysis, chronic cough, caseating granulomas, and cavitary pulmonary lesions. Health care workers, immunocompromised individuals, prisoners, and the homeless are at increased risk for contracting this disease.

○ *Gastroesophageal reflux (GERD)*: One of the leading causes for cough in the general population. It may be associated with frequent throat clearing, globus sensation, and a dry cough that is worse at night or when lying flat. Patients may also complain of both increased phlegm production and hoarseness that is more pronounced in the morning. GERD produces cough by stimulation of the receptors in the esophagus, irritation of the upper airways (laryngotracheal reflux), and microaspiration leading to irritation of the lower airways.

● **Neoplasm etiology**

○ Benign: *Adenotonsillar hypertrophy, vocal polyps* or *nodules*, and *bronchogenic adenomas* are occasionally associated with a dry cough.

○ Malignant: *Primary or metastatic carcinomas of the larynx, trachea, bronchi, or lungs* can lead to a chronic cough and hemoptysis. In cancers of the larynx and trachea, the patient may develop throat or ear pain, airway obstruction, and hoarseness due to direct extension of the tumor into the glottis or involvement of the recurrent laryngeal nerve. In the case of lung cancer, more pronounced symptoms of weight loss, anorexia, dyspnea, and chest pain are not present until late in the disease course in the majority of cases. Major risk factors are tobacco and alcohol.

● **Degenerative/deficiency etiology**

○ *Pulmonary fibrosis*: Development of progressive scarring in the lungs leading to a restrictive breathing pattern on pulmonary function tests. The cough is chronic, dry, and hacking.

○ *Chronic obstructive pulmonary disease (COPD)*: Leads to chronic dry cough, air trapping in the distal airways, and hypoxia. This can be due to two degenerative processes: *emphysema* and/or *chronic bronchitis*. Emphysema is the progressive, proteolytic destruction of the distal airspaces, leading to decreased elasticity, and therefore chronic, dry cough and air trapping. Chronic bronchitis is defined clinically by productive cough for 3 consecutive months in 2 consecutive years. Both subtypes of COPD are predominantly caused by long-term tobacco abuse; however, emphysema can be found in patients with *α-1 antitrypsin deficiency* syndrome.

● **Toxic exposure and medications etiology**

○ *Smoke*: Fire or tobacco exposure can lead to acute or chronic, dry or productive cough where prolonged contact can result in more systemic complications. In acute smoke exposure, such as a house fire, the examiner should look for signs of possible thermal airway injury, including singed facial hair or soot around the mouth or nose. Chronic smoke inhalation causes paralysis of the cilia of the airway, resulting in impaired mucociliary particle clearance. The characteristic chronic smoker's cough can be seen in the early morning and is associated with white-gray phlegm production.

○ *Inhalants*: Chemicals, perfumes, and cleaning agents can lead to an allergic reaction or exacerbate an underlying chronic systemic condition.

○ *Medications*: Angiotensin-converting enzyme inhibitors (ACE-I) are among the leading pharmacological agents associated with a cough. This drug leads to an increased production of bradykinin resulting in airway hyperreactivity, leading to a nonproductive, chronic cough in ~20% of users. Of interest, converting to an angiotensin receptor blocker can cure the cough.

- **Congenital etiology**

  ○ *Cystic fibrosis*: Caused by chloride channel gene mutation. It is often diagnosed in childhood and can lead to significant digestive, respiratory, and reproductive complications with reduced overall lifespan. The cough produces thick and copious secretions, and patients are prone to recurrent sinusitis and pneumonias.

  ○ *Bronchiectasis*: Irreversible dilatation of distal airways leads to impaired clearance of secretions, fluid entrapment, and recurrent infections. An associated chronic productive cough is exacerbated when the patient leans forward. The combination of bronchiectasis, situs inversus, chronic sinusitis, and ciliary dyskinesia is known as *Kartagener syndrome*.

  ○ *Tracheoesophageal fistula (TEF)*: An abnormal communication between the trachea and esophagus results in potentially life-threatening aspiration with coughing, choking, and cyanosis after eating. TEF may be congenital, associated with the spectrum of esophageal atresia, or acquired. The latter can be due to trauma, surgery, or prolonged intubation or tracheostomy tube use.

  ○ *Vascular ring*: These patients will have a characteristic high-pitched brassy cough and suffer from extrinsic compression of the trachea and bronchi leading to malacia, airway obstruction, and stridor.

- **Autoimmune/allergic etiology**

  ○ *Asthma*: One of the leading causes of chronic cough. This is a reactive airway disease resulting in inflammation and narrowing that lead to dyspnea, wheezing, and, during an acute exacerbation, even death. Some patients with asthma will also have associated nasal polyposis and aspirin sensitivity, known as the *Samter triad*.

  ○ *Angioedema*: Development of acute swelling below the dermis due to transient vascular leakage, which has a variable presentation of upper airway obstruction. It can be due to immunoglobulin E (IgE) or complement mediation, autoimmune disorders, infection, or hereditary C1 esterase inhibitor deficiency.

  ○ *Goodpasture syndrome*: Patients have autoantibodies to the basement membrane proteins and suffer from necrotizing lesions of the kidneys and lungs producing frank hemoptysis, cough, and renal failure.

  ○ *Granulomatous diseases*: Wegener granulomatosis and sarcoidosis are both multiorgan systemic conditions where airway manifestations can lead to recurrent or chronic sinusitis and a persistent cough, occasionally associated with bloody phlegm.

  ○ *Hay fever/seasonal allergies*: Pollen, mold, dust, pet dander, and environmental pathogens, among other agents, lead to increased IgE levels, eosinophilia, and increased levels of inflammatory mediators that affect the upper and lower airways. Postnasal drip and increased airway sensitivity lead to the development of a dry acute or chronic cough.

○ *Eosinophilic bronchitis*: There is an abundance of eosinophils and metachromatic cells, a lack of bronchial hyperresponsiveness, normal spirometry results, and adequate response to inhaled and systemic corticosteroids.

● **Trauma etiology**

○ *Foreign body*: Ingestion or aspiration of such matter can lead to irritation of the upper airway and vocal cords, resulting in an acute coughing episode. If the object is actually lodged in the distal airways, patients may have a "silent period" followed by chronic dry cough and wheezing.

○ *Pneumothorax/pneumomediastinum*: Accumulation of air in the intrapleural space or mediastinal structures, respectively, can lead to a dry, acute, or chronic cough associated with dyspnea, chest pain, and subcutaneous emphysema. In acute tension pneumothorax, patients will present with increased respiratory effort, hypoxia, and possibly tachycardia and hypotension. A history of COPD, trauma, or positive pressure ventilation may be present in patients with pneumothorax. Pneumomediastinum should raise suspicion for perforation of the esophagus.

○ *Blunt or penetrating trauma*: Various inciting events can lead to upper and lower airway injuries with a wide range of symptoms, including an acute dry or productive cough, blood-tinged sputum, to frank hemoptysis and airway hemorrhage. Patients warrant emergent airway evaluation because these events can often be fatal.

● **Endocrine etiology**

○ *Thyroid goiter*: With a substernal gland, one can develop compressive symptoms leading to a chronic cough, shortness of breath, and dysphagia. Malignant tumors can invade the recurrent laryngeal nerve leading to vocal cord paralysis.

● **Other etiologies**

○ *Psychogenic*: Frequently seen in the adolescent population and is a diagnosis of exclusion. These patients will have no cough during sleep, are not awakened by cough, and do not cough when enjoyable distractions are available.

○ *Otogenic*: Occurs with stimulation of the Arnold nerve, a branch of the vagus nerve, supplying sensation to the external auditory canal and tympanic membrane. Patients can experience a dry cough during ear cleaning procedures and a persistent cough with external canal foreign bodies such as a piece of hair.

◆ Evaluation

The differential diagnosis of cough is quite extensive and is largely based on the temporal length of the patient's symptoms as well as the anatomical site involved (**Fig. 44.2**). The patient's history and physical examination are impera-

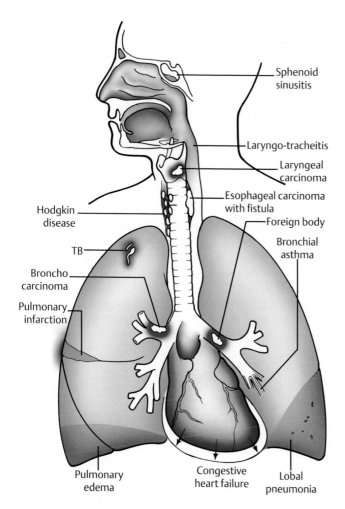

Fig. 44.2 Causes for cough in the upper and lower airway. Various ailments of particular anatomical subsites within the upper aerodigestive tract can lead to a cough.

tive for making a correct diagnosis. Tools to assist with the evaluation of particular complaints include imaging studies such as a chest x-ray; a computed tomographic scan of the sinuses, neck, or chest; a barium esophagram; ultrasonography; echocardiography; and angiography. Additional studies for aiding in diagnosis include pulmonary function tests, pH probe, laboratory tests, and upper aerodigestive tract endoscopies, such as nasopharyngoscopy, laryngoscopy, bronchoscopy, and esophagogastroduodenoscopy.

The care of the patient with a cough varies from supportive care and lifestyle modifications to aggressive surgical and medical care; a brief discussion is provided in **Table 44.1**. Cough is a complex pathophysiological symptom that has a broad differential diagnosis yet one can narrow the etiologies based on the patient's history, physical exam findings, and pertinent studies.

Suggested Reading

Balter MS. Hemoptysis. In: Irwin RS, Curley FJ, Grossman RF, eds. Diagnosis and Treatment of Symptoms of the Respiratory Tract. Armonk, NY: Futura Publishing; 1997;155–197

Chung KF, Widdicombe JG, Boushey HA. Cough: Causes, Mechanisms, and Therapy. Malden, MA: Wiley-Blackwell; 2003

Irwin RS, Boulet LP, Cloutier MM, et al. Managing cough as a defense mechanism and as a symptom: a consensus panel report of the American College of Chest Physicians. Chest 1998;114(2, Suppl Managing):133S–181S

Irwin RS, Madison JM. The diagnosis and treatment of cough. N Engl J Med 2000;343: 1715–1721

Lasserson D, Mills K, Arunachalam R, Polkey M, Moxham J, Kalra L. Differences in motor activation of voluntary and reflex cough in humans. Thorax 2006;61:699–705

Simonyan K, Saad ZS, Loucks TM, Poletto CJ, Ludlow CL. Functional neuroanatomy of human voluntary cough and sniff production. Neuroimage 2007;37:401–409

Widdicombe JG. Neurophysiology of the cough reflex. Eur Respir J 1995;8:1193–1202

45 Airway Obstruction (Noisy Breathing, Stridor, Dyspnea)

Lindsay Lipinski and David Goldenberg

Functionally, the airway begins at the nares and mouth and continues into the thoracic cavity to the bronchioles. Along this passageway, therefore, there are several anatomical locations that can cause obstruction. The airway can be divided into extrathoracic (including supralaryngeal, supraglottic, glottic, and subglottic areas) and intrathoracic (the tracheobronchial tree). The location of the obstruction can often be determined by carefully noting the qualities of the sounds made by the obstructed patient during breathing. The site of obstruction also plays an important role in treatment. Thus the diagnostic approach detailed following here is based on airway anatomy.

The age of the patient may help in determining the diagnosis. **Pediatric** airway obstruction tends to be due to a **congenital** or **inflammatory** condition; in **adults**, obstruction is usually caused by a **neoplasm** or an **inflammatory** condition. In adults, airways are wider and can tolerate greater degrees of obstruction. Children, whose airways are much narrower, will become symptomatic more quickly. The glottis is the narrowest part of the adult airway, whereas the subglottis is narrowest in children, and even a minor degree of inflammation in this area can cause severe distress.

A thorough clinical history and a complete physical examination are major components in reaching the diagnosis. The onset, frequency, and duration of symptoms should be determined, as well as any associations (feeding position changes, exercise, sleep). Obstruction may also be classified by whether it is local or systemic, and associated symptoms (such as dysphagia, drooling, aspiration, cough, bleeding) may help to determine this. A history of previous surgery, intubation, tracheotomy, or trauma can help to localize the problem. For pediatric patients, a birth and developmental history should be obtained. Physical exam, including indirect laryngoscopy, will provide further information. In some cases, additional diagnostic testing, including radiography, pulmonary function testing, and airway visualization, may be necessary.

◆ Supralaryngeal (Associated Sounds: Stridor, Gurgling)

- **Congenital**: Defects in the complex formation and development of the oral cavity, nasal cavity, and pharynx can lead to a variety of malformations that can cause obstructive symptoms.

  - *Micrognathia*: This defect in the formation of the jaw is due to retarded growth of the mandible, causing the tongue to be relatively large for the oral cavity.

○ *Macroglossia*: The anomaly may be focal or generalized, and the enlargement of the tongue can prevent adequate airflow.

○ *Choanal atresia*: Caused by obliteration or blockage of the posterior nasal aperture, this malformation is often associated with bony abnormalities of the pterygoid plates and midfacial growth abnormalities.

○ *Lingual thyroid*: Ectopic tissue may be present at the foramen cecum, and this can be confirmed by radionuclide scanning.

○ *Nasal septal deformity*: This malformation is due to intrauterine pressure effects or intrapartum trauma, or occurs in association with other anomalies.

○ *Pyriform aperture stenosis*: Congenital stenosis of this opening due to bony overgrowth can cause airway obstruction in infants.

● **Infectious**: Several infectious processes should be considered in the supralaryngeal airway, especially in febrile or toxic patients.

○ *Retropharyngeal/peritonsillar abscess*: A complication of acute tonsillitis, abscesses are associated with trismus, severe sore throat, malaise, and dehydration.

○ *Mononucleosis*: This viral infection is characterized by a triad of fever, tonsillar pharyngitis, and lymphadenopathy; rarely, edema of the soft palate and tonsils may lead to airway occlusion.

○ *Diphtheria*: An acute infection with *Corynebacterium diphtheriae*, most commonly occurring in the tonsillopharyngeal region, can rarely lead to massive swelling of the tonsils and uvula and cause respiratory insufficiency.

○ *Ludwig angina*: An acute cellulitis resulting from infection in the oral cavity that progresses to the tissues of the neck; the patient is ill and toxic with indurated swelling of the submandibular and submental space.

● **Inflammatory**: Inflammation of the upper airway is a common cause of airway obstruction in both children and adults, and inflammation of any part of the mucous membrane in the pharynx is readily transferred to other areas.

○ *Allergic rhinitis*: This process is characterized by episodic sneezing, nasal blockage, and nonpurulent rhinorrhea; edematous mucosa may impair airflow.

○ *Angioedema*: Extravasation of fluid into the interstitium in response to an inflammatory cascade (allergic, autoimmune, and drug-related etiologies) can lead to localized swelling of mucous membranes.

● **Trauma**: A history of trauma is important to consider in patients with difficulty breathing because it provides an obvious mechanism for obstruction.

○ *Hematoma*: The mass effect of a retropharyngeal hematoma may compromise airway patency and should be considered in patients with a history of head trauma.

○ *Facial fracture*: Displaced fractures or posttraumatic swelling can impinge on the airway and prevent adequate airflow.

● **Neoplasm**: Tumors of the oral cavity or pharynx should also be considered, particularly in patients with a history of alcohol or tobacco use. Tumor type is almost exclusively squamous cell carcinoma, but lymphoma or benign lipomas or fibromas may occasionally occur in the upper airway.

- **Iatrogenic**: Manipulation associated with oral or nasal surgery can result in edema and can impair airflow.

◆ Supraglottic (Associated Sounds: Inspiratory Stridor)

- **Congenital**: Congenital anomalies in the supraglottic region are also a common cause of airway obstruction in pediatric patients.
  - *Laryngomalacia*: A common cause of congenital stridor, the stridor is often relieved by prone positioning and worse when the baby is active; diagnosis is confirmed by endoscopy.
  - *Supraglottic cyst*: Laryngeal cysts are a rare cause of obstruction but may significantly occlude the airway.
- **Infectious**: Infection of the supraglottic area can also lead to swelling of tissues that occlude airflow.
  - *Epiglottitis*: Acute infection, usually with *Haemophilus influenza*, can be life threatening due to rapid and severe swelling.
- **Inflammatory**: Obstruction due to an inflammatory condition in the supraglottic area is less common but can also be a cause of rapid and serious airway obstruction.
  - *Angioedema*: Although usually self-limited, angioedema of the larynx can progress to airway compromise and asphyxiation.
- **Trauma**: Iatrogenic trauma to the supraglottic airway can be a cause of obstruction.
  - *Intubation*: Traumatic or prolonged intubation can cause irritation and tissue damage to the area with subsequent swelling.
- **Neoplasm**: Again, *squamous cell carcinoma* and other *malignant and benign neoplasms* can occur in the larynx and progressively lead to airway compromise, though respiratory distress is a very late complication.
- ***Sarcoidosis***: This systemic disorder of unknown etiology is characterized by the formation of noncaseating granulomas, usually in the supraglottis, that can, in rare circumstances, disrupt airflow.

◆ Glottic (Associated Sounds: Inspiratory or Biphasic Stridor, Hoarse/Breathy Voice)

- **Congenital**: Congenital anomalies at the glottis often present at birth and can be quickly fatal if not treated early.
  - *Glottic web*: Failure of resorption of the epithelial layer in the laryngeal opening results in incomplete separation of the vocal folds, leading to a rare cause of obstruction.

- ○ *Laryngeal atresia/stenosis*: Failure of recanalization during development in the region of the glottis can cause asphyxia early in life.
- **Infectious**: Though rare, infections of the vocal cord can cause airway obstruction along with hoarseness.
  - ○ *Tuberculous laryngitis*: Laryngitis is a rare presentation of miliary tuberculosis leading to hoarseness and mobile but edematous and erythematous vocal cords.
  - ○ *Laryngeal diphtheria*: Acute infection with *Corynebacterium diphtheriae* can also affect the vocal cords and lead to swelling and obstruction.
  - ○ *Respiratory papillomatosis*: Due to infection with human papilloma virus 6 (HPV 6) or 11, children develop single or multiple benign squamous papillomas.
- **Trauma**: Trauma to the glottis in the form of fracture or through traumatic or prolonged intubation also threatens the patency of the airway.
  - ○ *Laryngeal fracture*: Fracture can occur following direct trauma to the neck region and may lead to life-threatening airway obstruction and therefore needs to be treated urgently.
  - ○ *Prolonged intubation*: Intubation for long-term airway management can cause hyperemia and edema due to mucosal irritation, as well as protruding granulation tissue.
- **Neoplasm**: *Carcinoma* of the glottis tends to present earlier, usually as hoarseness, and has a low incidence of metastatic lymphadenopathy and therefore has a higher cure rate than tumors in other locations.
- **Foreign body**: *Inhalation of a foreign body* is particularly common in children but also occurs less frequently in adults. Objects likely to be inhaled include nuts, seeds, and small toys; larger objects tend to lodge at the larynx, whereas smaller objects pass down to the mainstem bronchi. A foreign body can lead to acute airway distress or more subtle obstructive symptoms.
- *Vocal cord paralysis*: This condition has several etiologies, including surgical or nonsurgical trauma or tumor affecting the recurrent laryngeal nerve as well as direct mechanical fixation by tumor; bilateral paralysis in the adducted position can lead to severe stridor and emergency tracheostomy.
- *Laryngospasm*: Involuntary contraction of the adductor muscles due to increased sensitivity of the laryngeal mucosa can impede airflow. This condition often occurs during recovery from general anesthesia but can also occur spontaneously and paroxysmally, sometimes associated with gastric reflux.

◆ Subglottic (Associated Sounds: Biphasic Stridor, Barking Cough, Husky Voice)

- **Congenital**: Congenital anomalies also occur with frequency in the subglottic area due to the complex development of this part of the airway and surrounding structures.

- ○ *Vascular ring/aortic arch anomalies*: Abnormal development of the complex vascular modeling and remodeling process of the aortic arch can cause symptomatic compression of the trachea in neonates.
- ○ *Subglottic stenosis*: Narrowing of the lumen of the larynx may be congenital, due to failed recanalization, or acquired, secondary to trauma or instrumentation.

- **Infectious**: Infection in the subglottic airway can lead to obstruction via inflammation and edema of the mucosa.

  - ○ *Croup*: Most commonly caused by parainfluenza virus, it is usually a mild and self-limited illness, though severe inflammation can cause significant airway obstruction. Croup is most common in children but can also occur in adults.

- **Inflammatory**: Inflammation at the subglottic level and below can severely limit airflow in and out of the lungs.

  - ○ *Wegener granulomatosis*: Upper respiratory tract lesions, particularly the subglottis, occur in approximately one fourth of patients with Wegener granulomatosis, an immune-mediated disorder in which tissue damage results from an inciting inflammatory event and the subsequent immune response.
  - ○ *Asthma*: Asthma is a chronic inflammatory disorder of the airways that causes susceptible individuals to experience airflow limitation due to smooth muscle contraction and excess mucus production in response to particular triggers.

- **Trauma**: Intubation itself can have detrimental sequelae on the airway by impairing patency through mechanical trauma and the resulting tissue injury.

  - ○ *Prolonged intubation*: Intubation for long-term airway management can cause hyperemia and edema due to mucosal irritation and the formation of granulation tissue.

- **Neoplasm**: Neoplasms inside the subglottic airway (intrinsic lesions) can cause obstruction, whereas masses or tumors of the surrounding structures can cause extrinsic compression, allowing for a larger differential of masses in this area.

  - ○ Intrinsic/internal

    - — *Squamous cell carcinoma* is the most frequent intrinsic tumor that can obstruct the airway, though it is more frequent at or above the glottis.
    - — *Subglottic hemangioma*: Rapid proliferation of a hemangioma in an infant can lead to airway compromise and should be considered in any child who has a cutaneous hemangioma and develops progressive respiratory distress.

  - ○ Extrinsic: Compression of the airway by a tumor may be caused by a *thyroid mass (cancer or goiter), mediastinal tumor* such as *thymoma* or *metastasis,* or *massive lymphadenopathy.*

◆ Tracheobronchial (Associated Sounds: Expiratory Stridor, Wheezing)

- **Congenital**: Developmental anomalies in the lower airway are more frequent and should therefore be considered in young children with obstructive symptoms.
  - *Tracheoesophageal fistula*: Infants with an aberrant connection between the trachea and esophagus become symptomatic early after birth with drooling/choking and respiratory distress due to excessive secretions.
  - *Tracheomalacia*: This relatively common anomaly of the upper respiratory tract is characterized by dynamic collapse of the trachea during breathing.
  - *Bronchomalacia*: Also due to dynamic collapse of the airway, bronchomalacia can be caused by congenital absence of cartilage or acquired postinfectious narrowing.
  - *Bronchial stenosis*: Congenital narrowing of the bronchial tree can be focal or diffuse and causes refractory wheezing or recurrent pneumonia.

- **Infectious**
  - *Tracheitis*: Caused by a bacterial infection (as a complication of a viral infection or as a primary infection). Purulent exudate can accumulate and be a source of airway obstruction.
  - *Bronchitis*: Acute bronchitis is usually caused by a virus leading to a self-limited inflammation of the bronchi and a productive cough.

- **Neoplasm**: Tumors arising from the mediastinum, trachea, or bronchus can all cause lower airway obstruction in a progressive fashion.
- **Foreign body**: If *foreign bodies* pass through the larynx into the lower airway, they are likely to lodge in the wider and straighter right mainstem bronchus, where a foreign body can cause more subtle symptoms of obstruction such as a persistent wheeze.

Suggested Reading

Goldenberg D, Bhatti N. Management of the adult airway. In: Cummings CW. Otolaryngology–Head and Neck Surgery. 4th ed. Philadelphia: Mosby 2005

46 Snoring and Other Breathing Problems During Sleep

James J. Kearney

The symptoms of snoring and sleep breathing problems can be due to airway obstruction at multiple levels from the entry of the nose to the trachea. The obstruction can be a fixed anatomical problem or a variable problem due to positioning, inflammatory issues, or muscle tone issues. It is common to have multiple levels of obstruction with a combination of fixed and variable problems. This makes it challenging to diagnose the etiology of snoring and sleep breathing problems. Snoring can be a sign of clinically significant sleep apnea. If sleep apnea is suspected based on history or physical examination an overnight sleep study (polysomnogram) should be ordered to quantify the severity of the problem.

It is important to differentiate between simple snoring and varying degrees of obstructive sleep apnea (OSA), which can be life threatening. Patients often underestimate the severity of their condition because they are asleep when the symptoms occur. Moderate to severe sleep apnea has been associated with hypertension, elevated rates of cardiac disease, right-sided heart failure, and early mortality.

Defining the difference between simple snoring and sleep-disordered breathing is important. The first is a condition that causes relationship disharmony or embarrassment, but the latter can significantly affect the chance of early mortality. A thorough history and good physical exam help guide when to refer the patient for a formal sleep study to quantify the problem. Once the degree of the sleep disturbance is quantified the foregoing differential is helpful in determining the level of obstruction.

Also, obesity is associated with OSA, although not required for the diagnosis. Many normal-weight patients have OSA. However, obesity causes generalized tissue fat deposition, even in the airway, so even without an identified single obstructing lesion, an obese patient can have upper airway obstruction during sleep.

- **Nasal obstruction** (see Chapter 27)
  - Fixed (anatomical)
    - *Nasal septal deformity*
    - *Turbinate hypertrophy*
    - *Nasal polyposis*
    - *Neoplasm of the nose or sinus,* such as *inverted papilloma* or *esthesioneuroblastoma*
    - *Nasal valve collapse*: Frequently seen after prior rhinoplasty but can be spontaneous.
    - *Nasal synechiae*: Typically due to prior surgery or a prolonged indwelling nasal tube.

- — *Cyst*
- — *Venous* or *lymphatic malformation*
- ○ Variable (infectious/inflammatory)
  - — *Rhinosinusitis*
  - — *Allergic rhinitis*
  - — *Vasomotor rhinitis*
  - — *Rhinitis medicamentosa*
  - — *Sarcoidosis*
  - — *Wegener granulomatosis*

Nasal obstruction alone does not usually cause snoring or sleep apnea, but it can contribute to or worsen the underlying problem. Usually there are also obstructions at the level of the palate, tongue base, or hypopharynx. Use of topical oxymetazoline or an external or internal stenting device, such as a Breathe-Rite strip, with observation by the bed partner for a night or two can be helpful in determining whether an improvement in the nasal airway will improve the symptoms.

- **Nasopharyngeal Obstruction**
  - ○ Fixed (anatomical)
    - — *Adenoid hypertrophy*: Seen primarily in younger individuals, often associated with enlarged tonsils, can be seen in older adults with HIV.
    - — *Neoplasm*
    - — *Cyst*
    - — *Venous* or *lymphatic malformation*
    - — *Nasopharyngeal stenosis*: Can be seen after adenoid or palate surgery, or with pemphigoid. It is fairly rare.

- **Oral Cavity/Oropharynx**
  - ○ Fixed (anatomical)
    - — *Mandibular hypoplasia*: Appearance of a "weak chin." The jaw doesn't project far enough anteriorly to keep the tongue from prolapsing into the oropharynx. This can be observed head on, but also from a profile view.
    - — *Macroglossia*: Can be quantified by use of a Mallampati or Friedman scale. This is most commonly due to a congenital disproportion of tissue. It can rarely be caused by amyloidosis.
    - — *Thick, low-hanging soft palate*: The soft palate is commonly the structure that vibrates to cause snoring. Chronic trauma to the palatal tissues from snoring perpetuates the cycle, causing edema of the tissues due to the trauma from the snoring.
    - — *Enlarged uvula*: This can be seen as an isolated idiopathic enlargement without associated palatal findings, but it is more commonly seen with an elongated, thick soft palate.
    - — *Tonsil hypertrophy*: Can be graded (1+ to 4+), and is primarily seen in younger age groups. Incidence decreases as patients age.

— *Neoplasm*: Carcinoma and lymphoma can affect the oropharynx and oral cavity. They are typically associated with significant asymmetry of the tonsils.
— *Cyst*
— *Venous* or *lymphatic malformation*

○ Variable (positional)

— *Tongue falls posteriorly* in the supine position: A very common scenario. Patients with this condition don't snore much when lying in the prone position or on their side.
— *Poor muscle tone*

  ○ Alcohol or drug induced: Many individuals experience an exacerbation of their snoring problems when under the influence of alcohol or a sedating medication.
  ○ Congenital: Some individuals do not maintain good tone in their tongue and pharyngeal muscles when they fall asleep, which allows collapse of the airway.

● **Hypopharyngeal**

○ Fixed (anatomical)

— *Tongue base hypertrophy*: Due to an increase in the lymphoid tissue of the tongue base; can be seen in the absence of tonsil hypertrophy.
— *Posterior hypopharyngeal lymphoid hypertrophy*: Often accompanies tonsil and adenoid hypertrophy
— Posterior external impingement by *cervical spine osteophytes (Forestier disease)*: primarily a condition of the elderly
— *Neoplasm*
— *Venous* or *lymphatic malformation*

● **Laryngeal**

○ Fixed (anatomical)

— *Supraglottic edema*

  ○ *Sarcoidosis*: The epiglottis is an uncommon but not a rare site of involvement.
  ○ *Radiation-induced edema*: Persists well beyond the end of radiation and can be permanent.

— *Impaired vocal cord movement*: Can cause stridor. This is usually a *bilateral vocal cord* involvement, which usually causes a good voice but an inadequate airway. Unilateral impaired mobility usually causes a breathy voice, but not a compromised airway.
— *Neoplasm*
— *Venous* or *lymphatic malformation*
— *Glottic* or *subglottic stenosis*: Can be induced by several conditions, such as prior intubation, prior tracheotomy, or laryngeal trauma, or it can be idiopathic.

- **Trachea**
  - Fixed (anatomical)
    - *Tracheal stenosis*
    - *Neoplasm*
    - *Venous* or *lymphatic malformation*
    - *Tracheomalacia*: Not commonly seen in adults. It can be caused by relapsing polychondritis or radiation-induced weakening of the cartilage.

Suggested Reading

Lieberman JA III. Obstructive sleep apnea (OSA) and excessive sleepiness associated with OSA: recognition in the primary care setting. Postgrad Med 2009;121:33–41

Ramachandran SK, Josephs LA. A meta-analysis of clinical screening tests for obstructive sleep apnea. Anesthesiology 2009;110:928–939

Stuck BA, Maurer JT. Airway evaluation in obstructive sleep apnea. Sleep Med Rev 2008;12:411–436

47 Odynophagia

Jeremy D. Richmon and James Rocco

The term **odynophagia** derives from the Greek roots *odyno-* (pain) and *-phagein* (to eat) and refers to the symptom of painful swallowing. This is different from **dysphagia**, which refers to difficulty swallowing. Although both symptoms are often present together they each may present separately as well and should not be confused. *Odynophagia* is a broad term that may refer to a myriad of symptoms and disease processes. The key distinguishing characteristic in odynophagia is **onset** (sudden or immediate, rapid, or slowly progressive). Other important aspects of the history include duration (hours, days, months, or years), clinical course (progressive, resolving, constant, or fluctuating), severity (mild vs severe), location (oropharyngeal or retrosternal), and exacerbating factors such as immunosuppression or other systemic diseases. The differential diagnosis of odynophagia is vast (**Table 47.1**). Therefore, the most critical element in patient evaluation is a thorough and directed history to narrow the differential diagnosis. After a thorough history, a complete head and neck examination including indirect laryngoscopy (unless epiglottitis is suspected in a pediatric patient) should further limit the differential of odynophagia.

Sudden or immediate-onset odynophagia is usually caused by an **iatrogenic** or **traumatic etiology**. The presentation of symptoms can usually be related to a particular circumstance, such as having finished a meal, taking a specific medicine, or experiencing trauma or a trip to the operating room.

- **Iatrogenic**: A recent history of upper aerodigestive tract manipulation followed by odynophagia should lead one to suspect a mucosal tear, muscular injury, and perforation, with mediastinitis being the most feared complication. Although odynophagia is common after intubation as a result of mild mucosal trauma and inflammation from the endotracheal tube, one must suspect more serious injury if pain is not resolving by postoperative day 2, is worsening, or is accompanied by systemic signs/symptoms such as leukocytosis, fever, tachycardia, chest pain, dysphagia, and sepsis. Traumatic esophagitis can also occur after nasogastric tube placement or after esophageal or gastric suctioning.

  - *Arytenoid subluxation*: Malpositioning of the arytenoid cartilage. It is usually the result of upper airway instrumentation (postintubation), although it can result from external trauma to the neck. It typically presents with hoarseness along with dysphagia, odynophagia, and cough. Diagnosis can be established by the clinical timing, laryngoscopy, and computed tomography (CT) of the larynx with spiral CT.

- *Traumatic*: Similarly, odynophagia associated with a recent history of trauma should result in a thorough evaluation to distinguish between sim-

Table 47.1 Causes of Odynophagia

Vascular	Carotidynia
Infectious	Tonsillitis/adenoiditis/pharyngitis Esophagitis Epiglottitis/supraglottitis
Iatrogenic	Aerodigestive tract manipulation/perforation, arytenoid subluxation
Inflammatory	Eosinophilic esophagitis Gastroesophageal reflux Laryngopharyngeal reflux Eagle syndrome
Neoplastic	Malignancy of oropharynx, hypopharynx, larynx, esophagus (squamous cell, adenoid cystic, adenocarcinoma, lymphoma, sarcoma)
Drugs/toxins	Caustic ingestion Pill esophagitis Mucositis secondary to chemotherapy or radiotherapy
Autoimmune	Scleroderma Systemic sclerosis Mixed connective tissue disease Polymyositis/dermatomyositis Crohn disease Pemphigoid/Stevens-Johnson syndrome/pemphigus Rheumatoid arthritis
Trauma	Blunt (tear, hematoma) Penetrating (laceration or perforation) Whiplash Foreign body (fish or chicken bone, food impaction, coin, toy, battery)
Other	Rings/webs/stricture Esophageal motor disorders (achalasia and diffuse esophageal spasm) Plummer-Vinson syndrome Eagle syndrome

ple muscular strain and more serious vascular, cervical, esophageal, or laryngeal injury.

- *Caustic ingestion*: Ingested chemicals either by accident (children) or in suicide attempts (adults) can result in mucosal injury depending on the type, concentration, and volume of the ingested substance. Household and garden materials are usually alkalis and cause a deep liquefaction necrosis with fat and protein digestion. Acids are less frequently encountered and typically lead to a more superficial coagulation necrosis with eschar formation. Complications include hematemesis, perforation, peritonitis, mediastinitis, and late-developing stricture.

- *Foreign body ingestion*: In this setting, odynophagia often indicates a sharp object that has penetrated the oropharyngeal mucosa, typically fish or chicken bones, toothpicks, needles, and dental bridgework. Blunt foreign body ingestions, on the other hand, often present with dysphagia or complete obstruction. Because many foreign bodies are radiolucent, endoscopy is required when imaging studies fail to reveal an etiology. Three narrow areas of the digestive tract tend to trap foreign bodies: (1) the cricopharyngeus muscle, (2) the middle third of the esophagus, and (3) the lower esophageal sphincter.

    o *Pill esophagitis*: Odynophagia commonly results when pills get stuck in the esophagus and dissolve, and may be secondary to dysphagia, structural abnormalities, or decreased saliva production. This condition, known as pill esophagitis, most commonly occurs with antibiotics, potassium chloride, nonsteroidal antiinflammatory drugs (NSAIDs), quinidine, emperonium bromide, and Fosamax. The degree of mucosal injury depends on the chemical nature of the drug, solubility, contact time with mucosa, size, shape, and pill coating, amount of water swallowed, and preexisting esophageal pathology. A pill trapped in the esophagus may cause ulceration and esophageal perforation 24 to 48 hours after ingestion. Diagnosis is usually made by endoscopy where an ulcer surrounded by normal mucosa is found and should be pursued when symptoms progress or dysphagia is present.

- *Chemotherapy stomatitis*: The systemic effects of cytotoxic medications used in cancer therapy may also result in mucosal changes in both the pharyngeal and esophageal tract, resulting in a range of inflammation and ulceration known as stomatitis. Chemotherapy esophagitis often occurs with dactinomycin, bleomycin, cytarabine, daunorubicin, 5-fluorouracil, methotrexate, and vincristine.
- *Radiation mucositis*: Radiation therapy to the neck and chest results in a dose-dependent mucositis that may result in odynophagia severe enough to preclude oral alimentation. Doses over 30 Gy may result in mild, limited retrosternal burning and odynophagia; 40 Gy results in mucosal erythema and edema; and 60 to 70 Gy causes moderate-to-severe mucositis and may result in strictures, perforations, and fistulas. Radiation mucositis occurs within the radiation field and classically presents 2 to 3 weeks after the initiation of radiation treatment. It is estimated to occur in 80% of patients undergoing head and neck radiation. Four stages of radiation mucositis have been described: an inflammatory stage that presents with initial erythema, an epithelial stage in which pseudomembranes are formed, a bacterial stage in which there is gram-negative bacilli overgrowth, and a healing stage. Resolution and healing occur within 3 to 4 weeks of the last radiation dose.

Rapid onset of odynophagia in the absence of a discrete precipitating event is usually the result of an **infectious process** and can be caused by a large number of different infectious agents (**Table 47.1**). In addition, it is critical to elicit and identify a history of immunosuppression because it is a significant contributing factor to odynophagia resulting from viral or fungal esophagitis. Patients who present with odynophagia of infectious etiology typically describe quick onset, rapid progression, and severe intensity. Infectious pharyngitis is much more common than esophagitis, with the latter presenting more commonly in the immunocompromised population. Patients with infectious pharyngitis will usually present with systemic symptoms (such as fever) that are usually lacking in patients with traumatic, iatrogenic, or foreign body–related odynophagia. Physical exam may be notable for bilateral cervical lymphadenopathy, anterior neck tenderness to palpation, erythematous pharyngeal mucosa, tonsillar exudates (bacterial infection), supraglottic edema (epiglottitis), white plaques (*Candida*), unilateral tonsillar protrusion with uvular deviation (peritonsillar abscess), posterior pharyngeal bulging (retropharyngeal abscess), or mucosal ulceration and blistering (viral infection). One can often differentiate viral, bacterial, and fungal causes from the history and physical exam alone.

- *Bacterial pharyngitis*: Group A β-hemolytic streptococci (GABHS, 15% of all pharyngitis) is the most significant pathogen in that appropriate recognition and treatment are necessary to prevent complications such as scarlet fever and rheumatic fever. The classic clinical picture includes a fever, with temperature of greater than 101.5°F; tonsil and pharyngeal erythema and exudate; swollen, tender anterior cervical adenopathy; headache; emesis in children; palatal petechiae; midwinter to early spring season; and absent cough or rhinorrhea. Other bacteria include group C, G, and F streptococci (10%), *Arcanobacterium* (*Corynebacterium*) *haemolyticus* (5%), *Mycobacterium pneumoniae* and *Chlamydophila pneumoniae* (5%), *Neisseria gonorrhoeae*, and *Corynebacterium diphtheriae*.

  - *Peritonsillar abscess*: Typically occurs in young adults during November to December and again from April to May when the incidence of streptococcal pharyngitis and tonsillitis is highest. It is the most common deep infection of the head and neck. Group A *Streptococcus* remains the predominant organism. Patients present with fever, odynophagia, dysphagia, and otalgia. On clinical exam, trismus and a muffled voice ("hot potato voice") are common.
  - *Viral pharyngitis*: Unlike bacterial pharyngitis, viral cases tend to be less severe and have fewer physical findings and systemic symptoms. Common viral causes of pharyngitis include *adenovirus* (associated with conjunctivitis), herpes simplex (vesicular lesions), *coxsackieviruses* A and B (A16 may cause hand, foot, and mouth disease), *rhinovirus, corona virus, respiratory syncytial virus,* and *parainfluenza virus.* Epstein-Barr virus (EBV, infectious mononucleosis) and cytomegalovirus (CMV) may have a severe presentation identical to GABHS.
  - *Infectious mononucleosis*: Should be suspected in younger patients (10 to 30 years of age) who present with odynophagia, fatigue, cervical adenopathy, and palatal petechiae. The presence of atypical lymphocytes and a positive heterophile antibody test are often seen.

○ *Acute HIV-1 infection*: Associated with pharyngeal edema and erythema, common aphthous ulcers, and a rarity of exudates. Fever, myalgia, and lymphadenopathy are also found. An appropriate history of risk factors and clinical suspicion is critical to making the diagnosis.

● *Fungal pharyngitis*: A high index of suspicion must exist to appropriately diagnosis a patient with fungal pharyngitis because both symptoms and physical findings can range from minimal to severe. Patients tend to be immunocompromised, elderly, diabetic, or otherwise debilitated and have significant comorbidity.

○ *Candida*: Oral thrush is not uncommon in patients undergoing treatment for head and neck cancer with chemoradiation. It may be common in young, otherwise healthy, children. Pseudomembranous *Candida* is the most common form and easily diagnosed by the soft, creamy white to yellow, elevated plaques that are easily wiped off affected oral tissues and leave an erythematous, eroded, or ulcerated surface, which may be tender. However, *Candida* may also present as hyperplastic *Candida* (asymptomatic white plaques or papules that do not wipe off) and atrophic (erythematous) *Candida* (red patch or velvet-textured plaque).

Infectious esophagitis: In contrast to infectious pharyngitis, patients with infectious esophagitis more likely have a fungal or viral cause that is more likely to occur in the immunocompromised population.

● *Fungal esophagitis*: *Candida albicans* is the most likely fungal pathogen and 25% of the time is not accompanied with oral thrush. It has a similar presentation as pseudomembranous thrush in the oral cavity, with patients often complaining of severe odynophagia out of proportion to findings on clinical exam. Some patients complain of retrosternal pain. Human immunodeficiency virus (HIV) infection is the most significant risk factor, although other conditions such as diabetes mellitus, alcoholism, and impaired esophageal motility (malignancy, scleroderma, achalasia) can predispose to infection. Increasingly, the use of inhaled corticosteroids can also result in esophageal *Candida* in healthy adults. Diagnosis of fungal esophagitis is made by endoscopy with brushings or biopsy.

● *Viral esophagitis*: Can be found in otherwise healthy adults during acute herpes simplex virus (HSV) infection where patients typically present with painful swallowing, nausea, vomiting, and fever. Concurrent orolabial lesions are only found in a small percentage of patients. CMV esophagitis tends to have a more gradual course than HSV; otherwise symptoms are similar to HSV esophagitis. CMV esophagitis is rarely seen in immunocompetent patients, and the odynophagia may be less severe. In acute HIV infection, esophagitis can be caused by HIV.

● *Bacterial esophagitis*: Extremely rare, occurring typically in immunosuppressed patients. Granulocytopenia is the most significant risk factor. Infectious agents include normal flora, *Mycobacterium tuberculosis*, and *Mycobacterium avium-intracellulare*.

● *Parasitic esophagitis*: Infections may also occur with *Chagas disease, Trypanosoma cruzi, Cryptosporidium, Pneumocystis, Leishmania donovani*. Risk factors include travel to endemic areas and immunosuppression.

Infectious laryngitis: Infections of the larynx often present acutely and in the vast majority of cases are viral. The presentation is similar to that of viral pharyngitis with the addition of dysphonia and occasionally stridor. In contrast, epiglottitis or supraglottitis is often bacterial in nature, and patients appear acutely ill. Odynophagia is present in nearly all patients, sometimes to the degree that they are unable to swallow.

Oropharyngeal tuberculosis: A rare disease and usually secondary to laryngeal involvement in pulmonary tuberculosis. The major symptom in such patients is odynophagia. These lesions can be difficult to distinguish from carcinoma so a biopsy is often necessary to establish the diagnosis. HIV coinfection is commonly seen.

Slowly progressive or **chronic odynophagia** can be caused by several persistent and unremitting conditions (**Table 47.1**). With rare exceptions these tend not to be infectious, although there can be considerable overlap in symptoms in some cases.

- *Laryngopharyngeal reflux (LPR)*: When acid ascends above the upper esophageal sphincter (UES) and contacts pharyngeal or laryngeal mucosa it may cause various symptoms, including odynophagia. Laryngopharyngeal reflux differs from gastroesophageal reflux disease (GERD see below) in that it is often not associated with heartburn and regurgitation symptoms. Reflux of acid above the UES is not physiological (as opposed to reflux within the esophagus) and can rapidly lead to mucosal irritation and inflammation. Indirect laryngoscopy may reveal erythematous vocal cords and arytenoids, edematous mucosa, pseudosulcus, posterior laryngeal mucosal thickening, and granulation tissue or granulomas. LPR is a diagnosis of exclusion in that no definitive exam finding or test can confirm the diagnosis without ruling out other causes of pharyngitis beforehand.
- *Gastroesophageal reflux disease (GERD)*: In patients with GERD, distal esophageal inflammation results when gastric and duodenal fluids, including gastric acid, pepsin, trypsin, and bile, are regurgitated into the esophagus to a greater than physiological degree. A decrease in the lower esophageal sphincter (LES) tone and altered motility, which increase esophageal clearance time, cause GERD. Esophageal inflammation can further induce both mechanisms, creating a vicious cycle.
- *Head and neck cancer*: Tumors growing in the oral cavity, oropharynx, hypopharynx, larynx, and esophagus may all present with odynophagia. Whereas benign growths frequently present with discomfort, globus, and dysphagia, invasive malignant tumors are more likely to result in progressive, deep, boring, or sharp pain that may become incapacitating. Additionally, the tumor mass may result in an obstructive dysphagia, especially in the hypopharynx, or esophagus. Pain may be referred to the ear via CN IX.
- *Eagle syndrome*: An elongated styloid process or calcified stylohyoid ligament may result in recurrent throat pain or foreign body sensation, dysphagia, or facial pain that may be positional. Patients may have atypical facial pain and headaches with pain radiating to the ipsilateral ear. Impingement on the carotid artery can cause carotidynia. Diagnosis can usually be made on physical examination with pain elicited by digital palpation of the styloid process in the tonsillar fossa.

- *Plummer-Vinson syndrome*: Also called sideropenic dysphagia, this syndrome is linked to severe, long-term iron deficiency anemia, resulting in dysphagia due to esophageal webs. In addition to dysphagia, it can be associated with throat pain and a burning sensation during swallowing. Middle-aged women are at highest risk, and due to an increased risk of esophageal squamous cell carcinoma it is considered a premalignant process.

Systemic diseases: Multiple systemic disease processes may result in odynophagia. These may be of a generalized inflammatory nature as in *rheumatoid arthritis* or a collagen-vascular disorder such as *scleroderma*. Odynophagia is unlikely to present in an isolated manner, however, and the overall clinical picture should indicate a systemic process. The exception may be skin disorders with mucosal involvement (*epidermolysis bullosa, pemphigus vulgaris, bullous pemphigoid, cicatricial pemphigoid,* and *drug-induced skin disorders*) where painful ulcers and odynophagia may present in the absence of other symptoms. Other systemic diseases with pharyngeal and esophageal mucosal involvement include *Crohn disease, polyarteritis nodosa, sarcoid,* and *polymyositis*.

Suggested Reading

Akhtar AJ. Oral medication–induced esophageal injury in elderly patients. Am J Med Sci 2003;326:133–135

Alcaide ML, Bisno AL. Pharyngitis and epiglottitis. Infect Dis Clin North Am 2007;21: 449–469, vii

Ebell MH. Epstein-Barr virus infectious mononucleosis. Am Fam Physician 2004;70: 1279–1287

Farrokhi F, Vaezi MF. Laryngeal disorders in patients with gastroesophageal reflux disease. Minerva Gastroenterol Dietol 2007;53:181–187

Mupparapu M, Robinson MD. The mineralized and elongated styloid process: a review of current diagnostic criteria and evaluation strategies. Gen Dent 2005;53:54–59

Rabeneck L, Popovic M, Gartner S, et al. Acute HIV infection presenting with painful swallowing and esophageal ulcers. JAMA 1990;263:2318–2322

Sack JL, Brock CD. Identifying acute epiglottitis in adults: high degree of awareness, close monitoring are key. Postgrad Med 2002;112:81–82, 85–86

Sulica L. Laryngeal thrush. Ann Otol Rhinol Laryngol 2005;114:369–375

Volpato LE, Silva TC, Oliveira TM, Sakai VT, Machado MA. Radiation therapy and chemotherapy-induced oral mucositis. Rev Bras Otorrinolaringol (Engl Ed) 2007;73:562–568

48 Dysphagia

Natasha Mirza

Dysphagia is defined as difficulty in transporting food from the oral cavity to the esophagus. It is to be differentiated from odynophagia, which is painful swallowing. Dysphagia leads to high morbidity, mortality, and cost. It is very common in the chronic care setting and is seen in more than half of all patients who reside in nursing homes. Consequences of dysphagia involve poor nutrition and weight loss and also aspiration, which can lead to pneumonia. It is important to investigate the cause of dysphagia to rule out malignancy and nutrition and improve an individual's quality of life. Detailed examination of the anatomy and physiology of each stage of deglutition is necessary to effectively diagnose and treat dysphagia.

◆ Anatomy and Physiology

Normal swallowing is a complex cascade of events involving many levels of the central nervous system and voluntary and involuntary muscles in the head and neck. The neural control is in the motor nuclei of cranial nerves V, VII, IX, X, and XII. There are three phases of swallowing, each involving a particular subset of anatomical structures and muscle activity. These phases are the (1) oral phase, (2) pharyngeal phase, and (3) esophageal phase. The following structures are involved in the oropharyngeal aspect of swallowing:

- Lips
- Dentition and muscles of mastication
- Tongue with both intrinsic and extrinsic muscles
- Palate
- Salivary glands, including the parotids and submandibular and sublingual glands
- Pharyngeal muscles consisting of the superior, middle, and inferior constrictor muscles

◆ Mechanism of Swallowing

Oral Phase

This consists of the oral preparatory stage and the actual oral stage, which involves the intake, mastication, and transfer of the food bolus from the mouth to the pharynx. Control of the swallowing mechanism is in the higher centers of the cortex and involves stimulation by the sight, smell, and taste of food. Respiration is inhibited centrally during the process of swallowing.

Preparatory stage: The first steps involve biting, lip closure, chewing (jaw motion and tongue movement), lubrication, and some digestion by saliva. The larynx and pharynx are at rest during this phase. The airway is open and nasal breathing continues until the voluntary swallow is initiated.

Oral stage: A bolus of suitable size and consistency is created and then transferred posteriorly from the oral cavity to the pharynx.

Pharyngeal Phase

The pharyngeal phase of swallowing is involuntary and under reflex control. Normally during this transit through the pharynx the bolus does not hesitate and a smooth movement is observed. It consists of two periods: (1) the early nasopharyngeal and oropharyngeal protective period whereby the bolus is prevented from regurgitating back into the oral cavity and (2) the later laryngeal protective period. This consists of laryngeal elevation, the folding backward of the epiglottis, and the activation of the laryngeal sphincters, including the adduction of the true vocal cords followed by adduction of the false cords and the aryepiglottic folds. The bolus is thereby diverted into the lateral piriform recesses. At rest the cricoid lamina touches the posterior pharyngeal wall at the level of the cricopharyngeal region. This position of the cricoid maintains closure of the upper esophageal sphincter (UES). As the larynx elevates and moves anteriorly during the swallow, extrinsic stretch is placed on the cricopharyngeus muscle and its adjacent fibers. The bolus is now cleared by the stripping action of the superior, middle, and inferior constrictor muscles. There is resetting of the larynx, and the upper esophagus now opens by the relaxation of the cricopharyngeus muscle.

Esophageal Phase

This phase involves active peristalsis or sequential contraction from top to bottom in two waves, primary peristalsis and secondary peristalsis. The esophageal phase is under involuntary neural control. At the base of the esophagus the lower esophageal sphincter (LES) is a circular muscular valve that opens to allow the passage of food but is otherwise closed to prevent gastroesophageal reflux.

◆ Clinical Presentations of Dysphagia

Manifestations include poor oral control of food and saliva and present as drooling, speech disorders, nasal regurgitation, coughing, and choking spells with aspiration pneumonia and weight loss.

◆ Etiologies of Dysphagia

The etiologies of dysphagia have for the sake of simplicity been divided into neurological causes, structural causes, and systemic causes (**Fig. 48.1**).

Neurological Causes of Dysphagia

These neurological conditions can involve the sensory or motor components of each stage of swallowing from the oral preparatory stage, the tongue movements, the pharyngeal swallow, and the upper esophageal stage. Neurological conditions are usually manifest as premature spillage, nasal regurgitation, and penetration and aspiration with a cough and choking, and patients have difficulty handling liquids.

- **Central causes**: There are various causes of central neurological problems, including stroke, palsy, tumors, and neurodegenerative conditions.
  - *Strokes* involving the posterior inferior cerebellar artery or vertebrobasilar artery lead to a palsy of several cranial nerves, including the trigemi-

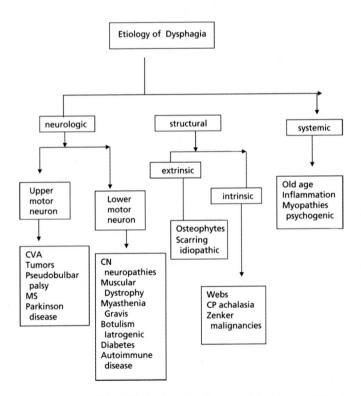

Fig. 48.1 Diagram showing the etiologies of dysphagia. CN, central nervous; CP, cricopharyngeal; CVA, cerebral vascular accident (stroke); MS, multiple sclerosis.

nal, glossopharyngeal, vagus, and accessory nerves. These result in poor velar closure and diminished laryngeal elevation. Aspiration occurs when both the superior and the recurrent laryngeal nerves are involved. There can be oral apraxia, which involves impaired voluntary movement of the bolus in the mouth and delay in bolus transfer, especially in left hemispheric lesions.

- ○ *Pseudobulbar palsy* leads to atrophy of the pharyngeal muscles and a decrease in mucosal sensitivity.
- ○ *Brainstem tumors* affect the swallowing centers in the brainstem and impair the initiation of swallowing.
- ○ *Neurodegenerative conditions* like *Parkinson disease, amyotrophic lateral sclerosis, multiple sclerosis,* and *familial dysautonomia* affect cognition and generally impair the oral phase of swallowing. The prevalence of Parkinson disease is ~10 to 450 per 100,000 of the population and appears to be increasing with age. It is generally slowly progressive and is usually accompanied with deficits in cognition along with dysarthria and dysphonia. Patients experience difficulties with the oral, pharyngeal, and esophageal phases of swallowing. There are problems in bolus preparation due to the tongue tremor and vallecular stasis of the bolus. Volitional cough is impaired. There is marked difficulty in switching between the voluntary and involuntary phases of swallowing. The loss of sensation in the pharynx leads to poor oropharyngeal protection and an increased risk for aspiration. In fact pneumonias secondary to aspiration are the major cause of morbidity and mortality in this population.

- **Peripheral or lower motor neuron diseases**: These conditions affect any location between the central nuclei and the myoneural junctions.

  - ○ *Myasthenia gravis* has a bimodal peak of incidence between the ages of 21 and 30 years and then again between 61 and 70 years. There is a decrease in acetylcholine release from the neuromuscular junction leading to fatigability and hypotonicity. This is manifest by poor initiation of swallowing, decreased tongue movement, and pooling of secretions. Dysarthria and weakness of the chewing muscles are present in more than 50% of individuals.
  - ○ *Amyotrophic lateral sclerosis (ALS)* is a motor neuron disease.
  - ○ *Multiple sclerosis (MS)* is a motor neuron disease that often follows an erratic course but can cause dysphagia.

- **Iatrogenic causes** include surgeries in the vicinity of the pharynx that damage the pharyngeal plexus or the superior or recurrent laryngeal nerves. Also included are the *neuropathies* induced by thyroid surgeries, cervical spine surgeries through an anterior approach, radiation damage, and skull base operations.

Structural Causes

These can be intrinsic within the lumen of the pharynx and esophagus or extrinsic and can coexist with other sensory or motor deficits. Symptoms are primarily related to solid food dysphagia and occasional regurgitation.

- **Extrinsic causes**
  - *Osteophytes* of the cervical spine (*Forestier disease*) can compress the esophagus from the outside and lead to dysphagia.
  - *Congenital craniofacial syndromes*: These conditions lead to nasopharyngeal and oropharyngeal obstruction secondary to abnormalities of the mandibular–hyoid relationship and a large tongue.
    - *Pierre Robin syndrome*
    - *Apert syndrome*
    - *Treacher-Collins syndrome*
  - *Tracheostomy* impairs deglutition by preventing laryngeal elevation and by anchoring the larynx to the superficial cervical soft tissues.
  - Vascular anomalies can also compress the esophagus.
    - *Aberrant aorta (dysphagia lusoria)*
    - *Aortic aneurysm*
  - Other causes include *compression by malignancies* of the thyroid or larynx.

- **Intrinsic causes**
  - *Esophageal web*: These are often associated with the *Plummer-Vinson syndrome*.
  - *Malignancy*
  - *Cricopharyngeal achalasia* is associated mainly with gastroesophageal reflux or central causes like strokes, poliomyelitis, myopathies, oculopharyngeal muscular dystrophy, postlaryngectomy, Parkinson disease, and amyotrophic lateral sclerosis.
  - *Zenker diverticula*: Normally the upper esophageal sphincter should relax during swallowing. When the sphincter closes prematurely, part of the bolus is trapped between the closing sphincter and the oncoming peristaltic wave. Eventually this leads to a weakening of the hypopharyngeal wall at the triangle of Killian (above the cricopharyngeus), at the triangle of Laimer (below the cricopharyngeus) or at the posterior pharyngeal wall. A protrusion of mucosa occurs leading to the formation of a Zenker diverticulum.
  - **Muscular pathologies**
    - *Diffuse esophageal spasm,* also known as *"nutcracker esophagus"*
    - *Incomplete muscular relaxation*
    - *Presbyesophagus*

Systemic Etiologies

This group of conditions includes problems related to the aging process, inflammatory conditions (e.g., esophagitis), myopathies, and psychogenic conditions.

- *The aging process*: Patients over the age of 70 often develop some abnormalities of the oral and pharyngeal phases of swallowing. These difficulties may be related to changes in dentition, poor oral hygiene, xerostomia, and general weakness.

- **Inflammatory causes**

  - ○ **Acute inflammatory conditions** are usually of infectious etiology and include *Ludwig angina, acute tonsillitis,* and *peritonsillar abscesses.*
  - ○ **Chronic inflammation** can lead to dysphagia due to indirect neurological damage or xerostomia. Some systemic causes of this include *thyroiditis, scleroderma, dermatomyositis* and *polymyositis, systemic lupus erythematosis, sarcoidosis, amyloidosis, rheumatoid arthritis,* and *postpoliomyelitis.*

- **Psychogenic causes** can be a side effect of neuroleptics that lead to decreased salivation. Anxiety can also lead to sensations that can mimic globus and difficulties with the oral phase.

◆ Investigations of Dysphagia

Barium Swallow and Modified Barium Swallow

The gold standard for diagnosing dysphagia is a barium swallow study. If there is a suspicion of oropharyngeal pathology then a videofluoroscopic modified barium swallow study in conjunction with a speech pathologist is required. This study provides information on bolus transport and safest consistency of bolus (honey, nectar, thin, pudding, puree, regular), and possible compensatory maneuvers that may facilitate swallowing.

Fiberoptic Endoscopic Evaluation of Swallowing (FEES)

A transnasal flexible laryngoscope is used to assess pharyngeal swallowing. The procedure is a sensitive technique to assess for laryngeal penetration, tracheal aspiration, and pharyngeal residue.

Swallowing Electromyography

Manometry: Helpful to assess motor function of the esophagus. A catheter with several electronic pressure probes is passed into the stomach to measure esophageal contractions and upper and lower esophageal sphincter relaxation in response to swallowing.

Esophageal pH monitoring: Esophageal pH monitoring is the standard criterion for diagnosing reflux disease.

Endoscopy: Gastroesophageal endoscopy enables the best assessment of the esophageal mucosa but does not detect esophageal function.

◆ Treatment

Swallowing therapy includes direct methods (including modifications of food consistency), indirect methods (including exercise regimens performed without food bolus and stimulation of the oropharyngeal structures), and adoption of behavioral techniques and postural changes. Electrical stimulation can be applied for dysphagia and has been found to be beneficial in neurological conditions. The Mendelson maneuver is used to improve laryngeal elevation and cricopharyngeal opening during the swallow. The Shaker exercise is a head lift designed to increase anterior movement of the hyolaryngeal complex and opening of the upper esophageal sphincter. Other techniques include biofeedback and are especially useful for oral motor and facial exercises. In patients who cannot achieve a safe swallow, alternate enteral feeding methods are instituted to bypass the oral cavity and pharynx (eg, nasogastric tube feeding and a percutaneous endoscopic gastrostomy).

Suggested Reading

Ertekin C, Aydogdu I. Neurophysiology of swallowing. Clin Neurophysiol 2003;114: 2226–2244

Logemann JA. Manual for the Videofluorographic Study of Swallowing. 2nd ed. Austin, TX: Pro-Ed; 1993

Logemann JA. Evaluation and Treatment of Swallowing Disorders. 2nd ed. Austin, TX: Pro-Ed; 1998

Paik NJ, Han TR. Critical review on the management for adult oropharyngeal dysphagia. Crit Rev Phys Rehabil Med 2002;14:247–272

Palmer JB, Drennan JC, Baba M. Evaluation and treatment of swallowing impairments. Am Fam Physician 2000;61:2453–2462

Spieker MR. Evaluating dysphagia. Am Fam Physician 2000;61:3639–3648

49 Aspiration

Craig H. Zalvan

Aspiration refers to the inhalation of particulate matter, fluid, or secretions into the trachea, bronchi, and lungs. It can be a process that is transient and short lived (acute) or can persist over time (chronic). The etiology of aspiration is highly variable and includes neurological conditions, mental status changes, anatomical changes, infection, ingestion of toxic substances, and traumatic or iatrogenic causes.

Symptoms of aspiration, many of which are nonspecific, can be obvious and clinically evident, or they can be silent. Typically, penetration and aspiration of contents through the vocal folds into the airway elicit coughing or choking. If normal protective mechanisms are impaired, this response is lost. Subclinical or silent aspiration refers to aspiration occurring without any outward sign or symptom of aspiration.

Aspiration, whether acute or chronic, can lead to significant morbidity, including pneumonia, pulmonary fibrosis, pulmonary hypertension, hypoxia, asphyxia, and death.

◆ Signs and Symptoms

As mentioned, the signs and symptoms of aspiration can be subtle and nonspecific. In cases of silent aspiration, there may be no indication of aspiration other than a comorbidity such as pneumonia or hypoxemia. The most common presentation of aspiration is coughing associated with oral intake, usually liquids. Many of the signs and symptoms associated with aspiration are associated with the underlying etiology, as opposed to the aspiration itself.

- **Esophageal**: Typically, esophageal signs and symptoms are associated with underlying esophageal dysmotility or obstruction leading to aspiration.
  - Dysphagia
  - Globus sensation
  - Odynophagia
  - Prolonged eating time
  - Regurgitation

- **Laryngeal**: The larynx serves several purposes, including phonation, respiration, and airway protection. Pathology that affects the larynx alters these processes, leading to several signs and symptoms.
  - Any change in voice: dysphonia, breathy voice, and the like
  - Throat clearing

- Weak, ineffective cough
- Dysphonia
- Globus
- Hiccups
- Laryngospasm
- Stridor

- **Pulmonary**: Pulmonary signs and symptoms are related to aspirated material causing irritation and infection of the airway and lung parenchyma.

  - Apnea
  - Hypoxia
  - Bronchitis
  - Bronchospasm/wheezing
  - Chest pain
  - Cough
  - Choking
  - Pneumonia
  - Pulmonary fibrosis
  - Pulmonary abscess
  - Tracheitis

- **General**: Symptoms associated with oral intake can discourage individuals from eating and lead to a general state of poor health and malnourishment.

  - Failure to thrive/weight loss
  - Fever
  - General malaise
  - Night sweats
  - Nocturnal fevers

◆ Causes

- **Acute**: Acute aspiration can be caused by sudden changes in status (such as mental status or anatomy), leading to a single event or a short time period of aspiration events.

  - Anatomical

    — *Foreign bodies*
    — *Tumors of the aerodigestive tract*
    — *Postsurgical alteration of the tongue base, palate, larynx, pharynx, or hypopharynx*

  - Infectious

    — *Viral*
    — *Fungal*

  - Neurological

- — *Cerebrovascular accidents*
- — *Traumatic head injury*
- — *Seizure*
- — *Vagus nerve injury/recurrent laryngeal nerve injury*
- — *Vocal fold paresis*

o Toxic

- — *Alcohol*
- — *Narcotics*
- — *Any drug with central nervous system (CNS) depression*

o Traumatic

- — *Nasogastric tube placement*
- — *Endotracheal intubation*
- — *Upper gastrointestinal endoscopy*
- — *Laryngeal trauma (external or internal)*

- **Chronic**: Chronic aspiration typically results from loss of airway protection and can be complicated by dysfunctional swallowing. Incidence increases with age, and depending on severity can be a significant source of morbidity and mortality. Chronic aspiration is most commonly caused by stroke; however, there are many nerve and neurological conditions that can lead to aspiration, including degenerative neuromuscular diseases, peripheral nerve disorders, and traumatic injury. Chronic aspiration can also result from anatomical structural alterations and related functional deficits, which disrupt normal swallowing or prevent adequate airway protection.

o Neurological

- — *Amyotrophic lateral sclerosis*
- — *Anoxic encephalopathy*
- — *Arnold-Chiari malformation*
- — *Cerebrovascular accidents*
- — *CNS tumors*
- — *Dementia*
- — *Guillain-Barré syndrome*
- — *Multiple sclerosis*
- — *Muscular dystrophy*
- — *Myasthenia gravis*
- — *Parkinson disease*
- — *Poliomyelitis*
- — *Progressive spinal muscle atrophy*
- — *Progressive supranuclear palsy*
- — *Traumatic head injury*
- — *Vagus nerve injury/recurrent laryngeal nerve injury*
- — *Vocal fold paresis/paralysis*

o Anatomical

- — *Achalasia*
- — *Caustic injury*

- *Cricopharyngeal dysfunction*
- *Esophageal neoplasm*
- *Esophageal strictures*
- *Head and neck radiation*
- *Laryngeal clefts*
- *Laryngopharyngeal reflux*
- *Tumors of the aerodigestive tract*
- *Postsurgical alteration of the tongue base, palate, larynx, pharynx, or hypopharynx*
- *Tracheoesophageal fistula*
- *Tracheotomy*
- *Vocal fold paresis/paralysis*
- *Zenker diverticulum*

Suggested Reading

Pletcher SD, Eisle DW. Chronic aspiration. In: Cummings CW, Haughey BH, Thomas JR, et al, eds. Otolaryngology–Head and Neck Surgery. 4th ed. Philadelphia: Elsevier Mosby; 2005:2077–2089

50 Throat Clearing and Globus Sensation

Keith G. Saxon and Jo Shapiro

The symptoms of throat clearing and globus sensation may be presenting complaints or may be associated with other presenting complaints either separately or together.

◆ Throat Clearing

Patients may be unaware of throat clearing even though it is obvious to those around them or present during their clinical exam. The act of throat clearing is a choice the patient makes as a response to a perceived sensation. The key differential points of throat clearing turn on the chronicity of the problem and the presence or absence of findings on laryngoscopic inspection, as well as associated history and symptoms. *Allergic rhinitis, chronic sinusitis, gastroesophageal reflux (GERD)/laryngopharyngeal reflux (LPR),* and *cough-variant asthma* account for the vast majority of throat clearing in nonsmokers with a normal chest x-ray.

Acute causes of throat clearing include the following:

- *Allergy:* Either as a result of alteration of secretions, inflammation of the mucosa, or sensory changes. Associated history and symptoms include seasonal occurrence, rhinorrhea, nasal congestion, and itchy eyes. Findings on physical examination may include turbinate hypertrophy, nasal mucosal edema, rhinorrhea, and the absence of laryngeal findings on endoscopy. There is often a response to antihistamines and topical nasal steroids.
- *"Postnasal drainage" (PND):* This term, although ubiquitous, is relatively meaningless. Normal nasal and sinus physiology assumes all patients have PND. However, when there are excessive posterior nasal secretions, it is usually due to rhinitis or sinusitis.
- *Rhinosinusitis/upper respiratory tract infection (URI):* Alteration in quantity and viscosity of secretions so that the patient may actually feel those secretions in the hypopharynx. Other systemic or focal symptoms, the presence of mucus in the middle meati, nasopharyngeal inflammation such as erythema, purulence or adenoid hypertrophy, or lymphoid hyperplasia of the oropharynx support this diagnosis.
- *Laryngopharyngeal reflux:* Single events of reflux may give rise to many days of symptoms, especially if the response of the patient is to throat clear. Direct laryngoscopic findings of inflammatory changes in the hypopharynx and esophageal introitus, and response to lifestyle changes, antacids, H2 antagonists, or proton pump inhibitors (PPIs) support this etiology.

- *Laryngotracheal bronchitis*: Usually this is viral and short lived. Persistent symptoms may be related to *Mycobacterium pneumoniae* or pertussis, especially if the cough is more predominant than throat clearing.

Chronic causes with **positive finding on laryngoscopy** include the following:

- **Mass**: *Benign or malignant neoplasm, granuloma, sarcoid, lingual tonsil hypertrophy,* or *amyloidosis.* Such entities may sometimes be associated with referred pain (especially to the ear), hemoptysis, or voice change. There may be a history of heavy smoking and alcohol intake, or LPR.
- **Ulceration**: *LPR, neoplasm, sarcoid, tuberculosis, pemphigus,* or *amyloidosis.* The presence of neck, lung, or skin manifestations or systemic symptoms can help in distinguishing etiology.
- **Secretions poorly cleared with swallow**: *Dysphagia* caused by *neuropathy, myopathy, Parkinson disease, myasthenia gravis, radiation therapy, cerebral vascular accident, Zenker diverticulum, cricopharyngeal dysfunction,* or *scleroderma.*
- **Mucous**: *Rhinosinusitis, tracheitis, bronchitis, cystic fibrosis, bronchiectasis,* or *dehydration.* In these cases, one might see thickened secretions in the hypopharynx.
- **Inflammation**: *LPR, fungal laryngitis, allergy, inhalation injury,* or *relapsing polychondritis.*

Chronic causes with **negative findings on laryngoscopy** include the following:

- *ACE inhibitor use*
- *Irritable larynx syndrome (ILS)*: Initiators include remote bronchitis and URI, LPR, allergy, sinusitis. There is sometimes an association with paradoxical vocal cord movement (PVCM), and laryngospasm. ILS is hypothesized to be a disorder of hypersensation that persists after the inflammation has resolved, or in the case of LPR is a consequence of continuing inflammation. It is a self-perpetuating problem because the patient's response of throat clearing or cough increases the sensitivity in the hypopharynx and larynx, making it more likely that the patient will cough or throat clear again. ILS is a diagnosis of exclusion made after the evaluation for other treatable causes has been completed. The mainstay of therapy, delivered by the speech-language pathologist, is interruption of the throat clear/cough response by increasing awareness of the sensations that come before a cough or throat tickle, and substitution of other behaviors. Swallowing instead of the throat clear is especially effective because it reflexively decreases sensation in the hypopharynx for a period of 5 to 15 seconds. Antitussives and drugs used to treat neuropathy are sometimes useful as adjunctive therapy with behavioral intervention.
- *Dysphagia*: If the patient has dysphagia caused by dysfunction at or distal to the cricopharyngeus, there may be difficulty moving secretions with a relatively normal laryngoscopic examination. Examples would include cri-

copharyngeal dysfunction or esophageal abnormalities, including esophageal dysmotility.
- *Non-acid reflux*
- *Asthma*
- *Congestive heart failure*
- *Psychogenic*

◆ Globus Pharyngeus

Globus is classically defined as the sensation of a mass or lump in the throat. Patients will most often define the globus sensation as being present at rest, sometimes worsening with a dry swallow, and generally lessening or transiently resolving during a bolus swallow. Dysphagia, the sensation of bolus obstruction or aspiration, throat pain, and odynophagia are *not* associated with globus. There is no known cause for globus. The symptom complex is often incorrectly referred to as *globus hystericus*, but there is no association with hysteria. Evaluation of globus patients should include a careful otolaryngologic and gastrointestinal history, especially to rule out neoplasia or infection, and with observation for sinusitis, lingual and palatine tonsil hypertrophy, LPR, or chronic laryngitis.

Certainly, if there are associated symptoms of concern such as throat pain, odynophagia, or dysphagia, other studies such as endoscopy and/or barium swallow should be performed depending on the associated history and physical examination.

- Associations with globus: Obsessive characteristics, neurosis, anxiety, depression, and introversion appear higher than in controls.
- Diseases purportedly associated with globus: *Malocclusion, lingual tonsillitis, chronic sinusitis,* and *cervical osteophytes.* Although these may occasionally occur in patients with globus, no convincing causal relationship has been shown.

Possible Etiologies of Globus

- *Upper esophageal sphincter (UES) hypertension*: Early studies showing elevated resting UES pressure in patients with globus have not been supported by more accurate manometric techniques.
- *GERD causing UES hypertension*, which may then cause globus sensation: There are studies both supporting and refuting this theory.
- Globus associated with more distal gastrointestinal lesions: These include *Barrett esophagus, ulcers, gastritis,* or *gastric cancer,* but one would expect additional symptoms rather than isolated globus in these disorders.

Suggested Reading

Andrianopoulos MV, Gallivan GJ, Gallivan KH. PVCM, PVCD, EPL, and irritable larynx syndrome: what are we talking about and how do we treat it? J Voice 2000;14:607–618

Morrison M, Rammage L, Emami AJ. The irritable larynx syndrome. J Voice 1999;13:447–455

Saxon KG, Martin S, Goyal R, Shapiro J. Disorders of the upper esophageal sphincter. In: Freid MP, Ferlito A, Rinaldo A, Smith RV, eds. The Larynx. San Diego: Plural Publishing; 2008

Saxon KG, Shapiro J. Paradoxical vocal cord motion. In: Rose, BD, ed. UpToDate, Waltham, MA: Up To Date, Inc.; 2008. www.uptodate.com

51 Regurgitation/Hematemesis

Christopher L. Oliver and Stephen Y. Lai

Hematemesis is literally translated as *bloody vomit* and refers to the clinical regurgitation of blood from the upper gastrointestinal/respiratory tract, which includes the nose, mouth, pharynx, esophagus, stomach, and small intestine. Regurgitation is the movement of contents within the upper gastrointestinal tract in a retrograde manner. Because there is limited overlap regarding the causes of hematemesis and regurgitation, they will be considered separately in this chapter.

◆ Hematemesis

The initial consideration when evaluating a patient with hematemesis is hemodynamic stability. In the face of acute large-volume hematemesis immediate airway protection and the initiation of the ABC (airway, breathing, circulation) resuscitation algorithm is required. It should also be noted that without (and occasionally, with) endoscopic evaluation one may be unable to differentiate hematemesis from hemoptysis. Dedicated endoscopic evaluation of the upper aerodigestive tract can separate the sources of hematemesis into those above and those below the esophageal inlet, and therefore into the general purview of the otolaryngologist versus the gastroenterologist, respectively.

- Systemic causes
  - Any systemic cause of *coagulopathy* can increase bleeding from various sources.
    - *Platelet dysfunction*
    - *Excessive anticoagulation*
    - *Von Willebrand disease*
    - *Hemophilia A and B*
    - *Idiopathic or thrombotic thrombocytopenic purpura*
    - *Medication,* such as *aspirin*
  - *Acquired or congenital vascular pathology* can cause bleeding.
    - *Hereditary hemorrhagic telangiectasia*
    - *Collagen-vascular disease*
    - *Vascular aneurysm* or *pseudoaneurysm*

Above the Esophageal Inlet

Hematemesis originating above the esophageal inlet tends to be bright red (unless secondarily regurgitated), and can be caused by the following (from superior to inferior):

- **Nose**
  - *Epistaxis*: Any cause of epistaxis can potentially result in hematemesis primarily or secondarily through regurgitation. Epistaxis is discussed in detail in Chapter 29. Due to anatomical constraints as well as volume characteristics, posterior epistaxis is more likely to result in clinical hematemesis than anteriorly based bleeds. Maxillofacial trauma can cause anterior or posterior nasal bleeding. A history of recurrent epistaxis in addition to hematemesis is suggestive of a nasal source. A recent history of nasal surgery, endoscopic or open, may also suggest a possible nasal source.

- **Nasopharynx**
  - *Trauma*: Recent surgery with nasotracheal intubation could suggest nasopharyngeal laceration.
  - *Surgical bleeding*: Recent adenoidectomy should prompt investigation for bleeding in the surgical bed; postadenoidectomy bleeding is usually less profuse than posttonsillectomy bleeding and can be intermittent. Any recent nasal, skull base, or endonasal neurosurgical procedure should raise the question of postsurgical bleeding. Recent ear surgery can result in hemotympanum and passage of blood from the middle ear to the nasopharynx through the eustachian tube.
  - *Neoplasm*: The most common lesions include *nasopharyngeal carcinoma* or *juvenile nasopharyngeal angiofibroma*. Nasopharyngeal neoplasms may present with a history of unilateral epistaxis, increasing nasal congestion, and/or other nasal complaints.
  - *Internal carotid aneurysm* may rarely be responsible for massive nasopharyngeal bleeding.

- **Oral cavity/oropharynx**
  - *Trauma*: Recent trauma with mucosal laceration is a common cause of oral bleeding that is usually spotty rather than profuse.
  - *Gingivitis*: In adults, severe gingivitis can lead to diffuse bleeding.
  - *Surgical bleeding*: History of tonsillectomy, dental work, or other recent oral cavity procedures should prompt investigation. Posttonsillectomy bleeding may be profuse or intermittent; a clot may be visible over the surgical site.
  - *Other*: *Neoplasm, vascular malformation, and foreign body* are other uncommon causes.

- **Hypopharynx/larynx**

  - *Laryngeal sources of hemorrhage*: These sources are very rare and are more likely to cause intermittent hemoptysis than hematemesis.
  - *Trauma*: Recent intubation or alternate mechanism of injury should be considered, and may be suggested by patient history.
  - Other: *Malignancy, recent laryngeal/hypopharyngeal surgery*, or the presence of a *hemangioma* may indicate the bleeding source.

Below the Esophageal Inlet

Causes of hematemesis originating below the esophageal inlet tend to produce more coffee-ground products and tend to be expelled in intermittent discrete episodes. Patients being treated for presumed bleeding below the esophageal inlet where a source cannot be identified should undergo endoscopic evaluation by an otolaryngologist if they fail to respond. All patients presenting with hematemesis from below the esophageal inlet should be referred for esophagogastroduodenoscopy (EGD). Blood is a gastric irritant and causes emesis; bleeding from below the esophageal inlet tends to fill the stomach and be expelled in discrete episodes. Of note, 50 to 80% of hematemesis is secondary to peptic ulcer disease and/or liver disease. Causes of hematemesis originating from below the esophageal inlet include the following:

- **Esophagus**

  - *Varices*: The most common cause of esophageal bleeding, these are usually a result of portal hypertension.
  - *Trauma*: Recent history of blunt or penetrating trauma. A history of severe retching/vomiting can suggest *Mallory-Weiss syndrome* and hemorrhage from esophageal tears. Although it may not present with hematemesis, the recognition of esophageal rupture (*Boerhaave syndrome*) is critical.
  - *Surgical bleeding*: A history of recent esophageal surgery can suggest postsurgical bleeding. This is often noted through an indwelling nasogastric tube.
  - *Esophagitis*: Can result in erosions and bleeding. These are best treated with endoscopic means.

- **Stomach**

  - *Peptic ulcer disease (PUD)*: The most common cause for gastric bleeding, followed by gastritis. Patients often have a history of peptic ulcer and are best diagnosed with endoscopy.
  - *Gastritis*: Acute superficial gastric erosions are usually multiple, begin in the fundus, and progress toward the antrum.
  - *Gastric varices, neoplasia, Dieulafoy lesion, angiodysplasia*, and *aortoenteric fistula*: Other causes of bleeding.

- **Upper gastrointestinal tract**
  - *Duodenal ulcer*
  - *Neoplasm*
  - *Angiodysplasia*
  - *Hemobilia*
  - *Pancreatic pseudocyst*
  - *Pancreatic pseudoaneurysm*
  - *Aortoenteric fistula*

◆ Regurgitation

The relationship between the stomach, lower esophageal sphincter (LES), and esophagus was elegantly described by Stein in 1992 as a simple plumbing unit; the esophagus functions as an anterograde pump, the LES as a valve, and the stomach as a reservoir. Any condition that interferes with the function of a single unit can increase the likelihood of clinical regurgitation and can include conditions less familiar to the otolaryngologist. In some cases regurgitation can be nonpathological, such as during infancy, if unassociated with failure to thrive or other pathology. Of primary importance in successfully treating regurgitation is properly identifying the level of pathology (ie, esophageal vs gastric).

- **Oral/Pharyngeal**: Difficulty executing an efficient swallow can lead to oral/nasal regurgitation of contents.
  - *Cerebral vascular accidents, age*, and neuromuscular disorders such as *Parkinson disease, amyotrophic lateral sclerosis, myasthenia gravis*, or *oculopharyngeal muscular dystrophy*: All can lead to oral and pharyngeal swallowing difficulties and regurgitation.
  - *Salivary changes*: *Xerostomia, Sjögren syndrome, medications*, or *head and neck radiation* may make bolus formation and propulsion difficult.
  - *Cricopharyngeal dysfunction*: Has been reported to be the primary, or contributing, cause for dysphagia in 5 to 25% of symptomatic patients. These patients commonly complain of a "lump in the throat" as well as a need for forceful swallowing. Cricopharyngeal dysfunction can be idiopathic or caused by several neuromuscular disorders.
  - *Zenker diverticulum*: A pharyngeal pouch originating just superior to the cricopharyngeus from the area of the Killian triangle (**Fig. 51.1A,B**). Patients can experience regurgitation of undigested food upon palpation, lying prone, or bending over. Recurrent aspiration pneumonia and cough are common.
  - *Foreign body impaction*: Usually occurs in younger children. Choking, coughing, dysphagia, regurgitation, and vomiting all may occur.
- **Esophageal**: Decreased motility and/or anatomical obstruction can increase the incidence of regurgitation.

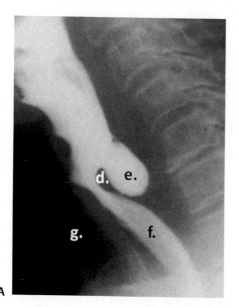

A

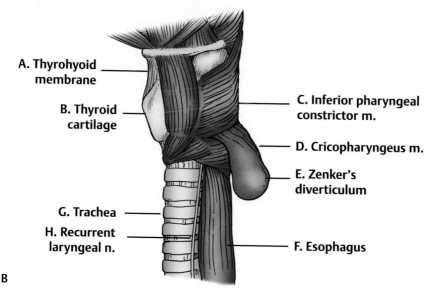

B

Fig. 51.1 Anatomy of a Zenker diverticulum. **(A)** Lateral view contrast fluoroscopy demonstrating a Zenker diverticulum. **(B)** Drawing of laryngopharyngeal anatomy including a Zenker diverticulum: (A) thyrohyoid membrane; (B) thyroid cartilage; (C) inferior pharyngeal constrictor; (D) cricopharyngeus; (E) Zenker diverticulum; (F) esophagus; (G) trachea; (H) recurrent laryngeal nerve.

- *Esophageal diverticulum*: Presents with similar symptoms to *Zenker diverticulum* but with fewer aspiration episodes.
- *Esophageal ring/stenosis/web*: Usually do not cause regurgitation but can classically present with meat impaction.
- *Foreign body impaction*: See earlier discussion.
- *Esophageal motility disorders*

— *Achalasia*: Progressive dysphagia for both solids and liquids is a hallmark of achalasia. In retrospect, symptoms are typically present an average of 6 years prior to diagnosis. Regurgitation of food from the proximal dilated esophagus is common, especially during recumbency. Weight loss is common with achalasia, but it is usually insignificant.

— *Spastic esophageal motility disorders*: Chest pain is the hallmark of spastic esophageal motility disorders. Intermittent dysphagia for both solids and liquids is common. Besides regurgitation, patients commonly report heartburn.

— *Scleroderma esophagus*: Scleroderma involves the esophagus in more than 75% of patients, regardless of clinical type. The main symptoms of dysphasia, reflux, and regurgitation are due to diminished esophageal peristalsis and erosive esophagitis.

— *Dermatomyositis*

— *Mixed connective tissue disease*

— Uncommon causes of decreased esophageal motility and regurgitation

   ○ *Chagas disease, familial adrenal insufficiency with alacrima, pseudoachalasia*, and *diffuse esophageal spasm*

○ *Esophageal atresia*: Can occur in infants with or without tracheoesophageal fistula. Drooling, choking, and regurgitation will occur with the first feeding. Maternal history of polyhydramnios is common. Diagnosis is made by attempting to pass a catheter into the stomach.

○ *Abnormal patency of the LES, or gastroesophageal reflux*: Can result in regurgitation of gastric contents into the esophagus, larynx, and/or pharynx. Patients may also have voice change and/or episodes of nocturnal coughing/choking episodes, and usually have variable symptoms of classic "heartburn." Certain foods and drink (eg, coffee, alcohol), medications (eg, nitrates, calcium channel blockers, β-blockers), and/or hormones (eg, progesterone) can decrease the pressure of the LES.

Suggested Reading

Alper C, Myers EM, Eibling DE, eds. Decision-Making in Ears, Nose and Throat Disorders. Philadelphia: WB Saunders; 2001

Bailey BJ, Johnson JT, eds. Head and Neck Surgery–Otolaryngology. 4th ed. Philadelphia: Lippincott Williams & Wilkins; 2006

Cerulli MA. Upper Gastrointestinal Bleeding. 2008. Available at: http://www.emedicine.com/med/topic3565.htm

VIII Differential Diagnosis of the Adult Skin, Face, and Neck, Including the Thyroid and Parathyroid

Section Editor: *Jason G. Newman*

52 Rash or Itching

Joslyn Sciacca Kirby and Christopher J. Miller

Rash is a nonspecific term used to describe any inflammatory reaction of the skin. Inflammation of any component of the skin, including the epidermis, dermis, or subcutaneous fat can cause a rash. Rashes that involve the epidermis usually manifest surface changes, such as pustules, vesicles, or scales (**Table 52.1**). By contrast, inflammation of the dermis and subcutaneous fat may change the color (usually red or purple) or thickness of the skin without surface changes.

A vast array of immunologic, infectious, genetic, and nutritional etiologies can cause rashes of the face and neck. For practical purposes, this chapter limits discussion to common rashes of the face and neck. Uncommon etiologies that mimic more common rashes are discussed selectively. Identifying the primary morphology of the rash (eg, papule, plaque, blister), distribution, and secondary changes of the skin (eg, scaling or crusting) will assist the practitioner in distinguishing among the many rashes that can occur on the face and neck. This chapter is divided into three sections: (1) scaling papules, plaques, and patches; (2) vesicles, bullae, and pustules; and (3) swelling.

◆ Scaling Papules, Plaques, and Patches (Table 52.2)

- **Eczematous rashes/dermatitis**: The term *eczema* describes rashes whose primary histologic feature is intercellular edema of the epidermis. These eczematous rashes are often itchy and have a wide range of presentations.

  ○ *Contact dermatitis*: A form of eczema due to a substance that causes either an irritant or allergic response when applied to the skin. Irritant contact dermatitis results when substances, such as acids or alkalis,

Table 52.1 Terms of Morphology

Term	Description	Size
Papule	Raised lesion	< 5 mm
Patch	Flat, broad lesion	> 5 mm
Plaque	Raised, broad lesion	> 5 mm
Vesicle	Small blister with clear fluid	< 5 mm
Bulla	Large blister with clear fluid	> 5 mm
Pustule	Small blister with cloudy fluid	< 5 mm

Table 52.2 Scaling Rashes

	Morphology	Configuration	Distribution	Symptom
Contact dermatitis	Early: erythema, blisters Late: erythema, scaling	Shape of allergen: lines, circles, squares	Localized or diffuse	Pruritic
Atopic dermatitis	Erythema, scaling, rarely blisters	Patches, raised plaques	Eyelids, neck, extremities	Pruritic
Seborrheic dermatitis	Greasy scaling, erythema	Patches	Scalp, brows, alar crease, and ears	Asymptomatic or pruritic
Psoriasis	Silvery scaling, erythema	Papules or raised plaques	Scalp, ears, trunk, or extremities	Pruritic
Tinea	Minimal scaling, erythema	Annular patches	Scalp, face, or body	Asymptomatic or pruritic
Drug reaction	Intense erythema, scaling later	Patches, plaques, or hives	Diffuse	Asymptomatic or pruritic

cause a direct toxic effect to the skin. Irritant contact dermatitis usually results within hours of the insult. By contrast, allergic contact dermatitis represents a delayed type IV hypersensitivity immunologic response from contact with any number of potential allergens. The immunologic response requires at least 1 to 4 days after contact before a rash arises. Common allergens causing dermatitis on the head and neck include topical antibiotics (**Fig. 52.1**), nickel in costume jewelry, and fragrances. Contact dermatitis frequently itches. **Acute** rashes usually present with small or large blisters, juicy papules, and crusting on a background of redness. **Chronic** dermatitis can progress to thick scaling plaques after frequent rubbing and scratching. Sharp delineation of the edges of the rash, geometric or linear configuration, and correlation with a known irritant or allergen may help diagnose contact dermatitis. Both irritant and allergic dermatitis will improve by avoiding the insulting agent.

○ *Atopic dermatitis*: A chronic, itchy rash often associated with allergic rhinitis and asthma. Family history may reveal a genetic predisposition for atopic dermatitis, allergic rhinitis, and asthma. Atopic dermatitis often starts in childhood and can improve with age. Patients usually present with skin that has grown thicker and has increased skin markings and scaling due to frequent rubbing and scratching. The distribution commonly includes the face, neck, and upper chest. Involvement of the flexural folds of the extremities may aid in the diagnosis.

● **Seborrheic dermatitis**: A chronic, common inflammatory dermatitis that waxes and wanes. The rash manifests as pink or red patches with greasy yellow scaling. The distribution is bilateral and symmetrical and typically

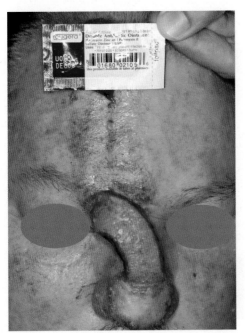

Fig. 52.1 Allergic contact dermatitis, due to a topical antibiotic, demonstrating rectangular erythema, swelling, and oozing where medication was applied to a dressing.

involves the scalp (dandruff), eyebrows, nasolabial fold (**Fig. 52.2**), and ears. Less commonly, the rash may also involve the sternal chest, inframammary folds, axilla, and gluteal crease.

- *Psoriasis*: A chronic inflammatory dermatitis that causes pruritic, red, sharply demarcated plaques that classically are covered in thick, silvery scale. Removal of the scale results in pinpoint bleeding (Auspitz sign). Psoriasis is often bilaterally symmetric and favors the scalp, ears, elbows, and knees. Changes of the fingernails (eg, pits, yellowish discoloration, or thickening) may help to confirm the diagnosis. This immune-mediated condition may also cause arthritis.
- *Tinea*: Commonly known as "ringworm." Tinea is an infection of the skin by a group of fungi, termed *dermatophytes*. The rash classically presents as a pruritic, scaling, annular or ring-shaped, pink patch. Involvement of the scalp (tinea capitis) usually presents with a scaling plaque with or without loss of hair. Advanced infection of the scalp can lead to red, boggy, and swollen places with pustules and scale. Involvement of the skin of the face (tinea faciei) is more subtle and presents as a slightly scaling, pink patch or slightly elevated plaque that may have indistinct borders. One clue to the diagnosis may be exacerbation or failure to respond to topical steroids, which will usually improve a case of dermatitis with a similar presentation.
- *Discoid lupus erythematosus*: An immunologically mediated disease that may or may not be associated with systemic lupus erythematosus. The rash presents as purplish-red plaques (ie, broad, raised lesions) with an adherent scale. The distribution favors sun-exposed areas, such as the face, upper trunk, and arms.

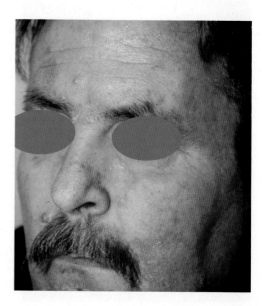

Fig. 52.2 Patient with seborrheic dermatitis demonstrating pink-red patches with fine white-yellow scaling in his brows and mustache as well as the glabella, cheeks, and beard area.

○ *Drug reactions*: Many prescription and over-the-counter medications can cause a rash. Many types of rashes can result from drugs and might include an asymptomatic or pruritic red rash on the neck and trunk, hives, or life-threatening blistering eruptions such as *Stevens-Johnson syndrome* or *toxic epidermal necrolysis*. Although most drug reactions are transitory, prompt recognition and discontinuation of offending agents can save the lives of patients presenting with diffuse blistering rashes accompanied by fever, flulike symptoms, or involvement of mucous membranes.

◆ Vesicles, Bullae, and Pustules (Table 52.3)

- *Folliculitis*: Small, red, pruritic, or painful follicle-based papules and pustules, distributed on the head, neck, and other hair-bearing areas. Most commonly due to bacteria such as *Staphylococcus* and *Streptococcus*. Folliculitis can also be caused by gram-negative bacteria, yeast, and fungus.
- *Pseudofolliculitis*: Small, flesh-colored to pink papules or pustules that most commonly occur on the cheeks and neck. The rash is thought to be secondary to hairs that become ingrown, causing irritation and inflammation. Men are affected much more commonly than women. However, women with hirsutism may also be affected. Black patients are affected more often, likely secondary to increased curling of the hair.
- *Acne*: Inflammation of the pilosebaceous units of the face and trunk resulting in comedones (blackheads and whiteheads) or inflamed red papules, pustules, or large, deep cysts and nodules. Inflammatory lesions may be mildly pruritic but are more commonly painful. Acne occurs primarily on the face, chest, and back, most commonly in adolescents and young adults. Women with hirsutism and masculinization of the voice may also develop acne as a result of a hyperandrogen state.
- *Rosacea*: A chronic inflammatory condition of the face (**Fig. 54.4**) that progresses from transient flushing and erythema of the face to persistent erythema, telangiectasias, and with or without papules, pustules, and nodules. Severe cases can lead to thick, oily skin of many parts of the face, especially the nose (ie, rhinophyma). Patients sometimes complain of burning in the skin or flushing or blushing of the skin with emotion, foods, or drinks. Rosacea often affects the forehead, cheeks, nose, and chin. Irritation of the eyes or lids can help to secure the diagnosis. Whereas acne most commonly affects adolescents, rosacea typically affects middle-aged adults.
- *Herpes simplex virus (HSV)*: A viral infection that causes painful vesicles at the site of inoculation by direct contact, usually at the vermillion border. Lesions begin as a group of painful vesicles or pustules on an erythematous base, then progress into eroded papules and plaques. The lesions are classically clustered or grouped together in one place, although more extensive lesions can be seen. In most cases the lesions are asymptomatic, although patients with recurrent HSV often describe a prodrome of tingling, itching, or burning sensation in the 24 hours prior to rash onset. The eruptions typically resolve without intervention within 3 weeks.

Table 52.3 Vesicles, Bullae, and Pustules

	Morphology	Configuration	Distribution	Symptom
Folliculitis	Red papules and pustules	Centered on follicles	Hair-bearing areas: trunk, buttocks, extremities	Asymptomatic, pruritic, or painful
Pseudofolliculitis	Flesh-colored to pink papules and/or pustules	Centered on follicles	Cheeks, neck, groin	Asymptomatic or pruritic
Herpes simplex	Early: vesicles Late: pustules or erosions	Grouped	Vermillion border, face, or neck	Pruritic or painful
Chickenpox	Vesicles	Come in crops	Generalized	Pruritic
Shingles (zoster)	Early: vesicles Late: pustules or erosions	Can be grouped	Dermatomal	Painful
Acne	Comedones, papules, and/or pustules	Not centered on follicles	Face, chest, and back	Asymptomatic or painful
Rosacea	Erythema, papules, and/or pustules	Not centered on follicles	Convexities of the face (forehead, cheeks, nose, chin)	Burning, flushing
Drug reaction	Early: vesicles or bullae Late: erosions	Target lesions, in some cases	Limited or generalized	Painful, can involve the mucous membranes
Autoimmune Blistering diseases	Early: vesicles or bullae Late: erosions	Target lesions, rare	Limited or generalized	Painful, can involve the mucous membranes

- *Varicella zoster virus (VZV)*: A viral infection that causes *chickenpox* and *zoster*. With either primary VZV infection or reactivation, the dermatitis is similar. There are vesicles in various stages of progression with surrounding erythema, classically described as a "dew drop on a rose petal."
  - *Chickenpox*: Occurs most commonly in children and is transmitted by direct contact or respiratory particles. Infants are currently vaccinated against VZV, so children may have atypical or attenuated infections later in life. The lesions favor the head and trunk and are very pruritic. Scarring is uncommon unless there is secondary infection or manipulation.
  - *Zoster* or *shingles*: Caused by reactivation of the VZV virus. The virus remains latent in sensory nerve ganglia after a chickenpox infection, and reactivation results in painful vesicles and erythema in the distribution of a sensory nerve. Zoster is most prevalent on the trunk; however, the trigeminal nerve and the cervical spinal nerves can be affected.
- **Others**: *Drug reactions* and *autoimmune blistering diseases* are uncommon causes of a blistering rash. Blistering drug reactions include *erythema multiforme* and the spectrum of *Stevens-Johnson syndrome/toxic epidermal necrolysis*. Examples of autoimmune blistering diseases are *pemphigus vulgaris* and *bullous pemphigoid*. Autoimmune blistering diseases and blistering drug reactions both cause generalized vesicles and bullae and can involve the mucous membranes.

◆ Swelling

- *Cellulitis*: A bacterial infection of the skin and subcutaneous fat. Clinically, this presents as tender, red, swollen patches in the affected area. There may be a history of preceding trauma or instrumentation.
- *Urticaria*: Also known as *wheals* or *hives*. Urticaria are pruritic, pink papules that can develop into ring-shaped plaques with a lighter pink or pale center. Individual lesions typically last less than 24 hours. Urticaria can be triggered by medications, foods, physical stimuli, and other causes. Chronic cases are often idiopathic.
- **Others**: Reactive conditions such as *Sweet syndrome* or *neutrophilic eccrine hidradenitis* can mimic cellulitis. *Lupus erythematosus* and *dermatomyositis* can cause swelling or a rash around the eyes.

Suggested Reading

Lookingbill and Marks. Marks JG, Miller JJ. Lookingbill and Mark's Principles of Dermatology. Available at: www.eMedicine.com

53 Ulceration

Thomas G. Takoudes

Ulcerated lesions of the skin of the face and neck occurs when there is loss of the epidermis and a portion of the dermis of the affected region. Lesions can be solitary or multiple, longstanding or new onset, painful or painless and may have secondary infection. They can be further described based on their size, location, color, symmetry, and border. Although there are exceptions, it is useful to categorize these ulcerations based on whether there are one or many lesions.

◆ Solitary Lesions

- *Basal cell carcinoma*: The most common skin malignancy. Typically caused by sun exposure, although genetics, trauma, and immunosuppression may play a role. More common in people with fair skin, former sunbathers, and the aging population. They are often painless.
- *Squamous cell carcinoma*: Second to basal cell carcinoma in incidence. Also associated with sun exposure, immunosuppression, and fair skin, although a non–solar de novo form exists. May arise from a long-standing actinic keratosis. Approaches basal cell carcinoma in incidence in people closer to the equator, secondary to long-term sun exposure. Much less common than basal cell carcinoma in less sunny locations.
- *Malignant melanoma*: Third most common skin malignancy, but more lethal than squamous cell and basal cell carcinomas. Often seen as a multicolored tumor with an irregular border. Typically arises in sun-exposed areas. Aggressive cancer that may metastasize to facial or cervical lymph nodes.
- *Keratoacanthoma*: Rapidly growing tumor usually in sun-damaged skin. Must be distinguished from carcinoma. Typically grows rapidly for up to 8 weeks, plateaus, and spontaneously regresses.
- *Merkel cell carcinoma*: Aggressive malignancy that arises from neuroendocrine cells in the dermis. Ultraviolet radiation may play a role because this generally occurs in the elderly Caucasian population. Begins as a purple-red nodule that may ulcerate as disease progresses.
- *Angiosarcoma*: Rare tumor that typically arises in the scalp or face of elderly Caucasian men. Usually presents as a painless purple-blue nodule and may ulcerate later.
- *Chondrodermatitis nodularis helicus (Winkler disease)*: Occurs on the pinna, usually the posterior/superior aspect of the helix and antihelix. It is a rapidly enlarging painful nodule that reaches a certain size then stops enlarging; usually in middle-aged to elderly men.
- *Trauma*: Burns and chemical injuries may lead to skin ulceration.

◆ Multiple Lesions

- *Pemphigus vulgaris*: Autoimmune-mediated disease characterized by blistering of the skin and mucous membranes. Typically develops between ages of 50 and 60; there may be a genetic component. The mucosa is usually involved as well.
- *Varicella zoster virus (VZV)*: Causes common childhood infection *chickenpox*. After years of lying dormant, VZV can reactivate to cause **shingles**, a painful unilateral rash characterized by vesicles that eventually rupture and ulcerate.
- *Discoid lupus*: Typical lesions are plaquelike and scaly, but a central ulceration may be present. Systemic lupus symptoms are uncommon.
- *Metastasis*: Primary skin or mucosal cancer may lead to facial and cervical adenopathy with involvement of the underlying skin in advanced cases.
- *Mycosis fungoides (cutaneous T cell lymphoma)*: Lesions are often confined to the dermis early in the disease, and histologic diagnosis is difficult. It may take years to obtain diagnosis after the first lesion appears. Epidermal involvement comes later in the form of a plaque.
- *Angiosarcoma*: See earlier description. Advanced tumors can present with multiple lesions.
- *Keratoacanthoma*: See earlier description. Keratoacanthoma can present as multiple lesions.
- Drug reaction: *Erythema multiforme, Stevens-Johnson syndrome*, and *toxic epidermal necrolysis* represent different manifestations of hypersensitivity. Lesions erupt rapidly and last 2 to 4 weeks.
- *Cutaneous porphyria*: Lesions are often blisters that develop into ulcerative scars. It is an inherited metabolic disorder that leads to overproduction of toxic heme precursors.
- Infection: There are many infectious diseases that cause cutaneous lesions with ulcerations.

  - *Anthrax*: Cutaneous anthrax occurs 1 to 7 days after exposure.
  - *Tuberculosis*: The typical lesion is 1 to 3 mm with central necrosis.
  - *Syphilis*: Tertiary ulcerative skin lesions (gummas) arise years after exposure.
  - *Parasitic*: This is not common in the United States.

Suggested Reading

Levene GM, Goolamali SK. Diagnostic Picture Tests in Dermatology. London: Wolfe Medical; 1991

Papel ID, Frodel JL, Holt GR, et al. Facial Plastic and Reconstructive Surgery. New York: Thieme; 2009

Swanson NA, Grekin RC. Recognition and treatment of skin lesions. In: Cummings CW, ed. Otolaryngology–Head and Neck Surgery. St. Louis: Mosby

54 Lesion (Nonpigmented or Pigmented)

Jacob D. Steiger

A thorough skin examination is an essential component of the complete head and neck evaluation. Whether the chief complaint or an incidental finding, the otolaryngologist often encounters cutaneous lesions and is faced with the diagnostic challenge. Care must be taken to differentiate benign skin lesions from premalignant or malignant lesions that require further attention. Cutaneous lesions may also alert the physician to a broader systemic illnesses or genetic condition.

In terms of physical findings, facial lesions can be broadly classified into pigmented and nonpigmented lesions. Examination involves observing the location, color, texture, consistency, and extent of the lesion. Palpation may reveal certain attributes regarding its subcutaneous extent, change in color with manipulation, and composition. All of these factors must be taken into consideration when making a diagnosis.

◆ Pigmented Lesions

Melanocytes give pigmented skin lesions their characteristic color. The melanocyte is a pigment-producing cell normally found in the basal layer of the epidermis. Pigmented lesions appear secondary to an increase in the number of melanocytes (melanocytic neoplasms) or through a change in melanin production. The majority of pigmented lesions are benign; however, care must be taken to rule out the possibility of malignant disease.

- **Melanocytic neoplasms**
  - *Malignant melanoma* (**Fig. 54.1**): Approximately 25% of melanomas are found in the head and neck. Suspicious lesions are defined by their physical appearance and growth characteristics. This constitutes the "ABCD" of melanoma. **Asymmetry**—If folded in half, the two halves wouldn't match. **Border**—Melanoma often has an irregular and scalloped border. **Color**—Presence of nonuniform pigment, with a variegated red, white, and blue color. **Diameter**—Enlarging pigmented lesions, and those greater then 6 mm must be scrutinized. Early diagnosis is paramount to the successful treatment of malignant melanoma.
  - *Nevocellular nevus*: Commonly referred to as moles, these benign lesions are histologically characterized by the presence of melanocytic nests. Nomenclature is based upon the histologic location of the nests within the skin.

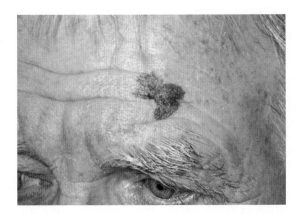

Fig. 54.1 Malignant melanoma.

- *Junctional nevus*: Located in the epidermal–dermal junction, these lesions are usually 1 to 6 mm flat to slightly raised, with symmetric borders and a uniform brown-black color. They are frequently found in children over the age of 2.
- *Intradermal nevus* (**Fig. 54.2**): Located within the dermis, these are the most common nevi seen on the adult face. Facial lesions are usually dome-shaped, smooth, and symmetric, and terminal hairs may grow through the nevi. They can be up to a few centimeters in size. Color may vary from a brown-black solid or speckled pigment to a translucent appearance. They are occasionally mistaken for basal cell carcinoma.
- *Compound nevus*: Located in both the epidermal–dermal junction and within the dermis, these nevi appear similar to intradermal nevi.
- *Blue nevus*: Located deep within or past the dermis, the pigment appears blue on the surface. They are less then 1 cm in size and are often indurated and palpable. They typically do not change appearance.
- *Spitz nevus*: A compound nevus most frequently found in children. It is commonly dome-shaped with a pink-red color. Histologically these may be difficult to distinguish from melanoma.

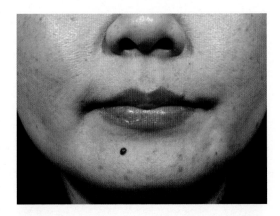

Fig. 54.2 Intradermal nevus.

- ○ *Congenital nevus*: Brown to black nevi that are present at birth. Giant congenital nevi are defined as being > 20 cm and carry a 5 to 20% risk of developing into a melanoma within the first 2 decades of life.
- ○ *Dysplastic nevus*: Larger then the typical nevi at 5 to 15 mm. May be associated with atypical nevus syndrome wherein a patient has greater than 100 nevi and is at a greater risk of developing melanoma. These patients must be referred to a dermatologist for annual examinations.
- ○ *Nevus of Ota*: A congenital macular brown-blue pigmentation of the skin and mucous membranes that follows the distribution of the first and second trigeminal nerve branches. Also known as nevus fusoceruleus ophthalmomaxillaris. This is most commonly seen in Asian patients.

- **Disorders of pigmentation**
  - ○ *Solar lentigo*: Often referred to as "liver spots," these lesions are dark, well circumscribed, and found on the sun-exposed skin of adults. They commonly present on patients with lighter complexions and increase in number with age. They are benign and not associated with malignant transformation.
  - ○ *Café au lait macule*: Tan to light-brown macules with uniform pigmentation that present in early childhood. They are benign, vary in size, and grow in proportion to the growth of the child. Identifying this type of lesion warrants full-body examination for additional spots. Patients with six or more may have *type 1 neurofibromatosis*. Other diseases that have been associated with café au lait macules include *McCune-Albright syndrome, Fanconi anemia*, and *tuberous sclerosis*.
  - ○ *Melasma* (**Fig. 54.3**): An acquired brown macular hyperpigmentation located on the face. Lesions are commonly found on the forehead, preauricular region, and malar eminence. They darken with sun exposure. These are often seen in pregnant women or those taking hormone replacement therapy.
  - ○ *Ephelides*: Commonly known as freckles, they present on sun-exposed skin of fair-skinned people. They are benign, small, well demarcated, and often darken with sun exposure. Presenting in early childhood, they tend to fade into adulthood.

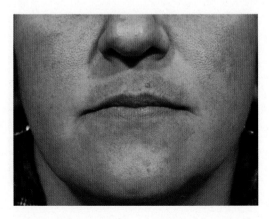

Fig. 54.3   Melasma.

○ *Postinflammatory hyperpigmentation*: PIH is an inflammatory dermatosis that arises from skin injury. The inciting factor is often obtainable in the history and involves inflammatory skin disease, trauma, and/or iatrogenic injury. It is commonly seen after skin resurfacing procedures.

○ *Vitiligo*: A chronic skin condition characterized by sharply demarcated, depigmented (white), and irregular patches. Lesions are commonly found on the neck and periorbital regions. There is a significant association with *thyroid disease* and *alopecia areata*.

◆ Nonpigmented Lesions

● Inflammatory

○ *Acne vulgaris*: Erythematous facial papules, pustules, nodules, and cysts that arise from inflammation within the pilosebaceous unit. *Propionibacterium acnes* overgrowth is seen within the obstructed follicles. Most commonly seen in adolescence.

○ *Seborrheic dermatitis*: Characterized by scaling and erythema of the scalp (dandruff), nasolabial folds, temples, feed edges of the eyelids, and hairline. Scalp lesions may be associated with alopecia.

○ *Acne rosacea* (**Fig. 54.4**): Patients have a characteristic erythematous flushing of the lower face. Close inspection may reveal small telangiectasias. A more severe form of this disease presents as *rhinophyma*.

○ *Morphea*: This is a localized form of scleroderma represented by hardened skin patches secondary to excessive collagen deposition.

○ *Atopic dermatitis*: Commonly seen in children as excoriating, pruritic, and erythematous lesions. It is associated with other atopic diseases.

● Viral infections

○ *Herpes simplex virus*: Frequently found in the perioral region but may occur in any location on the head and neck.

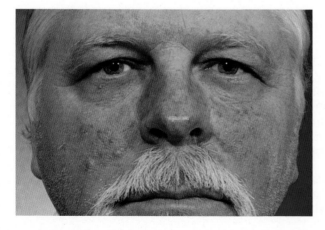

Fig. 54.4   Acne rosacea.

- ○ *Herpes zoster virus*: Exhibits a characteristic painful rash followed by a vesicular eruption that crusts over and may scar. Lesions typically appear in a dermatomal distribution.
- ○ *Verruca vulgaris (warts)*: May present anywhere on the head and neck and are caused by the human papilloma virus.
- ○ *Bacterial infection*: Cutaneous bacterial infections of the head and neck most frequently involving the staphylococcal and streptococcal species. Localized folliculitis is common in the hair-bearing skin and may give rise to a larger cellulitis or abscess.
- ○ *Epidermal inclusion cyst*: Also known as a sebaceous cyst, it is a true cyst lined by epidermis and filled with keratinaceous debris. They often present in the setting of an acute infection.
- ○ *Milia*: Small 1 to 4 mm superficial papules representing keratinaceous cysts. Milia are commonly seen on the face after epidermal injury from dermabrasion, surgery, or inflammatory skin conditions.
- ○ *Scars*: Develop as a result of intentional or accidental full-thickness cutaneous injury. An exaggerated fibrous response to injury may result in hypertrophic and keloid scars.

◆ Systemic Disorders

- ● *Sarcoidosis*: Skin lesions are observed in up to 25% of patients with sarcoidosis. The indurated, purple appearance of *lupus pernio* is the most characteristic. *Erythema nodosum* and rashes are also seen in this patient population.
- ● *Discoid lupus erythematosus*: Erythematous and scaly macular lesions most commonly seen on the malar areas and nasal dorsum. As lesions progress, they form a central region of depigmented scar. May occur in patients with systemic lupus, but less than 5% of DLE patients progress to systemic disease.

◆ Epidermal Neoplasms

- ● *Basal cell carcinoma (BCC)* (**Fig. 54.5**): The most common form of skin cancer, it manifests as a translucent papule with a raised pearly border. Patients often present with a nonhealing, bleeding lesion. Close inspection reveals superficial telangiectasias that blanch on palpation. They are most frequently found on sun-exposed areas but are also associated with immunosuppression, prior injury, and genetic diseases (basal cell nevus syndrome and xeroderma pigmentosa). BCC exhibits a slow, locally invasive growth pattern.
- ● *Squamous cell carcinoma (SCC)*: The next most common type of skin cancer presenting as a hyperkeratotic, scaly patch. More advanced forms appear as ulcerated nodules with rolled margins. SCC has similar risk factors and

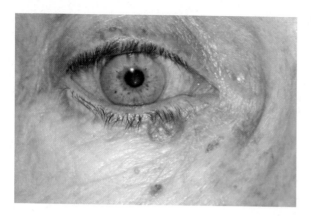

Fig. 54.5 Basal cell carcinoma.

genetic predispositions as for BCC. Cutaneous SCC has a slow growth rate and rarely metastasizes unless fairly large.

- *Bowen disease*: A distinct erythematous, scaly patch that is a variant of SCC. It represents the histologic appearance of full-thickness epidermal dysplasia.
- *Keratoacanthoma*: Another variant of SCC exhibiting a more rapid growth phase with a potential subsequent involutive phase.
- *Actinic keratosis*: Rough, scaly lesions most commonly found in sun-exposed areas. Palpable in the early stages, they exhibit a sandpaper texture and are often erythematous. Frequently seen in patients with a history of excessive sun exposure, they have up to a 20% risk of malignant transformation.
- *Seborrheic keratosis*: A benign, verrucous, usually tan-colored skin growth with a waxy "stuck on" appearance
- *Dermatosis papulosa nigra*: Benign brown, verrucous papules that appear in patients with dark skin types such as African Americans. They are a type of seborrheic keratosis.
- *Merkel cell carcinoma*: Actually a subcutaneous mass, but usually presents with overlying skin changes such as pink to purple discoloration and induration. Rapidly growing and aggressive, it will often metastasize early in the course. Typically presents in the elderly.

◆ Fibroadnexal Neoplasms

- *Atypical fibroxanthoma*: A malignant tumor presenting as a rapidly growing pink-red nodule. These are most frequently found in sun-exposed regions of the head and neck in the elderly population.
- *Neurofibroma*: Pink to brown pedunculated skin nodules, which may be pushed into the skin giving the classic "buttonholing" characteristic. Multiple lesions should alert one to the possibility of neurofibromatosis.
- *Syringoma*: A benign, flesh-colored papule representing an adnexal neoplasm formed by well-differentiated ductal elements.

- *Sebaceous hyperplasia*: Benign enlargement of the sebaceous glands most commonly seen on the forehead, cheek, and nose. These soft, yellow papules are most frequently seen in the elderly.
- *Hidrocystoma*: Benign eccrine or apocrine cystic proliferations that appear as solitary translucent nodules or papules with a cystlike consistency.
- *Xanthelasma*: Soft, yellow papules most frequently seen around the eyelids. Often associated with similar lesions in other portions of the body and elevated triglyceride levels.

Suggested Reading

Bolognia JL, Jorizzo JL, Rapini RP, et al, eds. Dermatology. New York: Mosby; 2003

55 Vascular Lesion/Birthmark

Stephen A. Goldstein

Vascular lesions of the head and neck region are relatively common when all groups are added together. They can be classified by several systems, but two broad categories of classification predominate and are easiest to remember:

1. Congenital versus acquired
2. Benign versus malignant

◆ Congenital

Congenital lesions have also been grouped in many ways over the years, but utilizing history and physical exam they can more readily be separated into hemangiomas or vascular malformations. At birth, 40% of hemangiomas are present, whereas 99% of vascular malformations are noted.

Hemangiomas

Hemangiomas are the most common benign vascular lesion of the head and neck. Hemangiomas can rarely be present at birth but are most notorious for their development after birth and rapid proliferation starting within the first 2 weeks of life. This rapid phase is followed by eventual involution, usually in the second year of life. These lesions may be divided into two subcategories depending on their location and histology.

- *Capillary hemangiomas*: "*Strawberry hemangiomas*" are superficial in the papillary dermis and noted to be red. They have a 3:1 female predominance. The proliferation of the endothelial cells results in either flat or nodular lesions with ill-defined pattern yet delineated appearance.
- *Cavernous hemangiomas*: "*Deep hemangiomas*" involve the reticular dermis and subcutaneous tissues. In the head and neck region mucosal surfaces are also at risk for involvement. These may appear as a pale, skin-colored blue or red mass. These too are ill defined in shape but well delineated. Hyperhidrosis over the area is common. Recurrent episodes of thrombophlebitis around the lesion can occur; however, most are asymptomatic.
- *Kasabach-Merritt syndrome*: A rare yet feared complication of large hemangiomas. The platelets and clotting factors are locally consumed within the hematoma, causing a consumptive coagulopathy. The patient will often present in disseminated intravascular coagulation (DIC), or rapid enlargement of the lesion or petechia, pallor, bruising, and prolonged bleeding from minor abrasions. It may also occur in adults.

Vascular Malformations

Vascular malformations are almost always present at birth (99%). Unlike hemangiomas, these grow in proportion to children as they age. They result from a genetic error in vascular morphogenesis. The most recognized is probably the "stork bite" or "salmon patch" typically located in the nape of the neck but may occur anywhere on the face. They present as red macular patches with irregular shapes. They are superficial within the dermis. On the face they will fade over the first year of life, whereas those on the neck often remain for life.

Nevus flammeus or *port wine stains* are another congenital malformation often involving the face and neck. These start as smooth, flat, red-purple patches in infants but with age will darken in color. Also with age these lesions tend to become papular. By the fifth decade of life, two thirds become nodular or hypertrophic. There are several syndromes with nevus flammeus that have a neurocutaneous component. *Sturge-Weber syndrome* is the most familiar, with its distribution following the dermatomes of the trigeminal nerve. These patients are often diagnosed at birth. Other syndromes that become evident in childhood include *Osler-Weber-Rendu disease, Cobb syndrome*, and *von Hippel-Lindau* disease.

Lymphangiomas range from localized lesions to larger cystic hygromas. Like hemangiomas they also have capillary, cavernous, or mixed forms. They have a proclivity for affecting the tongue and floor of the mouth. Unlike hemangioma they are colorless. In the buccal mucosa and oral cavity they can present as multiple white or brown blebs. They can be difficult to manage given their aggressive growth pattern, and slowly over time they can distort the bony skeleton of the face. Up to 60% are noted prenatally on ultrasonographic examination when affecting the head and neck. The potential for airway compromise is possible in larger lesions, and airway support may be required. Cystic hygromas tend to be poorly circumscribed and can extend deep into the soft tissue planes of the neck.

◆ Acquired

Acquired vascular lesions of the head and neck are predominantly benign.

- *Cherry angiomas*: These measure 0.5 to 5.0 mm and typically occur all over the body starting in the third decade of life. They are most prevalent over the trunk, especially in patients with liver disease. Pregnant women often develop them during pregnancy, and they involute postpartum.
- *Venous lakes:* These present as dark blue lesions. They will blanch with pressure unlike pigmented lesions. They represent dilated veins and are common in the sun-exposed surfaces of the face. They predominate at the vermilion border and on the ears.

Pyogenic granulomas are lobular capillary hemangiomas that often occur after localized trauma or infection. Patients will complain of persistent bleeding. The most common location of the hand and neck is the gingiva. They also present as skin lesions or may be found intranasally on traumatized mucosa as a small, raised punctate lesion causing recurrent epistaxis. Gingiva too are found in pregnant women subsequent to hormonal factors. *Pregnancy epulides* occur along the gingival as raised, lobulated, fleshy masses. The differential should include *Kaposi sarcoma, melanoma, angiolymphoid hyperplasia,* or *metastatic disease.*

Angiolymphoid hyperplasia with eosinophilia (pseudopyogenic granuloma) is a skin lesion of the face, ears, or scalp seen in adults. It presents as subdermal lesions up to 1 cm in size. These can be single or multiple erythematous or purple nodules, which may be crusted or even ulcerated in appearance.

Juvenile nasopharyngeal angiofibromas (JNAs) are found predominantly in adolescent males. These patients present with heavy, recurrent epistaxis and/or nasal obstruction. The lesion starts in the lateral wall of the nasopharynx and may extend into the pterygopalatine fossa and possibly intracranially.

Arteriovenous malformations (AVMs) of the head and neck often occur as a result of trauma or infection. They present as a painless mass with a pulsatile quality. Thrills and bruits and increased skin temperature may be found on clinical exams. They have been noted to have a growth phase with hormonal changes in pregnancy, puberty, or hormone replacement therapy. Profuse bleeding can occur, and embolization is often utilized to minimize blood loss before excision.

Telangiectasias or "*spider veins*" have been classified into primary (cause unknown) and secondary (associated with a known process). They are most commonly seen in healthy adults. They represent dilated capillaries or venules less than 1 mm in diameter. They emanate from a central vessel, which is helpful in diagnosis. When the central source is compressed the lesion goes away. Though most often benign and only causing cosmetic concern, they may be a clue to a larger underlying disease process. These lesions occur on both cutaneous and mucosal surfaces of the head and neck. The most common form, spider angiomas, present in 10 to 15% of healthy patients. Elevated levels of estrogen increase the prevalence in this group. They tend to regress after birth of the child. When mucosal involvement is seen, further examination is necessary to rule out a possible systemic syndrome.

Primary

- *Spider angioma*
- *Ataxia telangiectasia*: Typically presents with cerebellar ataxia in children. The syndrome includes recurrent pulmonary infections due to a hypogammaglobulinemia, immunoglobulin A (IgA). Telangiectasias can involve the conjunctiva, skin of the eyelids, ears, face, neck, and flexural surfaces of the limbs.
- *Hemorrhagic hereditary telangiectasia (HHT) (Osler-Weber-Rendu disease)*: is a systemic process. This most often presents with recurrent epistaxis at puberty. Punctate lesions on the septum and oral mucosa are visible. These lesions ulcerate and cause recurrent bleeding. They occur throughout the

mucosal surface of the gastrointestinal tract and viscera. Pulmonary involvement with arteriovenous fistulas typically occurs by the third to fourth decades of life. A family history is also common.
- *Generalized essential telangiectasia* (benign familial telangiectasia): Similar to HHT, without the bleeding history
- *Unilateral nevoid telangiectasia syndrome*: Numerous unilateral, threadlike telangiectasias along the dermatomes of either the trigeminal nerve or C3, C4. The congenital form is most common in males, whereas an increased prevalence is seen in women due to increased estrogen levels (acquired form). This process also occurs in alcoholic cirrhosis.

Secondary

- *Actinic damage*
- *Postsurgery*
- *Basal cell carcinoma*
- *Collagen vascular disease*
- *Scleroderma, systemic lupus erythematosus, dermatomyositis*
- *Cushing disease*
- *Estrogen elevation*
- *Pregnancy, oral contraceptive pills, cirrhosis*
- *Metastatic disease*
- *Poikilodermas*
- *Radiation damage*
- *Rosacea*
- *Steroid induced*
- *Xeroderma pigmentosa*

◆ Malignant Lesions

Malignant vascular tumors are relatively rare.
- *Angiosarcoma:* Arises from the endothelial cells. This can occur at any age but is most common in midlife. The scalp is the most common site of occurrence, with the neck, mouth, and antrum next in descending order. The clinical course is rapid and insidious. It is difficult to delineate margins given their spread down blood vessels. An intralumenal mass with thrombosis is common.
- *Hemangiopericytoma:* Arises from pericytes of veins. They occur in the nasal passages, oral cavity, and larynx. They have an insidious onset as painless blue, rubbery-appearing nodules.
- *Kaposi sarcoma (KS):* A tumor caused by herpes simplex virus (HSV) 8. It is not a true sarcoma but rather arises from lymphatic endothelium. These lesions present as nodules or blotches that may be red, purple, brown, or black, and are usually papular. It is commonly seen as a cutaneous process. In the head and neck it also presents in the oral cavity (palate and gums). Lesions are most common in patients with human immunodeficiency virus.

However, KS is also seen in patients with Mediterranean, eastern European, or Jewish ancestry—these forms are relatively indolent. An endemic variant has also been described in sub-Saharan Africans—this form is more aggressive. KS is also seen in immunosuppressed transplant patients.

Suggested Reading

Bailey B, Calhoun K. Head and Neck Surgery–Otolaryngology, Vol. 2. "Vascular Tumors of the Head and Neck." Philadelphia: Lippincott Williams & Wilkins; 2006
Bluestone C. Pediatric Otolaryngology. Philadelphia: WB Saunders; 2001
Cummings C. Otolaryngology–Head and Neck Surgery. 3rd ed. St. Louis: Mosby; 1998
Habif T. Habif: Clinical Dermatology. 4th ed. St Louis: Mosby; 2004

56 Facial Asymmetry (Including Paralysis)

Anthony Sparano

Facial asymmetry in the patient with normal facial nerve function is consequently due to mass effect. The causative factors in this subset of patients are infectious, inflammatory, and neoplastic. A specific focus can usually be identified fairly easily by history and physical examination of the facial skin and subcutaneous tissue, parotid glands, and maxillofacial skeleton. Occasionally, laboratory and radiographic imaging are necessary to make an accurate diagnosis.

More commonly, facial asymmetry results from paresis or paralysis of the facial nerve. Again, history and presentation are invaluable in making the correct diagnosis. The timing and course of progression, presence of associated symptoms, identification of inciting events, duration of noted abnormalities, and patient age and medical history are all necessary inquiries. An exhaustive list of potential causes of facial palsy can become tedious and impractical. The three most common causes—trauma, Bell palsy, and iatrogenesis—deserve further discussion, as do the additional causes listed below.

- **Trauma** is a common cause of *facial nerve palsy*, especially in the adult and neonatal (birth trauma) populations.

  - *Blunt injury* causing temporal bone fracture or fracture of the basilar skull adjacent to the stylomastoid foramen can account for facial palsy. As is the case with all potential etiologies, history, physical examination, and radiographic evaluation should attempt to identify complete facial paralysis of immediate onset versus delayed or progressive paralysis, to better direct the option of surgical repair.
  - *Penetrating injury* to the extratemporal portion of the facial nerve can also lead to abrupt complete paralysis from nerve transection versus delayed paralysis or paresis from associated inflammation.
  - *Birth trauma* is more commonly associated with unilateral facial palsy in the neonatal population. The underdeveloped mastoid process exposes the facial nerve for injury, especially during forceps delivery of the large neonate or neonate with arrested descent.
  - *Penetrating injury to the middle ear* can transect or injure the facial nerve along its horizontal course through the middle ear space.

- **Bell palsy**, also referred to as *idiopathic facial paralysis*, is a common cause of facial paralysis in all patient populations. It is thought to be caused by herpes simplex virus type 1 infection (either directly or reactivated from dormancy within the geniculate ganglion). Microcirculatory or autoimmune phenomena may also play a role. Bell palsy is a unilateral paralysis or paresis that manifests acutely (usually within 48 hours). By contrast, facial palsy that progresses over weeks to months suggests neoplasm. Most patients will report a variable prodrome or malaise in the days or weeks preceding onset if asked. Other causes must be excluded to make the diagnosis.

Most patients fully recover within 6 months, with the first signs of recovery usually within 3 weeks. Some patients never attain complete recovery, and late recovery beginning after 3 months is more commonly associated with sequelae (synkinesis, dyskinesis).

- **Iatrogenic injuries** to the facial nerve are most commonly encountered during otologic and parotid surgeries. The facial nerve is often dehiscent along its tympanic segment and thus injured as it traverses the middle ear space, or along its vertical segment during mastoid or neurotologic surgery. Cosmetic surgical rejuvenation of the brow (frontal branch) and rhytidectomy (frontal and marginal branches most commonly) place branches of the facial nerve at risk for injury. Similarly, dissection in the neck (marginal branch) and at the skull base (extratemporal trunk) merit careful attention to avoid injury to the facial nerve. Locally injected anesthetic agents frequently cause temporary loss of facial nerve function and should be noted and observed prior to additional evaluation and therapy.

- **Congenital** causes that should be considered include the following:

  - *Möbius syndrome*: with defects of the brain stem and neuromuscular system resulting in uni- or bilateral abducens and facial nerve palsies, and associated mental retardation, talipes equinovarus ("club foot"), hearing loss, auricular deformities, and tongue weakness.
  - *Albers-Schönberg disease*: with disordered bone metabolism potentially affecting the internal auditory canal with compression of cranial nerves VII, VIII, and sometimes III.

- **Neurological** causes that should be considered include the following:

  - *Stroke* usually presents acutely, spares the forehead musculature, and has additional qualifying neurological signs to help localize the site of the lesion.
  - *Myasthenia gravis* is an autoimmune disease affecting acetylcholine receptors at the level of the neuromuscular junction. It usually presents with progressive facial weakness, often associated with ptosis and difficulty speaking or chewing food.
  - *Guillain-Barré syndrome*, which presents as an ascending paralysis, affects the facial nerves bilaterally in an acute fashion.
  - *Multiple sclerosis* can present as slowly progressive facial nerve weakening, usually unilateral.

- **Infections** of various kinds can be associated with facial nerve palsy and include the following:

  - *Ramsay Hunt syndrome*, which is a primary or reactivated herpes simplex virus infection that causes acute facial palsy with associated painful vesicular lesions of the concha and external auditory canal, and bullae of the tympanic membrane. Patients may also have other associated cranial neuropathies and may complain of alterations in taste, difficulty hearing, or vertigo.
  - *Suppurative otitis media* presents with a progressive loss of facial nerve function from toxic effects unto the nerve sheath.

○ *Chronic otitis media with cholesteatoma* with a progressive loss of facial nerve function from compression by cholesteatoma.

○ *Necrotizing/malignant otitis externa* from associated temporal bone osteomyelitis.

○ *Lyme disease* from tick transmission of the spirochete *Borrelia burgdorferi.* Presentation can involve unilateral or bilateral facial palsy presenting weeks after the inciting tick bite with associated erythema migrans. Associated viral prodrome and arthralgias are not uncommon, and additional neuropathies, central nervous system infection, and cardiac conduction abnormalities may also contribute to the clinical presentation.

○ *Syphilis*

○ *Tuberculosis*

○ *Acquired immunodeficiency syndrome*

○ *Mononucleosis*

○ *Malaria*

● **Neoplasms** may cause either acute or progressive unilateral facial palsy and most commonly include the following:

○ *Malignant parotid neoplasms*, of which *mucoepidermoid carcinoma* and *adenoid cystic carcinoma* most commonly cause facial nerve dysfunction. These may be associated with pain and associated mass effect.

○ *Benign parotid neoplasms* very rarely present with associated facial nerve palsy, unless they are very large and compress a branch of the nerve, or rest adjacent to the nerve trunk as it exits the stylomastoid foramen at the skull base.

○ *Facial nerve schwannomas* uncommonly affect facial nerve function unless they are of significant size.

○ *Acoustic neuromas/vestibular schwannomas* uncommonly affect the facial nerve unless they are of significant size.

○ *Facial nerve hemangiomas* uncommonly affect facial nerve function unless they are of significant size.

○ *Glomus tympanicum/glomus jugulare* uncommonly affect facial nerve function unless they are of significant size.

○ *Meningiomas* uncommonly affect facial nerve function unless they are of significant size.

○ *Fibrous dysplasia*

○ *Melkersson-Rosenthal syndrome* is an idiopathic cause of recurrent uni- or bilateral facial paralysis or paresis with facial swelling beginning in childhood or young adult life. The earliest manifestations of the syndrome are sudden diffuse swellings of the lip or face. Fissuring of the tongue and cheilitis granulomatosa (generalized swelling of the lip) occur with chronicity. Facial palsy occurs in about one third of patients, and usually presents in intermittent fashion early but may progress to permanent dysfunction. Angiotensin-converting enzyme levels can be elevated during events. Lip or facial tissue biopsy shows lymphedema and perivascular lymphocytic infiltration during the early stages of disease and granulomatous changes in later stages. Chest radiography can help exclude sarcoidosis.

- **Metabolic** causes of facial palsy are uncommon, but when no clear etiology can be identified, consideration should be given to *diabetes mellitus, hyperthyroidism, malignant hypertension, acute porphyria,* or *vitamin A deficiency* as potential contributing disease processes.
- **Toxic** causes of facial palsy are uncommon, but when no clear etiology can be identified, consideration should be given to *arsenic intoxication, tetanus, ethylene glycol,* and *carbon monoxide poisoning.*

Suggested Reading

May M, Klein SR. Differential diagnosis of facial nerve palsy. Otolaryngol Clin North Am 1991;24:613–645

57 Swelling/Edema (Periorbital, Nose, Cheek, Jaw)

Jeffrey M. Shaari

Facial edema can have a variety of etiologies. It can represent local pathology or may be indicative of a systemic process. This section will focus on facial swelling and will be broken down into the following four facial regions: **periorbital, nasal and perinasal, cheek, and jaw**. Etiologies include infectious, inflammatory, neoplastic, traumatic, iatrogenic, and allergic, and some of these categories will overlap.

◆ Periorbital

The periorbital skin has low tissue resistance, making it particularly susceptible to fluid infiltration and subsequent edema. Generally speaking, local processes tend to cause unilateral edema, whereas systemic conditions tend to affect both periorbital regions.

Infectious

- *Superficial skin infection*: Most commonly caused by *Streptococcus* and *Staphylococcus* species, this typically causes a preseptal cellulitis with ipsilateral edema, erythema, and tenderness to the eyelids and periorbital skin. Examination of the conjunctiva and globe is usually normal because the infectious process does not usually cross the tough orbital septum. There may be a history of antecedent trauma or an insect bite.
- *Sinusitis*: Ethmoid and maxillary sinus infections may extend beyond the sinuses to cause periorbital edema. This may range from *periorbital cellulitis* to *cavernous sinus thrombosis*. With orbital involvement by infection, conjunctival edema, proptosis, ophthalmoplegia, and vision changes may be present. *Mucoceles* and *mucopyoceles* of the ethmoid and frontal sinuses can slowly expand to cause periorbital fullness and swelling, often with associated displacement of the globe.
- *Dacryoadenitis*: Inflammation of the lacrimal gland may be caused by viruses or bacteria. This usually causes swelling associated with tenderness centered about the upper lateral lid. Systemic conditions, such as *sarcoidosis* and *Sjögren syndrome*, should be considered when the swelling is chronic in nature and pain is absent.
- *Dacryocystitis*: Swelling centered about the medial canthus is typical for inflammation of the lacrimal sac. There is often associated tenderness and erythema, and pressure over the lacrimal sac may express purulence from the lacrimal puncta.
- *Anterior or posterior blepharitis*: Infection of the pilosebaceous unit of the eyelid will cause anterior *blepharitis* (*stye*), whereas dysfunction of the meibomian glands results in posterior blepharitis. Both processes can cause

eyelid edema, which is usually associated with erythema and a foreign body sensation from crusting on the eyelid margin.

- *Epstein-Barr virus (EBV) infection*: Seen early in the course of EBV infections, transient bilateral upper eyelid edema is rare and is known as the *Hogland sign*.
- *Chagas disease*: Insect bites near the eye that transmit the protozoan *Trypanosoma cruzi* (typically seen in South America) can cause unilateral periorbital swelling, known as the *Romaña sign*.
- *Trichinosis*: Seen in 80% of patients with trichinosis, periorbital swelling occurs from an increase in interstitial fluid.

Neoplastic

- *Primary or metastatic neoplasms*: Tumors of the globe, orbital contents, lacrimal gland, and lacrimal system can all cause secondary swelling of the eyelid and periorbital tissues.

Traumatic

- *Orbital and facial fractures*: Associated periorbital ecchymosis, paresthesias of V2, and extraocular muscle entrapment can be seen.
- *Carotid-cavernous fistula*: A rare cause of eyelid edema with associated pulsatile proptosis.

Iatrogenic

- *Endoscopic sinus surgery*: Violation of the lamina papyracea during endoscopic sinus surgery can lead to periorbital ecchymosis, crepitus, and swelling, particularly if the patient raises the intrathoracic pressure, as in a sneeze or cough.

Allergic

- *Angioedema* can cause periorbital edema with or without involvement of other areas of the face. There is often an associated medication or allergen exposure.

Other

A variety of inflammatory and autoimmune syndromes can cause periorbital edema. These include *systemic lupus erythematosis, dermatomyositis,* and *hypothyroidism. Renal failure, nephrotic syndrome*, and *cirrhosis* all involve a low albumin state that can cause an increase in interstitial fluid with subsequent periorbital edema. *Dermatochalasis* and *blepharochalasis* may be seen in older and younger patients, respectively. *Thyrotoxicosis* can cause unilateral or bilateral periorbital edema and is often associated with eyelid retraction and possibly exophthalmos. *Melkersson-Rosenthal syndrome*—the triad of relapsing facial and often lip edema, recurrent facial paralysis, and fissured tongue—is a rare cause of periorbital edema, but can be seen.

◆ Nasal and Perinasal

Infectious

- *Dacryocystitis*: See earlier discussion.
- *Sinusitis*: See earlier discussion.
- *Furunculosis*: Often caused by *Staphylococcus* and *Streptococcus* species. Infection of the vestibular skin may cause swelling of the nasal tip associated with erythema and tenderness.

Neoplastic

- *Lacrimal sac neoplasms*: Associated epiphora and the absence of tenderness (unless secondarily infected) over the lacrimal sac
- *Intranasal neoplasms*: Associated nasal obstruction and epistaxis.

Traumatic

- *Nasal and associated facial fractures*: Associated ecchymosis and tenderness may be associated with mobility or depression of the nasal and facial bones.

Congenital

- *Lymphovascular malformations*: sometimes seen at birth, these may also present later in life as a new or enlarging mass located anywhere on the face.

◆ Cheek

Infectious

- *Maxillary sinusitis*: See earlier discussion.
- *Dental infection*: Infection of the upper canine, premolar, and molar teeth may spread to cause cheek edema with associated tenderness.
- *Skin infection*: See earlier discussion.

Neoplastic

- *Maxillary sinus neoplasm*: Tumor that has eroded through or involves the anterior sinus wall may cause cheek fullness or secondary edema.

Traumatic

- *Zygomatic arch and other facial fractures*: The depressed zygoma may have superimposed swelling over the malar eminence. There may be associated trismus along with fractures of the maxilla and orbit.

Iatrogenic

- Recent **dental work** may cause swelling of the cheek.

◆ Jaw

Infectious

- *Parotitis*: Often seen in debilitated, dehydrated patients, can be caused by bacteria and viruses. Tenderness, swelling, and erythema over the angle of the mandible or the entire gland are typical for these infections. Purulence may be expressed from the Stensen duct. Bilateral parotid swelling can be seen in *mumps* infection.
- *Dental infection*: Dental infection or abscess of the lower teeth can lead to tenderness and swelling over the angle and body of the mandible.

Neoplastic

- *Parotid neoplasm*: Both benign and malignant lesions of the parotid gland can cause fullness either from the mass itself or from overlying edema. In human immunodeficiency virus patients, *lymphoepithelial cysts* can cause bilateral parotid swelling.
- *Oral cavity neoplasm* (alveolar ridge, retromolar trigone): Secondary swelling from underlying tumors can produce jaw swelling.

Traumatic

- *Mandible fracture*: Associated malocclusion, trismus, and V3 paresthesias may be seen.

Suggested Reading

Bluestone CD, Stool SE, Alper CM, et al, eds. Pediatric Otolaryngology. Philadelphia: Saunders; 2003

58 Facial Mass (Cutaneous, Subcutaneous, Periorbital)

Matthew C. Miller and David Rosen

Patients are often referred to otolaryngologists for evaluation of facial lesions. When confronted with a patient with a facial mass it is helpful to first determine whether the lesion is confined to the epidermis or whether deeper structures are involved. Further characterization among these groups will assist in narrowing the differential, guiding potential biopsy techniques, and ultimately making the correct decisions regarding treatment.

Cutaneous masses may be subcategorized based upon their general appearance as being nodular or papular, scaly, vascular, or pigmented. Masses confined to the subcutaneous tissues can be divided into those with and without overlying skin discoloration. Bony lesions represent a separate subgroup and may be suspected after simple palpation. Special consideration must be given to masses identified in the periorbital, perinasal, and preauricular regions because certain pathological processes have a predilection for these areas. Masses specific to these regions are listed under separate subheadings following here.

Facial masses encompass a wide variety of benign and malignant processes, many of which are discussed in detail elsewhere in this text. This chapter reviews many of those clinical entities and organizes them by appearance and location, rather than by pathology or etiology.

◆ Cutaneous Nodules and Papules

- *Skin tags (acrochordons)*: Small pedunculated lesions that are usually flesh colored. They often appear in clusters on the eyelids and in the periorbital region and are typically 1 to 2 mm in size.
- *Fibrous papules (angiofibroma/adenoma sebaceum)*: Smooth, tan to gray, dome-shaped papules measuring 1 to 2 mm in size. Typically seen on the nose and midface of middle-aged individuals. Usually, they are solitary but if multiple lesions are present, the diagnosis of tuberous sclerosis should be considered.
- *Senile sebaceous hyperplasia*: Yellow to tan papules that may become dome-shaped and umbilicated. May develop superficial telangiectasias, mimicking basal cell carcinoma. Common in the geriatric population.
- *Neurofibroma*: Soft, flesh-colored tumors that tend to invaginate into the skin surface when compressed. Multiple lesions should alert to the possibility of neurofibromatosis type 1.
- *Warts*
  - *Filiform*: Groups of fleshy, fingerlike projections that may emanate from a narrow base. Most commonly appear around the mouth, eyelids, and

nose. They may be spread to other regions of the face by shaving (ie, autoinoculation).

○ *Flat (verruca plana)*: Slightly elevated tan to yellow papules appearing in clusters on the forehead and shaved regions of the face. Tend to be less than 5 mm in diameter.

- *Hypertrophic scar and keloid*: Both appear as firm pink to tan masses in regions of previous trauma or surgical scar. Can be differentiated from one another by virtue of the fact that keloids are more often symptomatic (pain or itching), extend beyond the borders of the original scar, and are more common in blacks than in Caucasians.
- *Basal cell carcinoma (BCC)*: Most common malignant tumor in humans. Appearance varies based on histologic type, but the most common variant (nodular BCC) is a slow-growing papule with a pearly surface. Generally glistening and round with a telangiectatic surface.
- *Fibrosarcoma*: Firm, painless, fleshy mass that is tan in color. Patients may report a history of previous radiation exposure.
- *Pilomatrix carcinoma*: Most arise in preexisting pilomatrixomas. Tend to be asymptomatic, irregular, very firm masses with variable growth patterns. Generally appear as solitary tan, nodular masses.

◆ Scaly Cutaneous Masses

- *Actinic keratosis*: Premalignant lesions seen in areas of preexisting sun damage. More common in patients with low Fitzpatrick scores. Scaly, indurated lesions with yellow to tan coloration. Poorly demarcated from the surrounding tissues. Most are less than 1 cm in size.
- *Keratoacanthoma*: Rapidly growing mass seen in areas of previous sun damage. More common in the elderly population. Characterized by rapid growth phase, plateau, and subsequent involution over several months. May reach several centimeters in size and can appear as keratinized horns. In most cases they will develop a central crater during the involution phase. Difficult to differentiate clinically from squamous cell carcinoma.
- *Squamous cell carcinoma*: May present in a variety of ways, but typically appears as a scaly patch on an erythematous and often ulcerated base. They may arise in preexisting actinic keratoses.

◆ Cutaneous Vascular Masses

- *Pyogenic granuloma*: Bright red/yellow glistening lesions typically less than 1.5 cm in size. Often arise in regions of prior trauma. Hormone sensitive and may appear during pregnancy. May bleed profusely when traumatized.
- *Hemangioma*: Most hemangiomas are not present at birth, are not compressible, and exhibit proliferative growth that is not proportional to facial

growth (versus vascular malformations; see later discussion). They may appear as bright red macules with a glistening surface. Hemangiomas blanch with pressure. Deeper hemangiomas may be purple to blue in color. They are characterized by a rapid proliferative phase early in life and gradual involution over time (typically in the first several years of life).

- *Angiosarcoma*: Painless red to purple macule typically found on the forehead or scalp of elderly Caucasian males. May ulcerate or bleed in advanced or aggressive cases. Can be confused with benign lesions such as vascular malformations or even bruises.
- *Kaposi sarcoma*: Blue-red to violet nodules that may have superficial ulceration. Most often seen in association with human immunodeficiency virus/acquired immunodeficiency syndrome.

◆ Pigmented Cutaneous Lesions

- *Seborrheic keratosis*: The most common benign cutaneous neoplasms. Seborrheic keratoses have no malignant potential. They are generally well circumscribed lesions that may appear stuck onto the skin surface. They have a variable texture and are usually tan-brown in color with or without black and white keratin inclusions. They must be differentiated from malignant melanoma, which will most often have an irregular border and a smooth surface.
- *Common nevi (moles)*: Pigmented lesions that share the characteristic of melanotic pigmentation that is uniform in appearance. They may be flat or slightly elevated. Common nevi are of three types and must be differentiated from malignant melanoma.

  - *Junctional nevi*: Generally present beginning in childhood. They are flat to slightly elevated, brown to black in color, and hairless. They are rarely larger than 1 cm.
  - *Compound nevi*: Develop in adulthood. They are slightly elevated and light brown to tan in color and may contain hair. Generally smaller than 1 cm, they tend to become larger and more elevated with advancing age.
  - *Dermal nevi*: Most often raised, dome-shaped and brown in color. These often contain hair.

- *Malignant melanoma*: Pigmented lesions that may resemble benign nevi. Differentiated by the presence of asymmetry, irregular borders, variation in color, large diameter (greater than 6 mm), and elevation from the skin surface—a set of features referred to commonly as the ABCDE of melanoma.
- *Malignant fibrous histiocytoma*: Most common soft tissue sarcoma of the head and neck. When present on the face, it appears as a firm, tan to brown, slow-growing mass with a wide erythematous border. This is often difficult to differentiate from malignant melanoma.
- *Dermatofibrosarcoma protuberans*: Well circumscribed, painless mass covered by a thin layer of epidermis. It may or may not be pigmented or ulcerated, making the differentiation from melanoma and other pigmented lesions difficult.

◆ Subcutaneous Masses without Epidermal Discoloration

- *Lipoma*: Slowly growing, rubbery, subcutaneous masses. Generally, they are mobile and without symptoms other than localized mass effect and cosmetic deformity.
- *Lymphangioma*: Generally present as asymptomatic masses in the region of the parotid gland. Most often compressible and fluctuant. They are similar to lipomas in appearance and presentation, though the vast majority are diagnosed and definitively treated in early childhood. They may have rapid growth due to hemorrhage or infection.
- *Dermoid*: Congenital masses that develop at planes of embryonic fusion. They are typically seen in the periorbital region or nasal dorsum, though they may also be found in and around the parotid gland. They present as a painless swelling that is fixed to the overlying skin. They contain dermal appendages and will often possess a central sinus tract.
- *Epidermal inclusion cysts*: Cystic masses that may appear anywhere on the face or scalp. Compressible and rubbery, they may become fixed to overlying skin in the case of chronic or recurrent infection. Unlike dermoids, they do not contain skin appendages.

◆ Subcutaneous Masses with Discoloration of Overlying Skin

- *Vascular malformations*: All are present at birth and tend to enlarge proportionally with age, typically during or after puberty. Rapid enlargement may also be observed after trauma to the region. Four primary types are commonly seen.
  - *Capillary malformations*
  - *Venous malformations*
  - *Arteriovenous malformations*
  - *Lymphatic malformations*
- *Merkel cell carcinoma*: Rare tumors appearing in the sun-exposed areas of elderly patients. Rapidly growing and indurated, these are noncompressible subcutaneous masses with pink to purple discoloration of the overlying skin with or without telangiectasias.

◆ Bony Lesions

Bony masses of the face have similar presenting signs and symptoms, though vastly different pathologies and natural histories without treatment.

- *Fibrous dysplasia*: Slowly growing bony mass that most commonly presents as a painless asymmetric and nondiscrete swelling over the maxilla. This may blunt the nasofacial angle, giving the patient a catlike facial structure (called *leontiasis ossea*).
- *Osteoma*: Rare, slow-growing, discrete masses that may arise on the mandible or frontal bone. Benign and clinically differentiated from osteosarcomas by the absence of pain with growth.
- *Osteosarcoma*: Presents as an enlarging mass over the mandible or maxilla, though the growth is more rapid than in benign processes and is often associated with significant pain. Surrounding teeth may become loose with growth of these masses.

◆ Masses Specific to the Periorbital Region

- *Lacrimal gland neoplasm*: Typically present with swelling over the superolateral aspect of the orbit. Proptosis and downward and medial displacement of the globe may be observed.
  - *Pleomorphic adenoma*: Most common lacrimal gland neoplasm. Presents as a slowly progressive mass. It may recur if incompletely excised. There is a 10% risk of malignant degeneration over time.
  - *Adenoid cystic carcinoma*: Most common lacrimal gland malignancy. This often presents with pain secondary to perineural spread of tumor.
- *Malignant fibrous histiocytoma*: The most common nonepithelial malignancy of the orbit and most common radiation-induced sarcoma. Presents with pain, proptosis, excessive tearing, and a mass lesion in the region of the medial canthus. Consider this in patients with a history of previous radiation therapy.
- *Rhabdomyosarcoma*: Most common malignant orbital tumor in children. Presents as a superior orbital mass in ~25% of cases. Due to rapidly progressive lid edema, chemosis, and/or proptosis, this may be mistaken for infectious/inflammatory process.
- *Plexiform neurofibroma*: Most common benign peripheral nerve tumor of the orbit. Associated with neurofibromatosis type 1. Presents with eyelid swelling and thickening of the lid skin. These are likened to a "bag of worms" on palpation.
- *Lymphoid lesions*: May be benign, atypical, or frankly lymphomatous. Differentiated from one another by pathology and flow cytometry. They present as firm, rubbery masses, often in association with "salmon patches" on the conjunctiva.
- *Eosinophilic granuloma*: Orbital involvement in up to 20% of cases. Presents with painful mass and swelling over the superolateral orbit. There will often be surrounding erythema and induration.
- *Mucocele*: May arise from the ethmoid or frontal sinuses. Present as fluctuant masses along the medial or superior orbital rim. They may be seen in patients with a remote history of facial trauma (eg, nasoethmoidal com-

plex fractures or frontal sinus fractures), chronic sinusitis, or previous sinus surgery.

- *Pott puffy tumor*: Complication of acute frontal sinusitis. Defined as osteomyelitis of the frontal bone with subperiosteal abscess. These tend to be doughy masses centered over the frontal sinus with edema of the overlying skin. Patients will often report a recent history of acute purulent rhinosinusitis.
- *Dacryocystitis*: Painful palpable mass at the medial canthus. Represents obstruction of the nasolacrimal system with stasis, accumulation of debris, and eventually, superinfection.
- *Lacrimal sac tumors*: Rare. Most commonly present with epiphora, though a mass near the medial canthus is observed in up to one third of cases. Benign tumors are most frequently *squamous papillomas*. Lacrimal sac tumors may be malignant in nearly 50% of cases. The majority of these are *squamous cell carcinomas*.
- *Dermatochalasis*: Excessive skin and soft tissue in the periorbital region that may be mistaken for a mass lesion. More commonly involves the upper eyelid and may become severe enough to obstruct the patient's vision.
- *Hemangiomas*: May also present as periorbital masses. When present, these are most commonly seen on the medial aspect of the upper lid.

◆ Masses Specific to the Nasal and Perinasal Region

- *Rhinophyma*: Erythematous, irregularly swollen, and bulbous nasal dorsum and tip. This often contains widely dilated pores and follicles and is typically seen in older males.
- *Nasoalveolar cyst (Klestadt cyst)*: Cystic mass arising from the lowermost portion of the nasolacrimal duct or embryonic rests of ductal tissue. Expands subcutaneously and may displace the nasal ala or efface the nasolabial fold. More common in females.
- *Congenital nasal masses*: Typically observed in childhood, though some do not manifest until later in life. All present as midline masses, usually along the nasal dorsum.
  - *Dermoid*: Most common type. These present as cysts or draining fistulas. They may contain hair or skin appendages. Do not transilluminate or enlarge with Valsalva/jugular compression (negative Furstenberg sign).
  - *Encephalocele*: Soft, compressible, blue to purple in color. These transilluminate and have a positive Furstenberg sign.
  - *Glioma*: Firm, noncompressible, pink to red in color. These do not exhibit a Furstenberg sign.

◆ Masses Specific to the Preauricular Region

- *Parotid tumors*: See Chapter 59.

- *Preauricular adenopathy*: Seen in association with infectious and malignant conjunctival pathology. When present in the context of conjunctival inflammation, pretragal adenopathy is referred to as the oculoglandular syndrome of Parinaud.
- *First branchial cleft anomalies*: Suspect in patients with fluctuant swelling in the pretragal area with overlying skin erythema. May be accompanied by otorrhea. Variably present as a fistulous tract to the facial skin. Many will present having previously undergone attempts at excision, only to have the mass recur.
- *Sialadenitis*: Parotitis presents with acute onset of diffuse and painful swelling over the parotid gland. May be unilateral or bilateral. Suspect this in patients who are postoperative or who are otherwise at risk for dehydration and stasis of salivary flow.
- *Pilomatrixoma*: This has a predilection for the preauricular region.

Suggested Reading

Alsaad KO, Obaidat NA, Ghazarian D. Skin adnexal neoplasms, I: An approach to tumours of the pilosebaceous unit. J Clin Pathol 2007;60:129–144

Bailey BJ, Johnson JT, Newlands SD, eds. Head and Neck Surgery–Otolaryngology. 4th ed. Philadelphia: Lippincott Williams & Wilkins; 2006

Cummings CW, ed. Otolaryngology–Head and Neck Surgery, 4th ed. Philadelphia: Mosby; 2005

Habif TP, ed. Clinical Dermatology. 4th ed. Philadelphia: Mosby; 2004

Khanna G, Sato Y, Smith RJ, Bauman NM, Nerad J. Causes of facial swelling in pediatric patients: correlation of clinical and radiologic findings. Radiographics 2006;26:157–171

Sturgis EM, Potter BO. Sarcomas of the head and neck region. Curr Opin Oncol 2003;15:239–252

Yanoff M, ed. Ophthalmology. 2nd ed. Philadelphia: Mosby; 2004

59 Parotid Mass

Erica R. Thaler

The patient presenting with a parotid mass most often relates a history, long or short, of asymptomatic, unilateral, and progressive swelling. Uncommonly, there may be associated symptoms of pain, facial weakness or paralysis, or trismus. These accompanying symptoms usually, but not always, portend a malignant diagnosis. Absence of these symptoms does not confer a benign diagnosis. The vast majority of parotid masses are neoplastic. There are some nonneoplastic processes that may present as discrete lumps and should be considered in the differential diagnosis.

The most helpful ancillary test in the evaluation of a parotid mass is fine needle aspiration (FNA) biopsy. With the caveat in mind that FNA must be done by an experienced cytologist, it is ~85 to 90% accurate in making a histologic diagnosis. This can be quite helpful in treatment planning. Imaging, either computed tomography (CT) or magnetic resonance imaging (MRI), is also useful for treatment planning, particularly in considering the extent of surgery and whether or not facial nerve sacrifice may be likely prior to resection of a parotid malignancy. Definitive diagnosis is confirmed by surgical resection.

◆ Benign Neoplasms

Benign neoplasms comprise 85% of all parotid neoplasms and include the following:

- *Pleomorphic adenoma (benign mixed tumor)*: Most common of benign neoplasms, accounting for 53% of all parotid neoplasms. Pathology includes both an epithelial and a mesenchymal component. These tumors have incomplete encapsulation and pseudopod extension, therefore requiring wide surgical excision for margin, rather than "lumpectomy."
- *Warthin tumor (papillary cystadenoma lymphomatosum)*: Second most common benign neoplasm, accounting for 28% of all parotid neoplasms. Pathology reveals a papillary epithelium, lymphoid stroma, and cystic spaces containing thick, mucoid material. These are most commonly found in older men and have a 10% rate of bilaterality.
- *Oncocytoma*: An uncommon benign neoplasm of the parotid, accounting for less than 1% of all parotid neoplasms. These neoplasms have characteristic eosinophilic cells, packed with mitochondria.
- *Monomorphic adenoma*: Comprises a group of benign adenomatous neoplasms that are rare, nonaggressive, and well encapsulated.

◆ Malignant Neoplasms

Malignant neoplasms comprise 15% of all parotid neoplasms and include the following:

- *Mucoepidermoid carcinoma*: Most common of malignant neoplasms, accounting for 9% of parotid neoplasms. Aggressiveness depends upon grade, which is divided into low, intermediate, or high grade. Lower grade lesions tend to have more mucous cells and may contain mucinous fluid, whereas higher grade lesions have more epidermoid cells and are more solid. Treatment for lower grade and stage lesions is surgical alone, whereas for higher grade and stage lesions, adjuvant radiotherapy is necessary.
- *Adenoid cystic carcinoma*: Second most common malignant neoplasm, but only accounting for less than 1% of parotid neoplasms. It has a variety of histologic appearances, including cribriform, tubular, solid, and cylindromatous. Its cardinal pathological feature is perineural invasion, which can make surgical removal extremely challenging. Therefore, adjuvant radiotherapy is most commonly required. Distant metastasis to lungs and bone is common.
- *Acinic cell carcinoma*: Uncommon parotid malignancy, accounting for less than 1% of parotid neoplasms. Typical pathology includes cells with clear cytoplasm and serous acinar cells. Like Warthin tumors, these cancers may be multicentric. These are the most indolent of parotid malignancies.
- *Carcinoma ex-pleomorphic adenoma*: Rare parotid malignancy that arises out of the pleomorphic adenoma. Pathologically, there are benign components of the neoplasm, within which adenocarcinoma or adenosquamous carcinoma typically arises.
- *Squamous cell carcinoma*: Rarely primary to the parotid. The evaluation should include a careful search for a skin primary, with the parotid lesion representing an intraparotid nodal metastasis.
- *Adenocarcinoma*
- *Lymphoma*
- *Metastasis* from other primary sites

◆ Nonneoplastic Processes

Non-neoplastic processes may sometimes be confused with true neoplasm on presentation. The best way to make this distinction prior to surgery is by FNA. Some such diagnoses in the differential include the following:

- *Reactive adenopathy* of the intraparotid lymph nodes
- *Intraparotid adenopathy associated with indolent infectious organisms* such as histoplasmosis, toxoplasmosis, or tuberculosis

- *Cystic lymphoid hyperplasia* associated with acquired immunodeficiency syndrome. Often multicentric. This diagnosis should be considered in any HIV positive patient.
- *Benign lymphoepithelial lesion*
- *Salivary cyst*
- *Salivary stone*
- *Sarcoidosis*: usually bilateral and diffuse but can present as an asymmetric mass. When associated with uveitis and fever, this is known as *Heerfordt syndrome (uveoparotid fever)*.
- *Benign sialosis (hypertrophy)*: Can rarely masquerade as a mass.

Suggested Reading

Kamal SA, Othman EO. Diagnosis and treatment of parotid tumours. J Laryngol Otol 1997;111:316–321

Pinkston JA, Cole P. Incidence rates of salivary gland tumors: results from a population-based study. Otolaryngol Head Neck Surg 1999;120:834–840

60 Neck Mass

Brian Burkey

The two most important features regarding the evaluation of a neck mass are the age of the patient and the location in the neck. In general, the differential diagnosis of a neck mass can be broken into three main categories—inflammatory, neoplastic, and congenital. For patients under the age of 15, inflammatory etiologies make up the majority of neck masses followed by congenital and neoplastic pathology. Into young adulthood, the frequency of etiologies in these categories remains similar to the pediatric population. As the patient approaches the age of 40, however, the concern for neoplastic etiologies becomes paramount. This is followed by inflammatory and, finally, congenital causes. After the age of the patient is considered, location of the neck mass serves greatly to narrow the differential diagnosis. **Table 60.1** presents a breakdown of the various inflammatory, neoplastic, and congenital neck masses based on location.

This chapter focuses exclusively on presenting symptoms and signs found on the patient's history and physical exam. Used in conjunction with an appreciation of the age and location in which neck masses present, the history and physical can aid the clinician greatly in narrowing the differential diagnosis and deciding on the next step in evaluation or treatment. Possible etiologies are described according to **characteristics** and **associated symptoms**.

◆ Characteristics

Size

Cervical lymph nodes that are under 1 cm are most often the result of a benign, inflammatory process. Lymph nodes greater than 1.5 cm generally require additional evaluation, particularly in the patient with risk factors for malignancy or systemic symptoms.

Mobility

Benign lymph nodes are mobile and not fixed to adjacent structures. Nodes that are immobile are more concerning for a malignant etiology. Assessing mobility is of great importance to the head and neck surgeon, both in determining the risk for cancer and in surgical planning. Masses that are fixed generally indicate more advanced disease and, at times, can even mean unresectability of a mass. A pathognomonic sign for a *thyroglossal duct cyst* on physical exam is vertical motion of a midline mass with swallowing or tongue protrusion. *Carotid and vagal paragangliomas* are mobile side-to-side, but they are immobile in the craniocaudal direction.

Table 60.1 Inflammatory, Neoplastic, and Congenital Neck Masses Based on Location

	Congenital	Inflammatory	Neoplastic	Other
Midline	Thyroglossal duct cyst Dermoid Laryngocele Plunging ranula Ectopic thyroid tissue	Adenitis	Thyroid	Prominent thyroid or cricoid cartilage
Anterior triangle	Branchial cleft cyst Thymic cyst	Thorotrast granuloma Sialadenitis (submandibular, parotid)	Metastatic disease • Face • Oral cavity • Oropharynx • Hypopharynx • Larynx • Thyroid • Nasosinal primary tumors • Carotid body • Glomus • Paraganglioma • Parotid tumors • Submandibular gland tumors	Atherosclerotic carotid artery Prominent hyoid
Posterior triangle	Lymphangioma	Adenitis	Metastatic disease • Thyroid • Nasopharynx • Scalp	
Any	Lymphangioma	Adenitis (viral, bacterial, or granulomatous)	Lymphoma Metastatic thyroid Lipoma	

Consistency

Soft

- *Benign lymph nodes* are soft and fleshy on exam. Cervical lymph nodes that are firm and matted are more concerning for a malignant etiology.
- *Lymphomas* are discrete, rubbery, and nontender. Systemic symptoms should be investigated in young adults with a neck mass concerning for lymphoma.
- *Lymphangiomas* are characteristically soft, doughy, and compressible with indistinct margins. These congenital masses can also be diagnosed by characteristic transillumination and should be evaluated with computed tomography (CT) or magnetic resonance imaging (MRI) to delineate the extent of disease.
- *Hemangiomas* are also soft and compressible but can be distinguished from lymphangiomas by their red or bluish color. They increase in size with straining, and sometimes a bruit may be auscultated. Again, imaging is valuable to appreciate the extent of disease.
- *Lipomas* are soft, ill-defined, subcutaneous masses that generally present in patients over the age of 35. Although CT imaging is helpful in the evaluation of this mass, the characteristic consistency of this lesion is often sufficient for diagnosis.
- *Thyroglossal duct cysts, branchial cleft cysts,* and *thymic cysts* are all congenital lesions that, in their chronic state, are soft and doughy. However, they often present acutely in the setting of a recent infection as a firm, swollen, and tender mass.
- *Ectopic thyroid tissue* can be found anywhere from the base of the tongue to the thyroid cartilage and is soft to palpation.

Firm

- *Lymph nodes* that are firm, fixed, and/or matted are more concerning for a *malignant or atypical inflammatory condition* and require further work-up. Fluctuance and induration are indications of infectious etiology such as *suppurative bacterial lymphadenopathy.*
- *Teratomas* are firm masses that are generally present at birth or in the first year of life. Heterogeneity and calcifications are generally appreciated on CT and MRI.
- *Hematomas* in the anterior neck following trauma (forceps delivery in newborns) are generally firm and in the area of the sternocleidomastoid muscle.
- *Congenital torticollis* is a firm lesion in the area of the sternocleidomastoid with associated range of motion limitation.
- *Neuromas* are firm masses generally found following surgery of the neck (neck dissection). They are very tender, slow-growing masses that are most often associated with the great auricular nerve.
- *Paragangliomas* can be soft but are generally elastic to firm. They are often pulsatile or associated with a bruit. Carotid and vagal paragangliomas are characteristically more mobile in the lateral direction than in the craniocaudal direction. Peripheral nerve manifestations are common.
- *Schwannomas* can be associated with cranial nerves, the sympathetic chain, cervical roots, or the brachial plexus. They are generally firm and have peripheral nerve manifestations.

Hard

- *Thorotrast granulomas* can develop from the antiquated practice of using thorium dioxide as a radiologic contrast (in use from 1920 to 1955). Lesions in the neck are stone hard and are often associated with a lack of carotid system pulsation.
- A prominent *thyroid cartilage, cricoid cartilage, or hyoid bone* can be confused for a neck mass in the thin patient.
- An *atherosclerotic and, sometimes, tortuous carotid artery* can often be concerning for a neck mass. Pulsation and appreciation of neck anatomy help to identify this normal variant in the thin, elderly patient.

Pulsatile

Any neck mass adjacent to the carotid artery can initially seem pulsatile; it is important to distinguish masses that are themselves pulsatile.

- All types of *paraganglomias* can be associated with pulsation. *Carotid paragangliomas (carotid body tumors)* and *vagal paragangliomas* are associated with pulsation and audible bruit on neck exam. The bruit heard with a carotid paraganglioma can decrease with compression of the distal carotid. *Jugular paragangliomas (glomus tumors)* can be associated with pulsatile tinnitus.
- *Hemangiomas* can have a bruit or thrill on exam. These lesions are compressible and may refill slowly as opposed to the rapid refill appreciated with *carotid paragangliomas*.
- *Pseudoaneurysms* are pulsatile lesions that can present after blunt trauma to the neck or after fine needle aspiration or incision and drainage of a lesion near a major vessel.
- *Congenital arteriovenous malformations* are generally found to have a thrill or bruit.

Duration/Progression

Understanding the duration for which a neck mass has been present and whether there is any fluctuation in size or character is extremely important in evaluating a neck mass. When working up a neck mass in an adult, slow increase in size is generally reassuring for a benign process, whereas masses that show rapid enlargement should be considered malignant until proven otherwise. Fluctuation in size with periods of near to complete resolution is particularly indicative of a benign process.

Congenital Masses (Present at or Near Birth)

- *Branchial cysts, thyroglossal duct cysts*, and *thymic cysts* may be appreciated from infancy and evaluated at this early age. However, it is also very common for patients with these congenital neck masses to present later in life as the masses become infected and enlarged in the presence of an upper respiratory infection. In these cases, patients present with a tender, fluid-filled mass in the midline (*thyroglossal duct cyst*) or anterior to the sterno-cleidomastoid (*branchial cleft cyst*) that may be associated with drainage and systemic signs of infection.

- *Hemangiomas* have a characteristic progression. Most are not seen at birth but appear by 6 months of age. They progress rapidly to the age of 12 months, then start slow regression over the next 5 to 8 years.
- *Vascular malformations (lymphatic, venous,and capillary)* are all present at birth and, unlike hemangiomas, grow along with the child.

Slow Growing

- A slowly growing, nontender mass in the submental region is suspicious for a *plunging ranula.*
- *Dermoid cysts* can have a similar presentation as a *plunging ranula* in the submental region.
- *Solitary fibrous tumors* are slow growing, asymptomatic masses that are most often found in the area of the thorax.
- *Neuromas* are tender, slow-growing masses, often found in the posterior triangle after surgery in the neck.
- Other benign lesions in the neck that grow slowly include *paraganglioma* and benign parotid tumors such as *pleomorphic adenoma* and *Warthin tumor.*

Rapidly Enlarging

- Patients with *human immunodeficiency virus (HIV)* or other immunosuppressed conditions can present with rapidly enlarging adenopathy secondary to opportunistic infections or malignancies.
- Congenital neck masses such as *lymphangiomas* or *branchial cleft cysts* can become rapidly enlarging masses in the setting of an infection.
- Again, malignant etiologies should always be considered in the presentation of a rapidly enlarging neck mass.

◆ Associated Symptoms

Fever and Chills

Infection

Infectious etiologies that can present with a neck mass and associated fever include *viral* or *bacterial lympadenopathy, acutely infected congenital lesions, cat-scratch disease, brucellosis, tularemia, mononucleosis,* and *toxoplasmosis. Suppurative bacterial lymphadenopathy* often presents with enlarged lymph nodes associated with fever, tenderness, fluctuation, erythema, and induration of the skin with systemic signs of infection.

Up to 45% of patients with *HIV* present with cervical lymphadenopathy and generalized symptoms as a result of either follicular hyperplasia or atypical infections such as *Mycobacterium tuberculosis* or *Pneumocystis carinii.*

Systemic Inflammatory Conditions

Patients with inflammatory conditions, including *Rosai-Dorfman disease, Kawasaki disease,* and *Castleman disease* (plasma cell variant) can present with a neck mass and associated fever.

Malignancy

A majority of patients with *Hodgkin lymphoma* will present with a neck mass; generally these patients have associated fevers, chills, and, sometimes, night sweats. Fever can also be present in patients with a neck mass secondary to various *solid malignant tumors.*

Pain

Benign masses resulting from inflammatory or infectious etiologies generally elicit pain with palpation. Masses that are painless, with or without manipulation, are often neoplastic in origin; other qualities such as location, duration, size, and mobility can help determine if these painless masses are benign or malignant. However, masses that are painful at all times, even without palpation, are more concerning for a malignancy and should be worked up appropriately.

Voice Change/Stridor

Change in voice in a patient with a neck mass requires comprehensive laryngeal evaluation including fiberoptic laryngoscopy; see Chapters 43 and 45 for more details. Other neck masses that can cause voice change include *paragangliomas* and *thyroid neoplasms* by affecting recurrent laryngeal nerve function.

Dermatologic Findings

Patients with *Kawasaki disease* present acutely with cervical lympadenopathy, erythema, edema, and desquamation of the hands and feet. These patients may also be found to have conjunctival injection and erythema of the lips and oral cavity.

Patients with massive nontender lymphadenopathy of the neck associated with fever and skin nodules should be investigated for *Rosai-Dorfman* disease.

Sweet syndrome (also known as acute febrile neutrophilic dermatosis) presents with fever, elevated white blood count, and erythematous, tender plaques and nodules with dermal inflammation, usually on the neck and face, although the back and arms can also be involved. It is most common in middle-aged women. It may be idiopathic or associated with some medication use, infection, or underlying malignancy.

Neurological Findings

Carotid, vagal, and *jugular paragangliomas* can all present with deficits in cranial nerves IX, X, XI, and XII and/or the sympathetic chain. Common symptoms include dysphagia, hoarseness, upper extremity weakness, or Horner syndrome.

Hoarseness secondary to recurrent laryngeal nerve compression or involvement can be found in patients with *thyroid neoplasms*. Nerve involvement is more concerning for malignant disease.

Suggested Reading

Brousseau VJ, Solares CA, Xu M, Krakovitz P, Koltai PJ. Thyroglossal duct cysts: presentation and management in children versus adults. Int J Pediatr Otorhinolaryngol 2003;67:1285–1290

Gujrathi CS, Donald PJ. Current trends in the diagnosis and management of head and neck paragangliomas. Curr Opin Otolaryngol Head Neck Surg 2005;13:339–342

Mass SC, Dunham ME. Head and neck masses in children. Curr Opin Otolaryngol Head Neck Surg 1997;5:348–354

McGuirt WF. The neck mass. Med Clin North Am 1999;83:219–234

Solem BS, Schrøder KE, Mair IW. Differential diagnosis of a mass in the upper lateral neck. J Laryngol Otol 1981;95:1041–1047

Trible WM, Small A. Thorium dioxide granuloma of the neck: a report of four cases. Laryngoscope 1976;86:1633–1638

61 Thyroid Abnormality

Richard O. Wein and Randal S. Weber

The clinical presentations of symptoms related to thyroid diseases are multiple. This chapter focuses on symptoms related to hypothyroidism, hyperthyroidism, and the presentation of a thyroid mass. Patients with **hypothyroidism** complain of weight gain, fatigue, cold intolerance, hair loss, rough skin quality, constipation, irregularity of menstrual cycle, change in voice, depression, and rarely the development of carpal tunnel syndrome. In contrast those with **hyperthyroidism** note heat intolerance, palpitations, atrial fibrillation, anxiety, unintended weight loss, amenorrhea, hair- and skin-related changes, muscular weakness, and sweating. A thyroid mass may produce symptoms of a foreign body sensation in the throat, dysphagia, hoarseness, hemoptysis, and dyspnea.

◆ Hypothyroidism

Besides surgical removal of the thyroid, other etiologies for hypothyroidism include the following:

- Late stages of *chronic lymphocytic thyroiditis (Hashimoto)*: Autoimmune lymphocytic infiltration of the thyroid gland. Diagnosis may be assisted with assay for antimicrosomal and antithyroglobulin antibodies.
- *Radiation*: External beam radiation therapy or radioactive iodine (I-131) can lead to progressive fibrosis with lack of adequate function of the gland.
- *Subacute thyroiditis*: Triphasic course: hyperthyroidism, followed by hypothyroidism, with return to euthyroid state. Etiologies are typically *viral*, or *granulomatous (de Quervain disease)*.
- *Reidel thyroiditis*: Chronic inflammatory disease of the thyroid characterized by dense "woody" fibrosis that extends beyond the thyroid capsule. Etiology is unclear.
- *Previously diagnosed hypothyroid patient who is noncompliant with thyroid hormone replacement*: Failure in medication compliance will result in an elevated thyroid-stimulating hormone (TSH).
- *Medication related*: *Lithium, amiodarone, interferon-α*, and *interleukin-2* can impair the thyroid's capacity to synthesize thyroid hormone.
- *Severe iodine deficiency*: Iodine is required for the synthesis of triiodothyronine (T3) and tetraiodothyronine (T4). Acute supplementation of large quantities of iodine can result in decreased iodination of thyroglobulin (Wolff-Chaikoff phenomenon) transiently impairing hormone production.
- *Injury to the hypothalamus or pituitary gland*: Surgery, medical condition, or radiation therapy. Patients undergoing surgical procedures for pituitary or intracranial pathology may experience interruption in the function of the hypothalamic–pituitary axis with resultant decrease in TSH production.

- *Infiltrative disorders*: *Amyloidosis* or *sarcoidosis* can result in replacement of the normal thyroid gland, resulting in a change in shape and texture. This may cause dysphagia or airway compression, in addition to hypofunction of the gland.
- *Congenital disorders* of the thyroid: Disorders associated with abnormal descent of the thyroid gland to its normal anatomical position may predispose to hypofunctional status. Disorders of thyroid metabolism may manifest in childhood as *cretinism* or later in life with features consistent with *Pendred syndrome* (goiter and sensorineural hearing loss).

Hyperthyroidism can be caused by the following:

- *Graves disease*: Autoimmune disease typically presenting in young women (age 20 to 40 years) characterized by circulating autoantibodies directed at the thyrotropin receptor. Approximately 25% of patients develop an associated ophthalmopathy.
- *Toxic adenoma*: The presence of a hyperfunctioning "hot" nodule is best assessed by radionuclide I-123 scintigraphy (ie, thyroid scan).
- *Toxic multinodular goiter (Plummer disease)*: More common in iodine-deficient regions. Functional autonomy of multinodularity develops in the setting of a sporadic diffuse goiter and generally presents in older patients.
- *Acute thyroiditis*: Transient painful inflammation of the thyroid gland considered to be viral in etiology.
- *Early stages of subacute or chronic thyroiditis*: Early increases in thyroid hormone levels are usually seen, often with neck pain. Etiologies are subacute granulomatous (de Quervain) thyroiditis or chronic lymphocytic (Hashimoto) thyroiditis. Presentation is usually self-limiting.
- *Overmedication with thyroid hormone replacement*: If a recent TSH level has not been assessed in a patient whose dose of thyroid hormone was recently increased, iatrogenic hyperthyroidism may occur.

A **thyroid mass** can represent the following:

- *Goiter*: Common in iodine-deficient regions, nontender diffuse enlargement may extend below the sternum and result in progressive airway compromise and dysphagia. Pemberton sign (elicited with the arms raised over the head), venous distention with transient worsening of dyspnea, may be seen with extension of goiter into the thoracic inlet.
- *Hemorrhage into an existing benign thyroid nodule*: Acute painful increase in size of a previously existing thyroid nodule is the hallmark presentation. It may occasionally result in airway compromise.
- *Benign thyroid cyst*: Cystic quality may be noted on palpation and confirmed by ultrasonography. Fine needle aspiration is necessary to distinguish from cystic degeneration of a malignancy.
- *Benign thyroid neoplasm*: Difficult to distinguish from malignancy without fine needle aspiration. Vocal cord function should be normal, and associated dysphagia should be limited.
  - Follicular adenoma
- *Thyroid malignancy*: Presentation of the size of the thyroid mass varies and may be associated with regional lymphadenopathy. Pretreatment hoarse-

ness, hemoptysis, and/or dysphagia require assessment for locally invasive disease. The malignancies include the following:

- ○ *Well-differentiated thyroid cancer: papillary and follicular*
- ○ *Medullary thyroid cancer*
- ○ *Anaplastic thyroid cancer*
- ○ *Lymphoma*

- *Metastasis* to the thyroid gland: Infraclavicular neoplasms that may spread to the thyroid include renal cell carcinoma and colon cancer.
- *Parathyroid carcinoma*: Although uncommon, if parathyroid carcinoma presents as a palpable mass associated with the thyroid bed, prognosis is often poor. Calcium is typically greater than 14 mg/dL in this setting.

Suggested Reading

Ark N, Zemo S, Nolen D, Holsinger FC, Weber RS. Management of locally invasive well-differentiated thyroid cancer. Surg Oncol Clin N Am 2008;17:145–155, ix

Devdhar M, Ousman YH, Burman KD. Hypothyroidism. Endocrinol Metab Clin North Am 2007;36:595–615, v

Nayak B, Hodak SP. Hyperthyroidism. Endocrinol Metab Clin North Am 2007;36:617–656, v

Netterville JL, Coleman SC, Smith JC, Smith MM, Day TA, Burkey BB. Management of substernal goiter. Laryngoscope 1998;108(11 Pt 1):1611–1617

Wein RO, Weber RS. Contemporary management of differentiated thyroid carcinoma. Otolaryngol Clin North Am 2005;38:161–178, x

62 Parathyroid Abnormality

Edmund A. Pribitkin and Jeffrey L. Miller

Parathyroid abnormalities may result in a broad range of symptoms secondary to a disruption in the body's calcium ion homeostasis. Primary increases in parathyroid hormone (PTH) secretion typically result in hypercalcemia, whereas secondary increases in PTH secretion may occur as a physiological response to response to depleted vitamin D stores or as a result of severe chronic renal failure. Similarly, primary decreases in PTH secretion (such as those occasionally seen following thyroid or parathyroid surgery) result in hypocalcemia, whereas secondary decreases in PTH secretion may be an appropriate physiological response to the hypercalcemia of malignancy and to hypercalcemia associated with excess ingestion of calcium carbonate (milk-alkali syndrome) or vitamin D intoxication.

◆ Primary Hyperparathyroidism

This is caused by elevated PTH, from *parathyroid adenoma* or *parathyroid hyperplasia*—usually of all four glands, although the degree of enlargement may be asymmetric. With the increased prevalence of serum calcium screening and the availability of serum PTH assays, the majority of parathyroid abnormalities are detected through serological testing rather than as a result of the classic clinical triad of "bones, stones, and groans." The number and severity of signs and symptoms experienced vary with the patient's age at presentation, the rapidity of the change in calcium homeostasis, and the body's compensating mechanism. Although asymptomatic hyperparathyroidism has become the rule, many patients note improvements in quality of life following treatment, indicating that subtle signs and symptoms may have been underappreciated. Conversely, 10 to 20% of hyperparathyroid patients may initially exhibit normal serum calcium concentrations, but they come to the clinician's attention through evaluations for low bone mineral density or other symptoms listed following here.

- **Elevated serum calcium concentration**: Found on routine health screening or during evaluation for an unrelated medical problem leads to discovery of hyperparathyroidism in at least 75% of patients diagnosed with primary hyperparathyroidism. As previously noted, classic symptoms and signs of hypercalcemia, such as radial band keratopathy (deposition of calcium phosphate in the exposed areas of the cornea) are rarely seen. The hypercalcemia of malignancy can be readily distinguished from that of primary hyperparathyroidism through the finding of depressed levels of intact PTH.

Other common causes of hypercalcemia include the *milk-alkali syndrome* seen in postmenopausal women due to *excessive calcium carbonate intake* and *familial hypocalciuric hypercalcemia*, which is characterized by a defective calcium sensing detector in the parathyroid glands and kidneys.

- **"Bones"** (*osteitis fibrosa cystica*): Radiographic signs include brown tumors of the long bones, cystic bone disease of the clavicles, subperiosteal bone resorption of the distal phalanges, and salt and pepper erosions on skull radiographs. These classic radiographic signs are seen in cases of prolonged hyperparathyroidism and hypercalcemia and rarely found in developed countries. Elevated PTH induces a catabolic resorption of cortical bone but protects against resorption at sites of cancellous bone. Consequently, hyperparathyroid patients demonstrate decreased bone density at the distal third of the radius, little or no reduction at the lumbar spine, and an intermediate reduction in the femoral head (mix of cortical and cancellous bone). This is a reversal of the pattern seen in postmenopausal women who generally experience a loss of cancellous bone density due to estrogen deficiency. Interestingly, retrospective and population-based studies on fracture incidence reveal conflicting results regarding the fracture risks associated with primary hyperparathyroidism—these issues are likely to be resolved only through large-scale site-specific prospective studies. Numerous studies have consistently shown that successful parathyroid surgery results in increased bone mineral density. Therefore, the 2002 National Institutes of Health (NIH) Workshop on Asymptomatic Primary Hyperparathyroidism recommended surgery in patients exhibiting bone density at the hip, lumbar spine, or distal radius greater than 2.5 standard deviations below peak bone mass.
- **"Stones"** (*nephrolithiasis*): Hypercalciuria-nephrocalcinosis-renal insufficiency. nephrolithiasis (typically calcium oxalate stones) occurs in 15 to 20% of patients with symptomatic hyperparathyroidism and is viewed as an indication for surgery. Nephrolithiasis may be aggravated by dehydration and by the concomitant use of thiazide diuretics. Hypercalciuria is seen in 40% of patients, and a urinary calcium excretion greater than 400 mg/day in asymptomatic patients eating their normal diet was felt to warrant surgery, according to the 2002 NIH Workshop on Asymptomatic Primary Hyperparathyroidism. Chronic renal insufficiency characterized by decreased renal tubule concentrating function may develop in cases of prolonged and severe hyperparathyroidism, and a creatinine clearance 30% or lower than that of age-matched normal subjects is also viewed as an indication for surgery.
- **"Groans"**

  - **Neuromuscular Dysfunction**: Patients often complain of weakness and fatigue in addition to more specific complaints of paresthesias and muscle cramps. When prolonged and severe, hyperparathyroidism may result in a myopathy characterized by atrophy of type II muscle fibers.
  - **Neuropsychiatric manifestations**: Depressed mood, intellectual weariness, cognitive difficulties, anxiety, and lethargy have all been described in patients with primary hyperparathyroidism, but the prevalence and severity of such symptoms have not been well defined due to the lack

of rigorous studies. Moreover, although numerous studies describe improvements in health-related quality of life following successful parathyroid surgery, few studies demonstrate objective improvements in cognitive function. Accordingly, neuropsychiatric symptoms are not included in the 2002 NIH Workshop on Asymptomatic Primary Hyperparathyroidism as recommended criteria for surgery.

○ **"Abdominal moans"** (*gastrointestinal manifestations*): Vague abdominal pain and constipation have long been associated with hyperparathyroidism.

◆ Primary Hypoparathyroidism

Acquired primary hypoparathyroidism most commonly occurs following thyroid surgery (1 to 2% of patients), parathyroid surgery, and radical neck surgery for head and neck cancer. Primary hypoparathyroidism may also be a feature of *autoimmune diseases* and familial syndromes such as *polyglandular autoimmune syndrome type I (hypoparathyroidism, mucocutaneous candidiasis, adrenal insufficiency)*. Decreased parathyroid hormone secretion typically results in hypocalcemia, which may be further aggravated by hypovitaminosis D. Decreased serum ionized calcium concentrations result in a plethora of neuromuscular, cutaneous, cardiac, and ophthalmological signs and symptoms.

● **Neuromuscular irritability (tetany)**: Patients typically present with circumoral numbness, paresthesias of the hands or feet, and muscle cramps, but they can also complain of fatigue, stiffness, clumsiness, hyperirritability, anxiety, or depression. Hyperexcitability is not limited to peripheral neurons but occurs at all levels of the nervous system and may progress to carpopedal spasm, laryngospasm, and focal or generalized seizures. Greater symptoms are generally associated with a more rapid onset and greater magnitude of hypocalcemia. Symptoms are also aggravated by alkalosis (eg, hyperventilation), epinephrine, hypokalemia, and hypomagnesemia. More chronic symptoms such as the movement disorders of parkinsonism may be seen in longstanding hypocalcemia. A **Trousseau sign** (carpal spasm) is elicited by inflating a sphymomanometer above systolic blood pressure for 3 minutes and occurs because the resultant ischemia increases the excitability of the nerve trunk under the cuff. A **Chvostek sign** (contraction of the ipsilateral facial musculature) is elicited by tapping an area of the face overlying the facial nerve, but a partial Chvostek sign (contraction of the upper lip musculature) may be seen in up to 25% of normal subjects. Although a Trousseau sign is considered more specific than a Chvostek sign, both signs may be absent in patients with hypocalcemia. Patients with severe hypocalcemia may also experience *papilledema*, which improves with calcium repletion.

● **Cutaneous manifestations**: Patients with longstanding hypocalcemia typically exhibit dry, puffy, and coarse skin and may have coarse, brittle hair and brittle nails with characteristic transverse grooves. All of these manifestations typically correct with calcium repletion. Mucocutaneous candidiasis is a feature of polyglandular autoimmune syndrome type I and persists despite restoration of normocalcemia.

- **Cataracts**: Frequently result from chronic hypoparathyroid-induced hypocalcemia, but their progression may be arrested by restoration of normocalcemia.
- **Cardiovascular disease**: Acute hypocalcemia following parathyroid surgery has been associated with *prolongation of the QT interval* in the electrocardiogram and with reversible myocardial dysfunction.

◆ Parathyroid Masses

Parathyroid Adenoma

Parathyroid adenomas represent over 90% of parathyroid masses and account for 80 to 88% of primary hyperparathyroidism. A thyroid scan using technetium-99 (^{99m}Tc) sestamibi in combination with a subtraction iodine-123 (^{123}I) may have a predictive value of 90 to 100% for solitary adenomas but less accurately detects multiple involved glands.

Parathyroid Carcinoma

Patients with parathyroid carcinomas are more likely to exhibit the symptoms of primary hyperparathyroidism noted earlier, including marked hypercalcemia and the classic triad of "bones, stones, and groans." Serum PTH levels typically exceed four times the upper level of normal, and patients may present in parathyroid crisis. Radiographic studies may reveal invasion of contiguous structures and either lymph node or distant metastases. Unlike benign parathyroid adenomas, both sporadic and familial parathyroid carcinomas exhibit intragenic mutations of the *HRPT2* gene on chromosome 1. Surgical management involves en bloc resection with avoidance of capsular violation or tumor spillage as well as management of cervical metastases. Unfortunately, the recurrence rate is high, and both radiation and chemotherapy are generally ineffective in controlling disease. Medical therapy generally revolves around controlling hypercalcemia, the carcinoma's primary source of morbidity and mortality.

Parathyroid Cysts

Parathyroid cysts may present as neck or mediastinal masses and are generally nonfunctional. Computed tomography, magnetic resonance imaging, ultrasonography, and 99m-technetium sestamibi scans are of limited utility in distinguishing parathyroid cysts from cystic thyroid masses, thyroglossal duct cysts, and branchial cleft cysts. Parathyroid cysts are diagnosed by assaying PTH levels on fine needle aspiration of cyst contents. Such aspiration may also prove curative. Rarely, functional parathyroid cysts present with severe hypercalcemia—

such pseudocysts likely represent cystic degeneration of parathyroid adenomas or carcinomas.

Suggested Reading

Agus AS, Fuleihan GH. Preoperative Localization and Surgical Therapy of Primary Hyperparathyroidism. Available at: www.uptodateonline.com

Bilezikian JP, Potts JT Jr, Fuleihan Gel-H, et al. Summary statement from a workshop on asymptomatic primary hyperparathyroidism: a perspective for the 21st century. J Clin Endocrinol Metab 2002;87:5353–5361

Fuleihan GH. Parathyroid Carcinoma. Available at: www.uptodateonline.com

Ippolito G, Palazzo FF, Sebag F, Sierra M, De Micco C, Henry JF. A single-institution 25-year review of true parathyroid cysts. Langenbecks Arch Surg 2006;391:13–18

63 Neck Pain/Torticollis

Kristin B. Gendron

Neck pain and torticollis (or "wry neck") can be a result of disease of the musculoskeletal system or multiple other organ systems and may occur separately or concurrently. Degenerative disease of the cervical spine, disk herniation, and muscular strain are common causes of neck pain, but it is important to keep in mind that infectious, rheumatologic, and neoplastic etiologies among others can cause similar symptoms. Important factors in distinguishing the origin and type of neck pain include history pertaining to the onset of the pain, severity, timing (daytime vs nocturnal), and associated symptoms (fevers, chills, neurological symptoms, throat pain).

Torticollis in adults is often due to abnormalities of the atlantoaxial (C1–C2) joint or adjacent tissues, in which case it is usually accompanied by neck pain. However, torticollis may also be due to a generalized or focal dystonia, pharmacological effects, or other causes.

Neck pain that is **aching** in quality, **worse with activity**, and associated with **decreased range of motion** can be caused by the following:

- *Cervical spondylosis (cervical osteoarthritis)*: May present as neck pain alone, with radiculopathy (arm pain due to nerve root compression, often relieved by placing the affected hand on the head), or with cervical myelopathy (loss of manual dexterity, palmar paresthesias, subtle gait disturbance, possible urinary incontinence)
- *Cervical disk herniation*: Presents in younger patients and may cause cervical radiculopathy
- *Cervical strain* (muscular or ligamentous): Presents with nonradicular, nonfocal neck pain anywhere from the skull base to the cervicothoracic junction. It may be associated with muscle spasms, occipital headaches, fatigue, irritability, and sleep disturbance.
- *Flexion-extension injury* ("whiplash"). Most commonly after car accident. Symptoms may present minutes to hours after injury.
- *Cervical spine fracture*: May be posttraumatic or secondary to tumors. Injuries causing fractures usually involve axial compression, hyperextension, or flexion-type trauma. It is important to consider malignancies that can metastasize to bone (breast, prostate, lung, kidney, stomach).
- *Atlantoaxial subluxation* with or without basilar invagination (brainstem compression). This may be seen with *trisomy 21 (Down syndrome), rheumatoid arthritis,* and *congenital odontoid anomalies.* May present as untoward amount of flexion, posterior skull pain, torticollis, and numbness and paresthesias in the ulnar distribution.

Neck pain with **morning stiffness that improves with activity** can be caused by the following:

- Rheumatologic disease: Autoimmune disease causing inflammation and eventual ersion of synovial membranes, ligaments, and cartilages.

  ○ *Fibromyalgia*: Pain tends to be more diffuse, though patients often have multiple tender points throughout their body.
  ○ *Polymyalgia rheumatica* (neck, shoulder girdle, and pelvic girdle pain and stiffness): Important to keep in mind because up to 15% of cases are associated with *temporal arteritis* (eg, *giant cell arteritis*), which warrants aggressive therapy with high-dose steroids due to the risk of blindness.
  ○ *Spondyloarthropathies* (ankylosing spondylitis, Reiter syndrome/reactive arthritis, psoriatic arthritis, enteropathic arthritis): Cervical spine involvement is uncommon and is generally preceded by lumbar and thoracic disease, though early involvement may be seen in women.

- *Crowned dens syndrome* (microcrystalline deposition in the cruciform ligament): Causes acute and chronic cervical pain and morning stiffness. Should be in the differential diagnosis for polymyalgia rheumatica. Computed tomographic findings are subtle, so high-resolution imaging of C1–C2 is recommended.

Neck pain in association with **dysphagia, sore throat** can arise from the following:

- *Cervical lymphadenitis* or *deep neck space infection* (parapharyngeal or retropharyngeal) secondary to pharyngitis
- *Carotid sheath infection*
- *Lemierre syndrome*: Pharyngitis followed by internal jugular vein thrombosis and septic emboli, caused by *Fusobacterium necrophorum.*
- *Eagle syndrome*: Elongated styloid process associated with oropharyngeal pain, dysphagia, foreign body sensation, and referred otalgia.
- *Retropharyngeal calcific tendinitis*: Calcium deposition in the longus colli tendon leading to acute odynophagia, neck pain, and retropharyngeal soft tissue edema.

Symptoms that should raise suspicion of a dangerous etiology of neck pain warranting expedited evaluation include nocturnal pain, unrelenting pain, fever, night sweats, chills, weight loss, and history of intravenous drug use or immunocompromised status (including sickle cell anemia).

Neck pain that is **nocturnal, not relieved by rest**, and associated with **constitutional symptoms** may be a red flag for a neoplasm:

- *Spinal bony tumor*: Pain secondary to spinal tumors is often poorly localized and not relieved by rest. Tenderness and muscle spasms are absent. These tumors may present as pathological fractures.
- Primary neoplasm

  ○ *Malignant: Chordoma, multiple myeloma, Ewing sarcoma* (young adults), *osteogenic sarcoma* (usually in children), *chondrosarcoma, fibrosarcoma, lymphoma, round cell sarcoma, malignant giant cell tumor*
  ○ *Benign: Osteoid osteoma, osteoblastoma, osteochondroma, osteoclastoma, aneurysmal bone cyst, hemangioma, eosinophilic granuloma*

- *Metastatic* (more common than primary tumors): Breast, prostate, lung, kidney, stomach

  o *Spinal cord tumor: Ependymoma, astrocytoma, hemangioblastoma* (associated with *von Hippel-Lindau disease*)
  o Tumors with **referred pain to the neck**: *Pancoast tumor of the lung*—look for Horner syndrome, smoking history, shoulder and arm pain in the ulnar nerve distribution

- *Osteomyelitis*: The cervical spine is the least common site for vertebral osteomyelitis. When present, it is usually due to hematogenous spread of bacteria from other sites (oral cavity, oropharynx, genitourinary, respiratory, or skin sources). Most common bacteria are *Staphylococcus aureus,* followed by *Streptococcus* and enteric gram-negative rods. *Candida* and *Pseudomonas* are seen in intravenous drug users. *Tuberculous osteomyelitis* (Pott disease) is also rarely seen.

Other causes of neck pain include the following:

- *Retained needles* may cause chronic pain in intravenous drug users.
- Neurologic: *Occipital neuralgia, brachial plexopathy*
- Skeletal: *Diffuse idiopathic skeletal hyperostosis (DISH), gout*
- *Carotidynia*: Tenderness, swelling, and increased pulsations over the carotid; should be self-limited and under 2 weeks in duration.
- Vascular: *Carotid* or *vertebral artery dissection*
- *Referred neck pain*: Cardiovascular (coronary artery disease, aortic disease), gastrointestinal (hiatal hernia/diaphragmatic irritation, gall bladder, pancreas), temporomandibular joint, central nervous system (posterior fossa tumors)

Neck pain with **torticollis**: Many of the previously mentioned disease processes can lead to torticollis. Inflammation of the atlantoaxial or upper cervical joints due to infectious or rheumatologic disease can cause ligamentous laxity and thus torticollis. Alteration of skeletal anatomy by masses or trauma can have a similar effect. Etiologies of neck pain and torticollis in adults include the following:

- Infection

  o *Grisel syndrome*: Atlantoaxial subluxation seen with nasopharyngitis or postadenoidectomy (uncommon in adults)
  o *Retropharyngeal* or *parapharyngeal space abscess*
  o *Epidural abscess*
  o *Carotid sheath infection*
  o *Cervical osteomyelitis*

- Neoplasm

  o *Spinal bony tumor*: See page 348.
  o *Spinal cord tumor*: See above.

- *Trauma*
- Rheumatologic disease: *Rheumatoid arthritis, ankylosing spondylitis*

- Musculoskeletal disorders (*see atlantoaxial subluxation, earlier*): *Trisomy 21, Marfan syndrome, congenital odontoid anomalies*

Torticollis is difficult to completely separate from neck pain because torticollis itself generally causes discomfort and pain. However, in addition to the disease processes already discussed, there are cases in which torticollis is the primary symptom and pain is secondary to muscle spasm. The etiology of torticollis can be musculoskeletal or nonmusculoskeletal.

Torticollis of **muscular origin**:

- *Spasmodic torticollis*: Spasms in the cervical musculature may occur as an isolated *dystonia* or in the setting of *generalized dystonia*.
- *Iatrogenic/drug-induced torticollis*: Extrapyramidal effects of neuroleptic medications. *Acute dystonia (buccolingual crisis, acute torticollis, oculogyric crisis, opisthotonos)* may occur any time during treatment.

Torticollis of **skeletal origin**: In most cases, neck pain is a prominent symptom. Remember that new-onset torticollis should prompt an evaluation for spinal tumors.

- *Atlantoaxial disease*
- *Trauma*
- *Spinal bony tumor*: See page 348.

Torticollis of **nonmusculoskeletal origin**:

- *Infection*: See page 349.
- *Trauma*
- *Neoplasm*: See page 349.
- *Rheumatologic disease*: See pages 347, 349.
- Neurologic: *Sellar tumor/optic chiasmal process, ocular torticollis* (altered head positioning to compensate for ocular dysfunction), *Chiari I malformation* (teens or early adulthood)

Suggested Reading

Meleger AL, Krivickas LS. Neck and back pain: musculoskeletal disorders. Neurol Clin 2007;25:419–438

Nakano KK. Neck pain. In: Kelley's Textbook of Rheumatology. Harris Jr. ED, Budd RC, Firestein G, et al. (eds). 7th ed. Philadelphia: Saunders; 2005

64 Neck Swelling/Edema/Erythema

Ray Gervacio Blanco

When confronted with a patient who has any combination of neck erythema, edema, and tenderness, obtaining a detailed history will narrow down the differential diagnosis. The important points that must be elicited in the history are the following: respiratory symptoms, localized pain, referred pain, recent dental procedures, dental infection, tooth pain, upper respiratory tract infection, recent or previous blunt or penetrating trauma, previous neck surgery, previous carotid surgery or stenting, odynophagia, dysphagia, clinical signs of sepsis, foreign body, instrumentation, and immunosuppression (HIV, cancer, steroids, chemotherapy).

During the physical examination, the following are important points to check: asymmetry of the neck, associated mass, displacement and or compressions of structures, trismus, presence of fluctuant mass, nerve deficits, fever, respiratory symptoms, previous surgery, venous catheters, and trauma.

The airway should always be evaluated and should be secured prior to proceeding to surgical drainage or sending the patient for computed tomography/magnetic resonance imaging (CT/MRI). Although CT and MRI show good anatomical details in regard to structures involved and the extent of the pathology, other imaging such as Panorex may assist in identifying dental infection. Lateral cervical films can evaluate retropharyngeal and pretracheal neck spaces, and a sonogram may be able to guide needle aspiration.

There is no identifiable cause in 22% of deep neck infections, and familiarity with the common oral pathogens and your institution's antibiotic sensitivity patterns is important in choosing the appropriate antibiotics. Appropriate referral to infectious disease service, vascular surgery, or other subspecialties should be done if clinically indicated.

The differential diagnosis for patients with erythema, edema, and tenderness of the neck can vary widely. For simplicity, this chapter divides patients into groups based upon involvement of superficial or deep spaces, and then the face/head, upper neck, and lower neck. Finally, other causes of erythema, edema, and tenderness are considered.

◆ Infection, Superficial—Face or Neck

- *Folliculitis*: Will present as a "whitehead" infection at the base of the hair.
- *Carbuncle*: Skin infection that often involves a group of hair follicles and may coalesce to form a mass under the skin.

- *Cellulitis*: Will present as a swollen, red area of skin that feels warm and tender and may spread quickly. Lymph nodes that drain the region may be enlarged.
- *Impetigo*
  - ○ *Nonbullous impetigo*: Will present as a small blister that develops honeycomb-like crusting.
  - ○ *Bullous impetigo*: Results in bulla formation secondary to the *Staphylococcus* toxin, which results in separation of the epidermis from the underlying layers.
- *Abscess*: Presents with erythema of the overlying skin with a tender and fluctuant mass just below. Deeper abscess may not have a fluctuant mass but may present with erythema and tenderness only.
- *Lymphadenitis*: May present with erythema overlying a swollen, tender lymph node or over the region of lymphatic drainage area.

◆ Infection, Deep Tissue

With deep tissue infections, the clinical presentation should be correlated to anatomical structures and neck spaces. Although deep neck infections can be classified based on the anatomical space, the symptomatology of one infected anatomical space may be similar or may overlap with infection in another space. The severity of the infection may also depend on the duration and the extension of the disease to other areas. For this reason, imaging is an important tool in localizing the site of infection, determining possible avenues of extension, and planning the surgical approach. In radiated patients, tenderness without skin erythema or a fluctuant mass may be the only findings due to the significant changes induced by treatment.

◆ Face and Head Areas

- *Buccal space infection*: May present with cheek tenderness.
- *Odontogenic infection*: The specific tooth may determine the location and extent of symptoms and findings.
- *Masseteric infection*: Often associated with trismus.
- *Temporal space infection*: Can present with proptosis and unilateral facial swelling.
- *Pterygoid space infection*: Can cause additional symptoms of dysphagia and odynophagia.
- *Parotid space infection*

◆ Suprahyoid Tissue

- *Submandibular sialadenitis/sialolithiasis*: Examination may reveal purulence from the submandibular duct.
- *Lymphadenitis*
- *Submandibular abscess or infection*

Involvement of this region can be an extension from a sublingual space infection:

- *Peritonsillar space infection*: Presentation typically includes swelling in the pharynx, soft palate, and uvular deviation, with trismus and odynophagia.
- *Lateral pharyngeal space infection*: Similar symptoms as peritonsillar infection. It may be primary or an extension from infections in other areas, including the pharynx, parotid, mastoid/middle ear, masticator space, and submandibular or sublingual spaces.
- *Odontogenic infection*
- *Ludwig angina*: May include significant swelling in the floor of the mouth, "brawny edema."
- *Necrotizing fasciitis*

◆ Infrahyoid Tissue and Anterior Visceral Space

- *Infected thyroglossal duct cyst*
- *Infected dermoid cyst*
- *Infected sebaceous cyst*
- *Lymphadenitis*
- *Acute suppurative thyroiditis*
- *Pyriform sinus or upper aerodigestive tract fistula/perforation*
- *Trauma/instrumentation/surgery*: Exam may include crepitus over the neck.
- *Laryngopyocele*
- *Laryngeal cancer* with superinfection, or surrounding inflammatory response

◆ Length of the Neck (Supra- and Infrahyoid)

- *Retropharyngeal space infection*: May be related to trauma, instrumentation, infection, or suppurative adenopathy. The patient will often have odynophagia, nasal obstruction and regurgitation, dyspnea, fever, tachypnea, and bulging of the posterior oropharyngeal wall.
- *Prevertebral space infection*: Same presentation as with the retropharyngeal space, but the prevertebral space has no midline raphe so radiologic findings will be midline.

- *Vertebral osteomyelitis*
- *Paraspinous abscess*: May descend into mediastinum.
- *Pott abscess*
- *Pharyngeal trauma*
- *Spine trauma*
- *Infection or anastomotic leak* after aerodigestive tract surgery
- *Carotid sheath infection*: Symptoms may include fever, chills, neck erythema, neck induration, tender sternocleidomastoid muscle, nuchal rigidity, contralateral torticollis, ipsilateral Horner syndrome, vocal cord paralysis, internal jugular vein thrombosis, carotid artery rupture, and sepsis.
- *Infected pseudoaneurysm of a great vessel*: May include a bruit over the area and possible neurological symptoms.
- *Mycotic aneurysm*: Fungal infection within the vessel wall. Symptoms may include tenderness over the carotid region, and the patient can present with symptoms of septic emboli.
- *Internal jugular vein thrombosis (Lemierre syndrome)*: Often caused by intravenous drug abuse or other vascular abnormalities. These patients often present with a palpable cord in the neck, along with increased intracranial pressure, fever, and sepsis.
- *Infected fourth branchial cleft cyst*
- *Infected tumor* or fistula-related to tumor
- *Superior vena cava syndrome*: Presents with neck and facial edema, with upper extremity edema and dyspnea; caused by malignancy, infection, and indwelling catheters.

Suggested Reading

Cummings CW, Flint PW, Harker LA, et al. Deep neck infection. In: Cummings CW, ed. Otolaryngology–Head and Neck Surgery. 4th ed. Philadelphia: Mosby; 2005:2515–2524

Kaviani A, Ouriel K, Kashyap VS. Infected carotid pseudoaneurysm and carotid-cutaneous fistula as a late complication of carotid artery stenting. J Vasc Surg 2006;43:379–382

Mueller DK, Dacey MJ. Internal jugular vein thrombosis. eMedicine. 2006; http://emedicine.medscape.com/article/461577-overview

Papadoulas S, Zampakis P, Liamis A, Dimopoulos PA, Tsolakis IA. Mycotic aneurysm of the internal carotid artery presenting with multiple cerebral septic emboli. Vascular 2007;15:215–220

Wang CP, Ko JY, Lou PJ. Deep neck infection as the main initial presentation of primary head and neck cancer. J Laryngol Otol 2006;120:305–309

65 Fistula (Neck or Face)

Paul J. Del Casino and Jason G. Newman

Fistulas in the neck and face can arise from a variety of sources and present with a multiplicity of symptoms. Alternatively, patients can have fistulas and remain largely unaware of their existence. Once a fistula is suspected by the clinician, a key method for establishing a diagnosis is to categorize them into congenital and inflammatory/infectious etiologies. A thorough patient history is crucial because fistulas are largely slow to develop and are often caused by events in the relatively distant past. Associated infectious symptoms such as fever or previous trauma to the area, as well as a history of similar occurrences as far back as childhood, can be helpful to the diagnostic process.

Imaging for fistulas from congenital sources by computed tomography (CT) or magnetic resonance imaging (MRI) is important when considering treatment. CT may be a useful method for visualizing the sinus or fistulous tract and for evaluating the extent of the lesion. Ultrasonography and fine needle aspiration biopsy may be useful in determining the cystic nature of the lesion in the cases of branchial cleft and thyroglossal duct cysts.

◆ Congenital Fistulas

- *Branchial cleft cysts*
  - *First branchial abnormalities* are usually detected in childhood and may present with mucoid discharge from sinus openings above or below the mandible or in the external auditory canal.
  - *Second branchial cleft cysts* are among the most common of congenital neck masses, usually occurring in the carotid triangle just below the angle of the mandible and accounting for ~90% of branchial cleft anomalies. They are bilateral in ~2 to 3% of cases. If infected, they may form a deep neck abscess or a draining fistula.
  - *Third or fourth branchial clefts* are rare but may also present as a fistulous tract into the lower neck.

- *Thyroglossal duct cysts*: Most thyroglossal duct cysts are found at the level of the thyrohyoid membrane, under the deep cervical fascia. They are remnants of the embryonic thyroglossal duct and may occur anywhere from the base of the tongue to the thyroid gland. They are midline or just off the midline and move up and down upon swallowing. Occasionally, a sinus tract is present in the midline without a visible cyst. This midline sinus tract represents the remnant of the thyroglossal duct. It may open into the region of the hyoid or lower, above the sternal notch.

- *Dermoid or sebaceous cyst*: Dermoid cysts are often superficial in the nasal region of the face and present in childhood. They are not attached to overlying skin but may invade deeper structures. They often have a rubbery feel. An inflammatory reaction can occur if the dermoid cyst is disrupted. Both dermoid and sebaceous cysts can form fistulas (usually superficially to the skin) when infected.

◆ Infectious Fistulas

Fistulas caused by infectious or inflammatory etiologies are more common than congenital anomalies. History of prior infection or trauma to the area is critical because many fistulas are a result of an inadequately treated cutaneous infection.

- *Abscess*: Abscesses remain one of the most common causes of cutaneous fistulas. The variety of circumstances under which abscesses and associated fistulae may arise warrant a meticulous history to determine the instigating factor. Often arising from a simple staphylococcal cellulitis, abscesses can form fistulas to adjacent areas if left untreated or following an incomplete incision and drainage. Fascial-plane infections, deep neck space infections, and osteomyelitis can cause cutaneous fistulas. Fascial-plane infections often begin as cellulitis and progress to fluctuant abscess formation. Fistula formation is more likely to occur in the presence of an abscess with existing undermining or sinus tracking subcutaneously, so proper tracking of the abscess with a swab or other probe is necessary. Folliculitis can be a precipitating factor, as can minor outpatient cosmetic procedures, certain hair-removal techniques, and general hygiene.
- *Acute sialadenitis/parotitis*: Acute bacterial infection of the salivary glands can rarely cause cutaneous fistulae. Viral sialadenitis is less common in adults than in children and usually presents in conjunction with an overlying viral infection such as mumps, coxsackievirus, Epstein-Barr virus (EBV), or human immunodeficiency virus (HIV). In bacterial sialadenitis, the parotid gland is most commonly affected and often presents with regional lymphadenopathy.
- *Cosmetic implant/hardware rejection*: Acute, subacute, or chronic rejection can occur following reconstructive or cosmetic surgery involving foreign body implants. Although hardware used in traumatic repair is relatively nonreactive, failure of cosmetic implants or perioperative infection coupled with natural shearing forces of many repair sites (nose, chin, jaw, etc.) can lead to dermal breakdown and fistula formation. As with most rejections, erythema, drainage, and pain at the site are noted, with possible extrusion of the implant.
- *Periapical dental abscess*: Acute pulpitis spreading beyond the tooth apex causes pus to accumulate and pressure to increase periapically. Over time, spontaneous drainage may occur through the mandible/maxilla adjacent to the root. Fistulas form near the roof of the mouth or on the gum and are difficult to detect. A fistula from a subperiosteal infection reaches the surface

of the mouth, presenting as a small pimple. This pimple usually ruptures to form an opening. Infection can spread to the skin if it is the path of least resistance. Fistulas usually occur in settings of periodontal decay, but recent dental work and immunocompromised status are also precipitating factors.

- *Salivary gland surgery/trauma*: Trauma, microorganisms, neoplasms, xerostomia, immunosuppression, and malnutrition are usually the cause of infections that result in fistulas from salivary glands. Iatrogenic causes include surgery and radiation therapy to the parotid. Several cases have been reported of fistulas arising from sialoliths migrating through adjacent tissue from the salivary gland. Traumatic fistulas may be due to injury or surgical repair in areas where mucosal and epidermal surface epithelia line the fistula wall. No inflammation is associated with this type of fistula unless an infection develops. In addition to penetrating injuries and fistulas as a result of skin breakdown, fistulas can form postoperatively from procedures such as parotidectomy and rhytidectomy. Postoperative sialoceles and fistulas draining saliva are complications associated with these surgeries. Most do not become infected and resolve with conservative therapy in a few weeks. Fistulas can also result from surgery of the mouth or upper aerodigestive tract. In the absence of a postoperative infection with tunneling and sinus formation, fistulae can be caused by exposure of operative sites to normal salivary secretions and their enzymatic activity. Fistulas often occur through an existing incision. Reconstructive surgery and trauma can also lead to salivary fistulas, or fistulas created from inflammation and pressure or necrosis of traumatized tissue.
- *Neoplasms*: Neoplastic fistulas result from the penetration of a neoplasm from the oral cavity, nasal cavity, sinuses, and larynx to the outlying skin. Fistulas are most commonly caused by squamous cell carcinoma and have a poor prognosis because of skin lymphatic drainage.
- *Lymphadenopathy*: Most lymph node pathology does not lead to fistula formation, so the differential list is small compared with other etiologies. Benign inoculation lymphoreticulosis or cat scratch disease should be considered in the differential diagnosis of sinus tracts from lymph nodes.
- *Scrofula*: More precisely, *cervical tuberculous* or *nontuberculous lymphadenopathy*, is most often observed in immunocompromised patients. The vast majority of scrofula cases in adults are caused by *Mycobacterium tuberculosis*, which is more unusual in children. The rest are caused by nontuberculous *Mycobacterium* (NTM) (eg, *Mycobacterium scrofulaceum*). With the marked decrease of tuberculosis in the second half of the twentieth century, scrofula became a very rare disease. With the appearance of acquired immunodeficiency syndrome (AIDS), however, it has shown a resurgence, and presently affects ~5% of severely immunocompromised patients. The most common presentation is a chronic, painless mass in the neck, which is persistent and usually grows with time. The mass is referred to as a "cold abscess" because there is no accompanying local color or warmth and the overlying skin acquires a violaceous rather than an erythematous color. NTM infections do not usually show other notable systemic symptoms. However, tuberculous adenitis is often accompanied by other symptoms of the disease, such as chills, fever, weight loss, and malaise in about half of

patients. As the lesion progresses, skin becomes adherent to the mass and may rupture, forming a sinus or an open wound.

◆ Other Causes of Fistulae

- *Osteomyelitis*: Chronic osteomyelitis of the paranasal sinus or facial bone is a rare complication of sinusitis. The obstructed secretions in the sinus may result in pressure necrosis, resulting in a persistently discharging fistula. In some cases, and largely dependent on individual anatomy, the fistula can drain cutaneously (frontal sinuses), but cases of fistulas draining into the oral cavity and orbit have been reported. Oroantral fistulas involve the maxillary sinus.
- *Radiation treatment*: Radiation is the primary cause of delayed fistulas, which can occur from 1 month to many years after the initial radiation treatment. Osteoradionecrosis and soft tissue fibrosis predispose the patient to fistula formation, with a direct correlation between radiation dosage and prevalence of fistula formation. Radiation therapy has been used to treat fistulas of the parotid into the external acoustic canal, but it is far more commonly used as postoperative cancer treatment. The immunocompromised status of many uncured cancer patients increases the possibility of fistula formation further out from the end of radiation therapy as the disease progresses.
- *Facial and upper aerodigestive tract surgery*
- *Trauma*

Suggested Reading

Bronstein SL, Clark MS. Sublingual gland salivary fistula and sialocele. Oral Surg Oral Med Oral Pathol 1984;57:357–361

Calhoun KH, Eibling DE, Wax MK. Expert Guide to Otolaryngology. Philadelphia: ACP; 2001

Cantatore JL, Klein PA, Lieblich LM. Cutaneous dental sinus tract, a common misdiagnosis: a case report and review of the literature. Cutis 2002;70:264–267

Lalwani AK. Current Diagnosis and Treatment—Otolaryngology: Head and Neck Surgery. New York: McGraw-Hill; 2008

IX Differential Diagnosis of Pediatric Skin, Face, and Neck Disorders

Section Editors: *Max M. April and Robert F. Ward*

66 Rash in Children

Adele K. Evans

The symptom of facial or neck rash requires careful description to approach the proper treatment plan. Rashes are described clinically by the **type, shape, margination, arrangement** and **distribution** of the lesions.

◆ Type

Rash types may be **papular** (consisting of fine raised lesions) or **macular** (consisting of wide, flat lesions). They may be restricted to an allergic-type **wheal-and-flare**. The type may be **nodular** (solid) or **cystic**. **Pustular** lesions consist of papule-like lesions filled with pus, whereas **vesicular** lesions are nonpustular and contain small volumes of liquid, and **bullous** lesions are blister-like and contain large volumes of liquid. The lesions may alternatively be erosive and **ulcerated**, scaly and **hyperkeratotic**, or heavily scarred and referred to as **sclerotic**, or the skin structures may be destroyed by the process characterized best as **atrophic**. The color, feel on palpation, response to heat or cold, tenderness, and tissue mobility are also used to characterize lesions.

◆ Shape

Descriptors of shape include **round, oval, polygonal, polycyclic, annular** (ring-shaped), **iris** (target), **serpiginous** (snakelike), or **umbilicated**.

◆ Margination

Margination describes the edges of the lesions, such as well defined versus ill defined.

◆ Arrangement

Arrangement describes grouped lesions such as **herpetiform** or **linear** patterns versus **disseminated** patterns with scattered discrete appearance or diffuse involvement.

◆ Distribution

Distribution descriptors include descriptors of *extent*, such as isolated, localized, regional, or generalized. Pattern descriptors include symmetrical, exposed areas, pressure sites, intertriginous areas, follicular localization, or random. There are many characteristic lesion patterns that are helpful descriptors as well, such as Lyme disease or Rocky Mountain spotted fever, varicella or erythema multiforme.

For differential diagnosis, we have grouped rashes based on associated findings and location.

◆ Rash with Fever

Rashes appearing on the face and presenting with fever include *measles, rubella*, and *varicella* (**Fig. 66.1**), although these are all less frequent today because of widespread vaccination. However, *fifth disease* remains common and is also known as slapped cheek disease due to the characteristic presentation of the cheek rash. This self-limited infection is caused by parvovirus B19, and is also called *erythema infectiosum*. It presents with a distinctive red cheek rash, which then spreads to the trunk, arms, and legs (**Fig. 66.2**). The rashes of *Rocky Mountain spotted fever* and *Lyme disease* are characteristic in appearance, endemic in certain regions, and associated with characteristic systemic findings, including fever. *Erysipelas* (a specific type of cellulitis caused by group A β-hemolytic

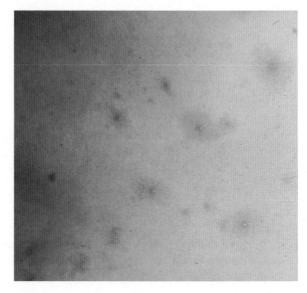

Fig. 66.1 Varicella's raindrop-on-a-rose-petal rash appears similar to the bite from a fire ant.

(Courtesy of Dr. Daniel Krowchuk.)

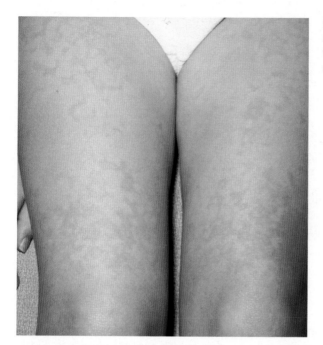

Fig. 66.2 Erythema infectiosum, the rash associated with fifth disease.

(Courtesy of Dr. Daniel Krowchuk.)

Streptococcus pyogenes) and other types of *facial cellulitis* also present with facial erythema, edema, and sometimes fever. Cellulitis may be a consequence of a dental infection, a sinus infection, or a secondary infection at the site of an underlying skin condition or excoriated insect bite, or it may spread from a nasal or scalp *folliculitis*. The classic rash of *lupus erythematosus* is a butterfly pattern across the midface, or "malar erythema." *Dermatomyositis*, which is rare in children, presents with a classic "heliotrope" rash that appears bright red or violaceous on the face, neck, and chest as though one were staring at the sun.

◆ Rash without Fever

Oral/Perioral Location

Herpetic blisters (**Fig. 66.3**) due to primary herpes simplex eruptions are common in young children. They result from exposures to older relatives with disease, to other children with disease, or to contaminated fomites, particularly in the toddler age group and the day-care setting. *Pemphigus* may present with multiple bullous lesions also present in the mouth. Ulcerative lesions such as *aphthous ulcers* may be idiopathic or may occur in association with *Crohn disease* or *Behçet syndrome*. Lips can be extensively involved in *erythema multiforme, Stevens-Johnson syndrome, graft-versus-host disease*, and *chemotherapeutic agent exposures*.

Fig. 66.3 Herpes labialis.
(Courtesy of Dr. Daniel Krowchuk.)

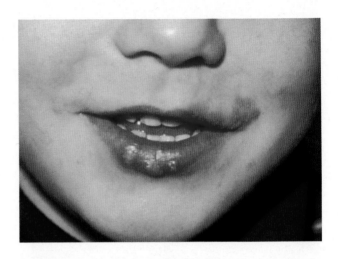

Facial Location

Eczematous dermatitis, as a result of a contact dermatitis, may present with a confluent weeping facial rash and pruritis due to the contact exposure. Similarly, atopic dermatitis or eczema is a similar rash resulting from allergic exposure but not necessarily due to contact. *Seborrheic dermatitis* is very common in early infancy and again around puberty and results in a nonpruritic erythematous, scale-forming rash. *Ichthyosis* may have associated areas of erythema with scale formation but is more likely than seborrheic dermatitis to include non-hair-bearing areas and have disseminated findings.

Pustular and Bullous Rash

Drug-associated reactions, acne vulgaris (**Fig. 66.4**), *pustular psoriasis* (**Fig. 66.5**), and *insect bites* can appear as pustular lesions. Associated pruritis or pain, distribution, and history of exposure can help determine the diagnosis. *Bullous pemphigoid* can present in children; it begins as urticarial lesions and develops over weeks to months into bulla. It requires treatment with steroids. *Bullous impetigo* is a disseminated bacterial infection (caused by *Staphylococcus aureus*) that results in the formation of bulla filled with serous or purulent fluid; these bulla spread rapidly and are painful, and the patient usually has systemic symptoms of infection. *Impetigo contagiosa* is the most common form of impetigo in children and is caused by *S. aureus* or *Streptococcus pyogenes*. Lesions are most common on the face, with bullous lesions and development of a characteristic golden crust.

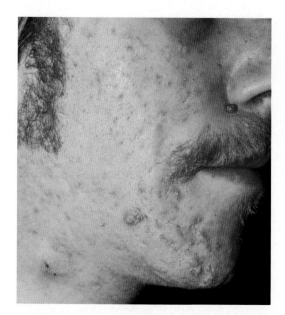

Fig. 66.4 Acne vulgaris (shown in an adult). (Courtesy of Dr. Daniel Krowchuk.)

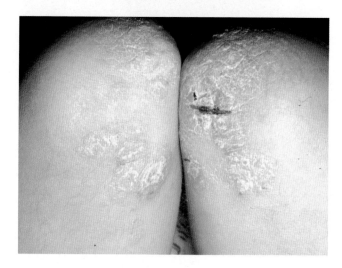

Fig. 66.5 Psoriasis.
(Courtesy of Dr. Daniel Krowchuk.)

Purpuric/Telangiectatic Rash

Thrombocytopenia (**Fig. 66.6**), either primary or as a result of leukemia, bacterial endocarditis, Henoch-Schönlein purpura, meningococcemia, gonococcemia, or disseminated intravascular coagulation, may present with varying appearance from flat to palpable purpura, as well as telangiectasia.

Fig. 66.6 Immune (idiopathic) thrombocytopenic purpura.

(Courtesy of Dr. Daniel Krowchuk.)

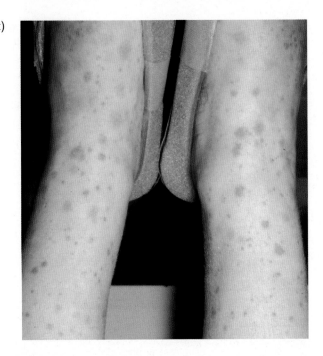

Suggested Reading

Fitzpatrick TB, Johnson RA, Wolff K, Polano MK, Surmond D. Outline of an approach to dermatologic diagnosis. In: Color Atlas and Synopsis of Clinical Dermatology. New York: McGraw-Hill Health Professions Division; 1997

67 Lesions of the Face and Neck in Children

Adele K. Evans

Facial lesions may be single or multiple, and multiple discrete lesions should be distinguished from a rash.

◆ Papular Clusters

Two common perinatal lesions are *neonatal acne* and *molluscum contagiosum*. The latter is due to a transient infection with a poxvirus that spontaneously resolves.

◆ Vascular Lesions

- *Hemangiomas* (**Fig. 67.1**) are benign vascular neoplasms that frequently present during the first few months of life grow rapidly during the first year of life. They begin to regress after 1 to 2 years of life and continue regression for as long as 5 to 10 years. Local tissue invasion can result in the destruction of cartilage and the deposition of fibrotic tissue.

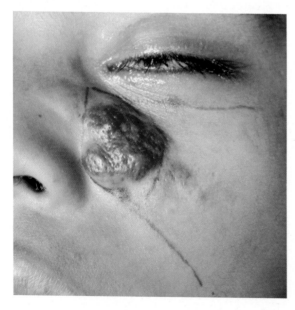

Fig. 67.1 Hemangioma in late childhood at time of surgical excision.

- *Vascular malformations* are present at birth and grow proportionately with the child. Rapid expansion may occur after infection or trauma. This class of malformation includes *arteriovenous malformation (AVM), capillary malformation* or *port wine stain* (commonly occurring in the midface region), *venous malformation,* and *lymphatic malformation (lymphangioma* or *cystic hygroma).* AVMs are more common intracranially than extracranially, but in the face are most common on the cheeks and ears. Capillary malformations can be associated with *Sturge-Weber syndrome.* Venous malformations are spongy compressible lesions that can often present in the lips and perioral region. Lymphatic malformations that occur in the neck below the mylohyoid tend to be less invasive, with larger fluid-filled compartments; lesions presenting above the mylohyoid tend to be invasive and often involve deep tissues, including the parotid.
- *Stork-bite,* or "salmon patch," is properly termed *nevus simplex* and is a collection of dilated vessels aggravated by Valsalva maneuver.

◆ Pigmented Lesions

- *Nevi* (**Fig. 67.2**) evolve during life with varying degrees of pigmentation. *Ephelis* is the medical term for freckles, or lightly pigmented small nevi. These result from rupture of melanocytes with spillage of the melanin. *Lentigo* represents the darker "mole," wherein the melanocytes produce increased quantities of pigment. *Congenital nevus* and *dysplastic nevus* have higher risks of the development of melanoma.
- The mildly pigmented *café-au-lait spot* (**Fig. 67.3**) may appear in isolation. If it occurs in a number greater than 6, in size greater than 15 mm in diameter in children over 5 years, or greater than 5 mm in children under 5 years,

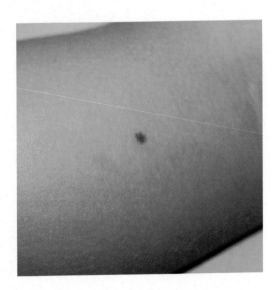

Fig. 67.2 Simple nevus.

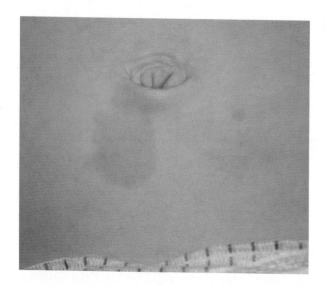

Fig. 67.3   Café-au-lait lesion.

in the axilla, or in the presence of skin tags, it may be a clue to the diagnosis of *neurofibromatosis type 1*. These isolated lesions are most prevalent in African Americans (18%) and least prevalent in Caucasians. They are the result of giant melanocytes.

- *Dermatofibromas* (**Fig. 67.4**) resemble dysplastic nevi. However, these lesions are benign cellular (presumably fibroblastic) proliferations that arise within the dermis of the extremities. Later in life, they may become inflammatory.
- *Facial angiofibroma*, or *adenoma sebaceum*, is a group of reddish spots or bumps, which appear on the nose and cheeks in a butterfly distribution.

Fig. 67.4   Dermatofibroma.

These lesions start to appear during childhood and are associated with tuberous sclerosis.

◆ Unpigmented Lesions

The differential diagnosis of unpigmented facial and neck lesions in children is much the same as in adults; see Chapter 54.

◆ Pruritic Lesions

- *Impetigo* may be a painful or pruritic isolated lesion resulting from systemic dissemination of bacteria, such as *Streptococcus*.
- *Insect bites* are significantly more common in children, and the original bite may be masked by excoriation as a result of pruritis. **Ants** inject formic acid with each bite, resulting in several days of pruritis and, frequently, formation of a small pustular head at the site of the bite. **Tick** bites can be intensely pruritic for weeks after the bite and are of particular concern because of the possibility of tickborne illness such as *Rocky Mountain spotted fever, Lyme disease, Lyme-like disease,* or *tularemia.* **Mosquito** bites are often pruritic and associated with a small erythematous and nonindurated mark that is easily masked by excoriation. **Flea** bites are less common on the face and can be frequently pruritic without associated erythema. **Spider** bites may be associated with findings of intense local tissue destruction, or systemic symptoms from toxin release such as generalized malaise.

◆ Inflicted Lesions

A sad yet crucially important aspect of pediatric care is the fact that *child abuse* or neglect may be the driving force for the presentation of a patient to the clinic, or signs may be noted during routine examination. Signs suspicious for abuse and/or neglect have many presentations. One is the scald lesion, which usually presents with erythema and possibly induration, desquamation, or bullous blister formation on the body part that has been dipped in scalding water. Facial exposures are possible and may present as a series of lesions, particularly if related to a hot-oil injury. The delicate skin of the infant is susceptible to scalding even at lower temperatures.

Regular centrally dark and dry lesions surrounded by erythema and smaller than a dime suggest cigarette burns. Ecchymotic lesions on the neck may suggest attempts at strangling. Bite wounds (**Fig. 67.5**) may present on the face or neck. They usually appear several hours after the injury, developing an erythematous impression of the biter's teeth for ~24 to 48 hours.

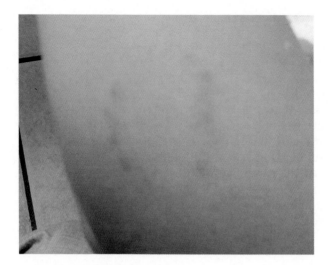

Fig. 67.5 Bite wound.

Suggested Reading

Friedman NR, Mitchell D. Congenital vascular lesions. In: Bailey BJ, Johnson JT, eds. Otolaryngology–Head and Neck Surgery. 4th ed. Lippincott Williams and Wilkins; 2006:1349–1357

McGill T. Vascular anomalies of the head and neck. In: Wetmore RF, Muntz HR, McGill TJ, eds. Pediatric Otolaryngology—Principles and Practice Pathways. New York: Thieme; 2000:87–101

68 Masses of the Face and Neck in Children

Adele K. Evans

There are a variety of head and neck presentations of a mass that may or may not be associated with surface findings such as a rash or lesion. These can best be grouped first based upon **location**, then based on characteristics on palpation. It is important to remember that at any site there can be presentation of a **solid organ tumor** involving the nerves, muscles, vascular, or connective tissue; **lymphoma** within or outside lymphoid tissue; and **leukemic infiltrate**, which may appear to be a solid organ mass but represents tissue infiltration by a circulating blood-cell neoplasm.

◆ Anterior Neck

Submental adenopathy (level I): Usually resulting from oral cavity soft tissue or periodontal infection, represents the most likely etiology of a submental neck mass. *Ranula, plunging ranula,* or *traumatic lymphocele* (**Fig. 68.1**) may also present in the submental region. These are likely to be unilateral, but they can extend across the floor of the mouth to present bilaterally. Ranula and plung-

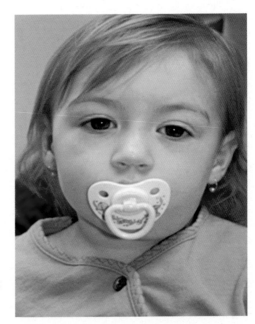

Fig. 68.1 Traumatic lymphocele in the left submandibular region.

(Courtesy of Dr. Daniel J. Kirse.)

ing ranula are likely to have an oral component (submucosal blue, soft mass), assisting in their diagnosis. The traumatic lymphocele follows a history of regional trauma, is often painless itself, and may have no intraoral component.

A *dermoid cyst* is a subcutaneous anterior neck mass, which is often adherent to the skin structures and is likely to have a tiny skin tract with hair emanating from the center. Dermoid cysts can present with infection of the contained debris. The presence of multiple dermoid cysts warrants consideration of *basal cell nevus syndrome* (*Gorlin syndrome*). Dermoid cysts may also present on the face, usually in the midline of the nose, and may have a tract with intracranial connection, so a suspected dermoid cyst involving the nose should have an appropriate radiologic evaluation.

A *thyroglossal duct cyst* (TDC) is another midline subcutaneous mass that can also present with a tiny skin pit. It may swell and become noticeable only after it becomes infected (usually associated with an upper respiratory infection). TDCs move with swallowing and are often near the hyoid bone, through which the cyst tracks developmentally. However, TDC can present as high as the submental space or as low as the thyroid gland isthmus. The clinician should investigate to ensure that the TDC is not the only functioning thyroid tissue in the patient.

Teratoma is likely to present in the midline, and often in the oral cavity/pharynx; it represents a tumor containing all three germinal cell lines. These are sometimes diagnosed prenatally on ultrasonography and can lead to congenital high-airway obstruction syndrome (CHAOS). Even if asymptomatic, teratomas should be excised to avoid potential degeneration to malignancy.

Thyroid nodule is much less common in children than in adults, but masses, when present, are more likely to be malignant in children than in adults. *Autoimmune* or *infectious thyroiditis* may present with a tender inflammatory mass in the anterior neck, even in children. Finally, an abnormally large *thymus* may present at the suprasternal notch.

◆ Lateral Neck

The lateral neck contains multiple lymph node groups (level IIa, IIb, III, IV, and V). *Enlarged lymph nodes* may present as isolated masses or in matted collections of nodes. They may be firm or fluctuant. In children, enlarged lymph nodes are much more likely to represent infection rather than metastatic malignancy.

Lymphatic malformations (**Fig. 68.2**) frequently present in the lateral neck and face. These are often multicystic and refractory to simple excision. They can be transilluminated with a light, using caution not to burn the delicate overlying skin with the light source. The macrocystic malformations are usually quite easily collapsed on palpation, and the overlying skin may appear very redundant once the cysts are collapsed. Microcystic malformations may be firmer. The unusual *lateral neck teratoma* may masquerade as a multicystic lymphatic malformation.

Fig. 68.2 Lymphatic malformation of the neck.

(Courtesy of Dr. Daniel J. Kirse.)

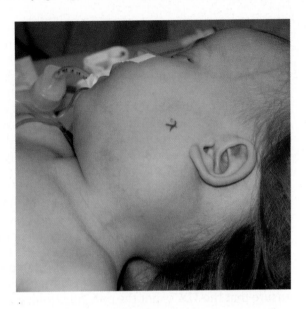

Venous malformations are likely to present in the lateral neck and usually have a bluish discoloration. *Mixed venous-lymphatic malformations* may also occur. The blood flow is low through lymphatic and venous malformations and is not usually evident on four-dimensional ultrasonography.

The *arteriovenous malformation*, on the other hand, has high blood flow and often a palpable thrill or auscultated hum. These can be further identified with arteriography or computed tomographic–virtual arteriography. These are uncommon primary lesions but may result from traumatic injuries to the head and neck.

A *branchial cleft cyst* (BCC), with or without fistula, is a somewhat challenging lateral neck mass that may present with an intraoral component in the pharynx or as a collapsible cystic neck mass. If the BCC has a connection to the skin it is called a branchial cleft fistula; all BCCs have a sinus connection internally to the aerodigestive tract, but in many cases that sinus is closed or has regressed by the time of presentation. Many times, BCCs present with acute swelling after an upper respiratory infection due to their respiratory epithelial lining. These may be mistaken for acute adenopathy in this setting. There are several types of BCC, named based on their presumed embryological derivation. If presenting as a mass (with or without fistula) around the earlobe, ear canal, or submandibular gland, it is referred to as a first branchial cleft cyst; these may include an ear canal duplication or intraparotid tract (first BCC—Work type I and Work type II). If presenting in the cervical region anterior to the sternocleidomastoid muscle in level 2, it is a second branchial cleft cyst; the internal sinus tract will terminate in the palatine tonsil region. Ninety-five percent of all BCCs are second BCCs. A third BCC will also present in the level of the neck, but the internal sinus tract will travel in a slightly different direction and terminate in the pyriform sinus. Fourth BCCs are very rare and can present in different locations in the lateral neck, including levels 3 and 4; based on embryological principles the tract should be similar to the path of the recurrent laryngeal nerve and extend into the chest.

A purely lateral firm mass within the sternocleidomastoid and the primary etiology of a neck mass in the neonate is the muscular knot of *fibromatosis colli (or sternomastoid tumor of infancy)*. This is completely within the belly of the sternocleidomastoid muscle and is classically associated with an ipsilateral tilt of the top of the head and contralateral turn of the face.

Neurofibromas present as large lateral deep neck masses in neurofibromatosis type 2. These may be extremely large and can extend from the skull base to the thoracic inlet. They are rarely painful but may result in physical limitation as a result of mass effect.

◆ Mandible

Benign and malignant tumors of the mandible may present as a facial or lateral neck mass. Fibroosseous lesions *fibrous dysplasia* or *ossifying fibroma* may appear as a mass and result in a slowly growing, firm distortion of the bone. *Ameloblastoma, odontogenic cysts, giant cell tumor, cherubism,* and *vascular malformations* of the bone may present as either firm or cystic lesions. Rarely in children, malignancies such as *Burkitt lymphoma, osteosarcoma,* or *metastatic neuroblastoma* may present as a jaw mass. Actinomycosis of the jaw can also present as a mandibular mass.

◆ Cheek, Face, and Other Skin

Many "parotid masses" in children are actually a first BCC, or an infectious process such as parotitis. The intraparotid lymph nodes are a common location for *nontuberculous mycobacteria adenitis* in children, with frequent characteristic violaceous change of the overlying skin. Benign and malignant neoplasms of the parotid can occur in children; the most common childhood parotid neoplasm is hemangioma (**Fig. 68.3**), and the differential diagnosis of other neoplasms is the same as that in adults; see Chapter 59.

Other soft tissue tumors, such as *rhabdomyosarcoma, lipoma, liposarcoma, atypical lipoma,* and *neurofibroma* may also present in the face or cheek, and often originate from the infratemporal/pterygopalatine fossa or paranasal sinuses.

Nasal dermoid, glioma, and *encephalocele* may present as expansile central nasal masses. Lacrimal duct cysts (*dacryocystoceles*) (**Fig. 68.4**) may present as unilateral or bilateral bluish paranasal masses with an intranasal component and nasal obstructive symptoms.

Fig. 68.3 Parotid hemangioma in an infant.

(Courtesy of Dr. Daniel J. Kirse.)

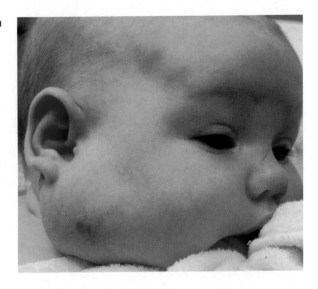

Benign *skin tags* are often specifically localized to skin involvement alone as a congenital mass. At the region of the auricle and tragus, congenital abnormalities of the development of the auricular hillocks may lead to skin or skin and cartilage tag formation, as well as a *preauricular pit, cyst, or sinus*. If seen in conjunction with *café-au-lait spots*, skin tags may be significant for *neurofibromatosis type 1* (von Recklinghausen disease). If seen in conjunction with neck sinus tracts, conductive hearing loss, or kidney abnormalities such as horseshoe kidney, these periauricular anomalies may be indicative of *branchio-otorenal* syndrome.

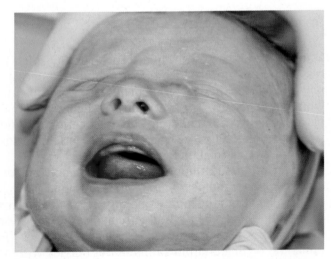

Fig. 68.4 A bilateral dacryocystoceles, external component is shown.

(Courtesy of Dr. Daniel J. Kirse.)

After enlarging and fading in their typical life cycle, hemangiomas may leave behind a calcified mass intimately associated with the skin. Similarly, *pilomatrixoma* may present as an intradermal or subcutaneous firm mass in the periauricular area with or without an associated skin lesion or calcifications.

Suggested Reading

Bent JB III, Herbert RL, Smith RFH. Pediatric neck neoplasms. In: Wetmore RF, Muntz HR, McGill TJ, eds. Pediatric Otolaryngology—Principles and Practice Pathways. New York: Thieme; 2000:993–1019

Bent JP, Sessions RB. Congenital anomalies of the nose. In: Bailey BJ, Johnson JT, eds. Otolaryngology–Head and Neck Surgery. 4th ed. Philadelphia: Lippincott Williams & Wilkins; 2006:1217–1227

Chung WL, Cox DP, Ochs MW. Odontogenic cysts, tumors and related jaw lesions. In: Byron J, Bailey BJ, Johnson JT, eds. Otolaryngology–Head and Neck Surgery. 4th ed. Philadelphia: Lippincott Williams & Wilkins; 2006:1569–1584

Cunningham MJ. Neoplasms of the ear and temporal bone. In: Wetmore RF, Muntz HR, McGill TJ, eds. Pediatric Otolaryngology—Principles and Practice Pathways. New York: Thieme; 2000:385–405

Friedman NR, Mitchell D. Congenital vascular lesions. In: Bailey BJ, Johnson JT, eds. Otolaryngology–Head and Neck Surgery. 4th ed. Philadelphia: Lippincott Williams & Wilkins; 2006:1349–1357

Gerber ME, Cotton RT. Pediatric malignancies. In: Bailey BJ, Johnson JT, eds. Otolaryngology–Head and Neck Surgery. 4th ed. Philadelphia: Lippincott Williams & Wilkins; 2006:1359–1369

Ibrahim HZ, Handler SD. Diseases of the salivary glands. In: Wetmore RF, Muntz HR, McGill TJ, eds. Pediatric Otolaryngology—Principles and Practice Pathways. New York: Thieme; 2000:647–656

Krowiak EJ, Grundfast KM. Congenital malformations of the ear. In: Wetmore RF, Muntz HR, McGill TJ, eds. Pediatric Otolaryngology—Principles and Practice Pathways. Thieme; 2000:249–250

McGill TJ. Vascular anomalies of the head and neck. In: Wetmore RF, Muntz HR, McGill TJ, eds. Pediatric Otolaryngology—Principles and Practice Pathways. New York: Thieme; 2000:87–101

McGill TJ. Soft tissue sarcoma in children. In: Wetmore RF, Muntz HR, McGill TJ, eds. Pediatric Otolaryngology—Principles and Practice Pathways. New York: Thieme; 2000:103–111

McGill TJ, Rahbar R. Neoplasms of the mid-face and anterior skull base. In: Wetmore RF, Muntz HR, McGill TJ, eds. Pediatric Otolaryngology—Principles and Practice Pathways. New York: Thieme; 2000:513–520

Ohlms LA. Neoplasms of the oral cavity, pharynx and upper alimentary tract. In: Wetmore RF, Muntz HR, McGill TJ, eds. Pediatric Otolaryngology—Principles and Practice Pathways. New York: Thieme; 2000:670–675

Wiatrak BJ. Clinical evaluation of the neck. In: Wetmore RF, Muntz HR, McGill TJ, eds. Pediatric Otolaryngology—Principles and Practice Pathways. New York: Thieme; 2000:931–948

Zur KB, Myer CM III. Salivary gland disease in children. In: Bailey BJ, Johnson JT, eds. Otolaryngology–Head and Neck Surgery. 4th ed. Philadelphia: Lippincott Williams & Wilkins; 2006:1241–1252

69 Skin Infection in Children

Adele K. Evans

In children, *cellulitis, abscess,* and *folliculitis* of the skin of the face and neck are quite similar to presentation in the adult (see Section VIII).

◆ Scalp

In addition to bacterial *folliculitis,* another common scalp infection is caused by the fungus *Trychophyton* spp., known as *ringworm, serpigio,* or *tinea capitis*; this involves a round reddish lesion usually associated with alopecia, which recovers after appropriate treatment. *Neonatal seborrheic dermatitis (cradle cap)* is very common and presents as scaly, dry, yellow-colored flaky scalp.

◆ Ear

Simple *otitis externa* (OE) is common in children. Treatment of OE with ear drops is sometimes complicated by *contact dermatitis* (neomycin is the most frequent culprit). This presents with erythematous, sometimes vesicular, glassy or desquamating lesions and can follow a pattern where the drops have rolled out of the ear canal, down the conchal bowl, and onto the ipsilateral neck skin.

◆ Nose

Acne is found quite commonly in the external paranasal and nasal regions. It is essentially a case of isolated follicular infection. The same process can occur internally on the skin-lined portion of the nose, called the nasal alar vestibule. Such folliculitides can be quite painful, and cellulitis rapidly ensues, producing *nasal vestibulitis.* Although painful, this infection is not serious, and simple treatment with appropriate anti-*staphylococcal* ointment is effective. However, venous drainage from the skin in this region occurs directly to the cavernous sinus, which can rarely result in central nervous system infection.

A slowly enlarging ruddy mass that often bleeds and may or may not be associated with discomfort is likely to be a *pyogenic granuloma (capillary hemangioma).* Although these often present during pregnancy, they can present in childhood as well. Common locations are the nose and lips.

◆ Periorbital

Periorbital erythema and edema are almost always due to *preseptal cellulitis* (**Fig. 69.1**), or infection of the preorbital septum soft tissue space, resulting from extension of rhinosinusitis. Patients with preseptal cellulitis can also have other orbital and periorbital complications of rhinosinusitis. Periorbital erythema can also be a primary cellulitis from local skin infection.

◆ Mouth/Lips

Red flaky lesions at the corners of the mouth may be a sign of *vitamin deficiency* (riboflavin, B2) or of chronic infection of the skin at the corners of the mouth with *Staphylococcus aureus* or *Candida albicans*. This is referred to as *angular cheilitis* or *perleche*.

Primary *herpesvirus* infections may result in satellite vesicular eruption around the mouth just past or adjacent to the vermilion. Reactivation herpes lesions are equally likely to contain virus and usually appear as single, large, crusty lesions just touching the vermillion border but not involving the wet vermillion.

◆ Neck

In children, infectious neck masses are most commonly *bacterial lymphadenitis*, usually caused by pharyngitis, oral cavity infection, or skin infection. Bacterial adenitis can progress to *neck abscess* or to *necrotic degeneration*.

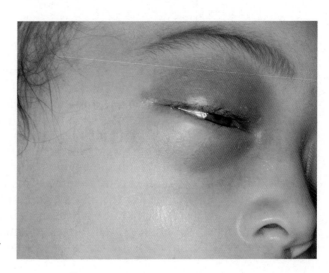

Fig. 69.1   Preseptal cellulitis.
(Courtesy of Dr. Daniel J. Kirse.)

Another common infectious cause of pediatric neck mass is *infection of a congenital anomaly*, for example, *branchial cleft cyst, thyroglossal duct cyst*, or *lymphangioma*. Findings of nodal involvement with heavily violaceous overlying skin change, and less local tenderness or systemic symptoms than you would expect given the size of the mass, is concerning for *tuberculous adenitis*—either *nontuberculous mycobacteria* (NTM) or *scrofula*. NTM usually presents with unilateral findings, anterior neck or periparotid involvement (**Fig. 69.2**), and no systemic symptoms or history of exposure to tuberculosis, in an otherwise healthy child. Scrofula usually involves bilateral, posterior neck nodes, with possible systemic manifestations and history of exposure to tuberculosis, or immunocompromise or human immunodeficiency virus infection.

Cat scratch disease (**Fig. 69.3**) usually presents similarly to bacterial adenitis, but with less tenderness. However, it does not respond to standard antibiotic treatment.

Neck or throat infection with soft tissue involvement and unilateral deep neck pain should be evaluated for *deep neck abscess* or *phlegmon* or *jugular vein thrombophlebitis (Lemierre syndrome)*. Other rare infections can present with cervical adenopathy, such as salmonella.

Molluscum contagiosum is a common, benign, self-limiting viral infection of the skin caused by a poxvirus. The lesions are multiple, dome-shaped, flesh-colored papules with a central depression, which usually present on the chest and arms but can extend to the neck. It usually affects children between ages 2 and 4 years. Molluscum is spread between people, and is more common with crowding, swimming together, and the like.

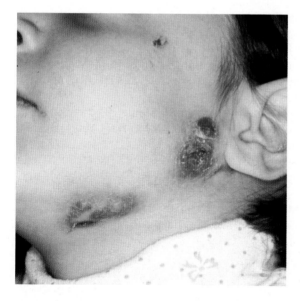

Fig. 69.2 Nontuberculous myco-bacterial cervical lymphadenitis in a toddler. (Courtesy of Dr. Daniel J. Kirse.)

Fig. 69.3 Cat scratch disease cervical lymphadenopathy. (Courtesy of Dr. Daniel J. Kirse.)

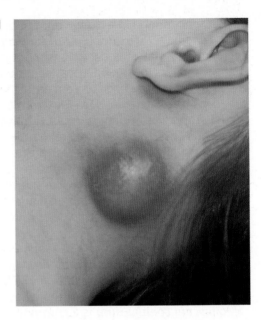

Suggested Reading

Clary RA. Acute inflammatory and infectious disorders of the nose and paranasal sinuses. In: Wetmore RF, Muntz HR, McGill TJ, eds. Pediatric Otolaryngology—Principles and Practice Pathways. New York: Thieme; 2000:472

Ibrahim HZ, Handler SD. Diseases of the salivary glands. In: Wetmore RF, Muntz HR, McGill TJ, eds. Pediatric Otolaryngology—Principles and Practice Pathways. New York: Thieme; 2000:647–656

Papsin BC, Friedberg J. Infectious and inflammatory disorders of the neck. In: Wetmore RF, Muntz HR, McGill TJ, eds. Pediatric Otolaryngology—Principles and Practice Pathways. New York: Thieme; 2000:949–968

Richardson MA. Regional and intracranial complications of sinusitis. In: Wetmore RF, Muntz HR, McGill TJ, eds. Pediatric Otolaryngology—Principles and Practice Pathways. New York: Thieme; 2000:487–490

Wetmore RF. Diseases of the external ear. In: Wetmore RF, Muntz HR, McGill TJ, eds. Pediatric Otolaryngology—Principles and Practice Pathways. New York: Thieme; 2000:253

Wiatrak BJ. Clinical evaluation of the neck. In: Wetmore RF, Muntz HR, McGill TJ, eds. Pediatric Otolaryngology—Principles and Practice Pathways. New York: Thieme; 2000:931–948

Zur KB, Myer CM III. Salivary gland disease in children. In: Bailey BJ, Johnson JT, eds. Otolaryngology–Head and Neck Surgery. 4th ed. Philadelphia: Lippincott Williams & Wilkins; 2006:1241–1252

70 Fistula/Sinus in Children

Adele K. Evans

Sinus tracts and fistulas in the pediatric face and neck are almost always congenital in origin, as opposed to adult patients in which they are usually related to infection, cancer, or trauma/iatrogenic. Sinus tracts and fistula are best diagnosed by their region of presentation and their location within the region.

◆ Ear

A sinus near the anterior root of the helix is a preauricular pit or sinus (**Fig. 70.1**). A sinus near the earlobe is usually a first branchial cleft sinus.

◆ Face

Sinuses on the face are usually from a *dermoid cyst*, which will typically have a tiny hair protruding from the sinus, or an *epidermal inclusion cyst*. An infected dermoid cyst is shown in **Fig. 70.2**.

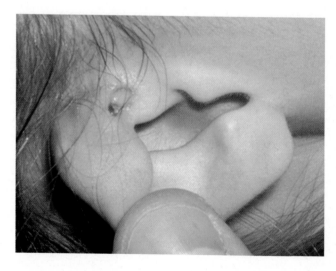

Fig. 70.1 Preauricular pit, draining.

(Courtesy of Dr. Daniel J. Kirse.)

Fig. 70.2 A nasal dermoid fistula, infected. (Courtesy of Dr. Daniel J. Kirse.)

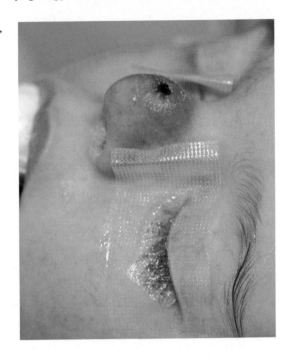

◆ Neck

Anterior neck pits, tracts, or fistulas in the midline of the neck may indicate a *thyroglossal duct anomaly* (**Fig. 70.3**), a *midline cervical cleft* (**Fig. 70.4**), or a *dermoid cyst*. Lateral neck fistulas are almost always a *branchial cleft sinus* (second, third, or fourth). **Figure 70.5** shows a second branchial cleft sinus.

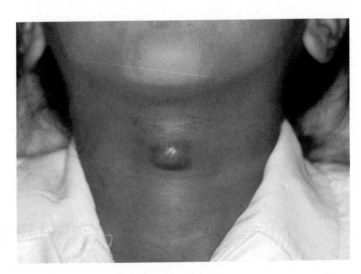

Fig. 70.3 Thyroglossal duct cyst, infected.
(Courtesy of Dr. Daniel J. Kirse.)

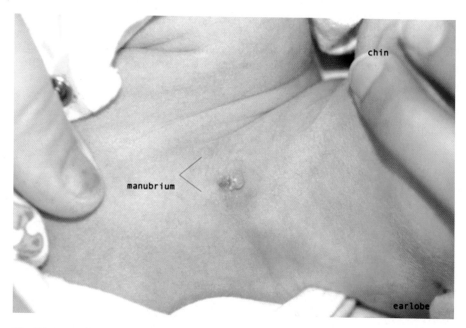

Fig. 70.4 Midline cervical cleft. (Courtesy of Dr. Daniel J. Kirse.)

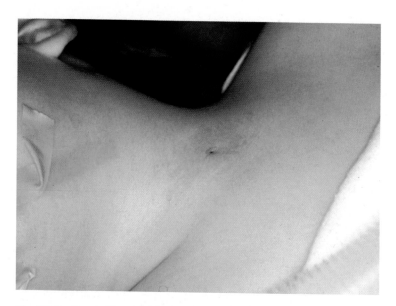

Fig. 70.5 Second branchial sinus tract, intraoperative.
(Courtesy of Dr. Daniel J. Kirse.)

Suggested Reading

Wiatrak BJ. Clinical evaluation of the neck. In: Wetmore RF, Muntz HR, McGill TJ, eds. Pediatric Otolaryngology—Principles and Practice Pathways. New York: Thieme; 2000:931–948

71 Facial Asymmetry in Children

Adele K. Evans

Facial symmetry can be a good indicator of an underlying syndromic diagnosis. Asymmetry may be created by clefting of the face, lip, or cranial vault; by early suture line closure; by eye/lid anomalies; by ear anomalies; and by facial growth restrictions.

◆ Lip/Nose/Face

The most common anomalies of the lip, nose, and face are those resulting from *cleft lip and palate*. Cleft lip (**Fig. 71.1A,B**) with or without cleft palate (**Fig. 71.2**) occurs in ~1/1000 births, and as lesions and defects are more severe, the proportion of male patients increases. Cleft lip and palate are associated with many other syndromes, including *Pierre Robin sequence* (see below), *ectrodactyly-ectodermal dysplasia-clefting (EEC) syndrome, ectrodactyly-cleft palate (ECP) syndrome, Bowen-Armstrong syndrome, Larsen syndrome, Van der Woude syndrome, velocardiofacial (Shprintzen) syndrome,* among many other more rare, and some lethal, syndromes.

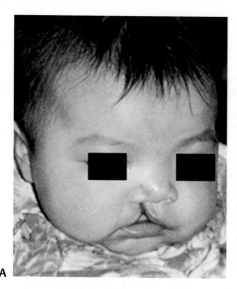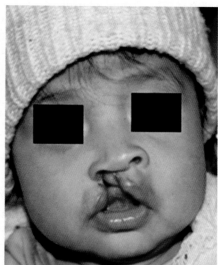

A   B

Fig. 71.1 (**A,B**) Unilateral cleft lip.

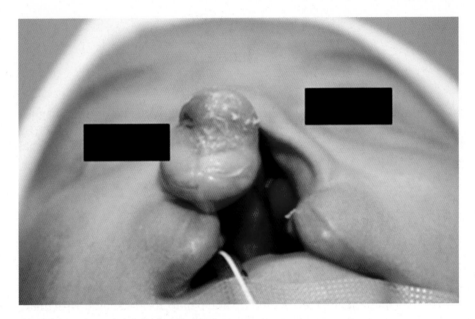

Fig. 71.2   Bilateral cleft lip (and palate).

Nasal asymmetry, the classic "*cleft lip nose*," results from a cleft lip and often persists despite efforts at repair of the lip, requiring reconstructive rhinoplasty for correction. *Primary nasal cleft* is much less common.

Midface growth restriction with or without cleft palate may occur in the setting of *autosomal dominant achondroplastic dwarfism*; with associated proptosis in *Crouzon syndrome*; or with syndactyly and proptosis in *Apert syndrome (acrocephalosyndactyly)*. Other rare syndromes causing midface hypoplasia are *Pfeiffer syndrome* (also has hypertelorism and downsloping palpebral fissures), and *Jackson-Weiss syndrome* (also has acrocephaly, hypertelorism, and proptosis).

◆ Cranial Vault

Primary cranial vault clefts can be simple, resulting in hypertelorism, or quite complex (**Fig. 71.3**), resulting in facial duplications associated with hydrocephalus. *Craniosynostosis*, or premature closure of the cranial suture lines, may occur spontaneously (idiopathic) or in conjunction with a syndromic diagnosis such as *Crouzon syndrome* or *Apert syndrome*. Cowlicks and whorls in the hair may be associated with underlying developmental disorders. The white forelock is classically associated with *Waardenburg syndrome*, which includes sensorineural hearing loss.

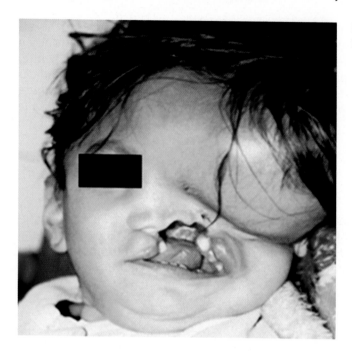

Fig. 71.3 Complex cranio-facial cleft.

◆ Ear Anomalies

In addition to the previously mentioned pits, sinuses, and fistulae of developmental anomalies of the auricular hillocks and branchial clefts, **microtia** and **anotia** may present unilaterally or bilaterally and may be balanced or unbalanced. These anomalies are very frequently associated with **aural atresia** of the external auditory canal, and with middle ear ossicular anomalies. Such findings may occur in an isolated fashion, or they may occur in conjunction with hemifacial and mandibular anomalies hence suggesting a syndromic diagnosis. A partial list of syndromes with auricular abnormalities includes *hemifacial microsomia* or *Goldenhar (oculoauriculovertebral) syndrome, Treacher Collins (mandibulofacial dysostosis) syndrome, Miller syndrome, branchio-oto-renal syndrome, cervico-oculo-acoustic syndrome* (often with Klippel-Feil anomaly of fused vertebrae), and *Bixler (hypertelorism-microtia-clefting) syndrome.*

◆ Eye/Lid Anomalies

There are multiple anomalies of the eyes that are helpful to the otolaryngologist. Classically, the slanted palpebral fissure of Down syndrome earned that genetic anomaly the early terminology, "Mongoloidism." The laterally down-slanted, sometimes almost "dripping," lateral canthus may be an early indication of *Treacher Collins syndrome*. Lid, iris, or retinal colobomas or clefts (the latter diagnoses with dilated retinoscopy) may be indictors of *CHARGE association* (coloboma of the eye, *h*eart anomaly, choanal *a*tresia, *r*etardation, and *g*enital and *e*ar anomalies). As previously mentioned, hypertelorism is often an indication of cranial vault cleft. Heterogeneous iris coloration is seen in *Waardenburg syndrome*. Proptotic or proptotic-appearing eyes are seen in *Crouzon syndrome* and *Apert syndrome*.

◆ Mandible

The small, posteriorly set mandible is a predominant feature of *Pierre Robin sequence*, which consists of micro- and/or retrognathia, varying degrees of palatal cleft, and glossoptosis. *Hemifacial microsomia* and other syndromes involving the face and ear are already listed and include *Goldenhar syndrome* and *Treacher Collins syndrome*.

◆ Neck

Vertebral body anomalies are found in *achondroplastic dwarfism, Apert syndrome, Crouzon syndrome, Down syndrome*, and *VACTERL association* (*v*ertebral, *a*nal, *c*ardiac, *t*racheal, *e*sophageal, *r*enal, and *l*imb). Such vertebral anomalies may become critical with neck hyperextension, so caution is advised in the operating room. Several syndromes have **neck webbing** (pterygium colli) with limitation of range of motion. *Klippel-Feil anomaly* is congenital fusion of cervical vertebral bodies. *Noonan syndrome* has neck webbing and chest wall abnormalities and is associated with pulmonic stenosis and sensorineural hearing loss. *Turner syndrome* is classically associated with a webbed neck in females.

Suggested Reading

Bent JB III, Herbert RL, Smith RFH. Pediatric neck neoplasms. In: Wetmore RF, Muntz HR, McGill TJ, eds. Pediatric Otolaryngology—Principles and Practice Pathways. New York: Thieme; 2000:993–1019

Bent JP, Sessions RB. Congenital anomalies of the nose. In: Bailey BJ, Johnson JT, eds. Otolaryngology–Head and Neck Surgery. 4th ed. Philadelphia: Lippincott Williams & Wilkins; 2006:1217–1227

Dyleski RA, Crockett DM. Cleft lip and palate: evaluation and treatment of the primary deformity. In: Bailey BJ, Johnson JT, eds. Otolaryngology–Head and Neck Surgery. 4th ed. Philadelphia: Lippincott Williams & Wilkins; 2006:1317–1321

Gorlin RJ, Cohen MM, Levin LS. Syndromes of the Head and Neck. 3rd ed. New York: Oxford University Press; 1990

Krowiak EJ, Grundfast KM. Congenital malformations of the ear. In: Wetmore RF, Muntz HR, McGill TJ, eds. Pediatric Otolaryngology—Principles and Practice Pathways. New York: Thieme; 2000:249–250

Lusk RP, Muntz HR. Introduction to pediatric rhinology. In: Wetmore RF, Muntz HR, McGill TJ, eds. Pediatric Otolaryngology—Principles and Practice Pathways. New York: Thieme; 2000:439–446

Sidman JD, Muntz HR. Cleft lip and palate. In: Wetmore RF, Muntz HR, McGill TJ, eds. Pediatric Otolaryngology—Principles and Practice Pathways. New York: Thieme; 2000:566–568

Tewfik TL, Manoukian JJ. The syndromal child. In: Bailey BJ, Johnson JT, eds. Otolaryngology–Head and Neck Surgery. 4th ed. Philadelphia: Lippincott Williams & Wilkins; 2006:1371–1387

Ward RF, April MM. Congenital malformations of the nose, nasopharynx and sinuses. In: Wetmore RF, Muntz HR, McGill TJ, eds. Pediatric Otolaryngology—Principles and Practice Pathways. New York: Thieme; 2000:453–463

Wiatrak BJ. Clinical evaluation of the neck. In: Wetmore RF, Muntz HR, McGill TJ, eds. Pediatric Otolaryngology—Principles and Practice Pathways. New York: Thieme; 2000:931–948

X Differential Diagnosis in Cosmetic and Plastic Surgery, Trauma, and Reconstruction

Section Editor: *Patrick J. Byrne*

72 Cosmetic Skin Lesion

Zayna Nahas and Nanette Liégeois

Skin cancer is the most commonly encountered malignancy in the head and neck. Although the vast majority of skin lesions are benign, early detection is the key to ensure good prognosis for potentially metastatic skin cancers. In skin cancers that are less frequently metastatic, early diagnosis and treatment are important to prevent invasion and destruction of underlying critical structures. Clinically distinguishing benign from malignant disease is an important skill for the otolaryngologist. Clinical findings on physical exam and knowledge of important risk factors are often sufficient to make the diagnosis. However, histological diagnosis remains the gold standard, and if any doubt exists about the diagnosis, a biopsy is warranted.

◆ Benign Skin Lesions

In general, these have well-defined edges, are symmetrical, and have uniformly distributed color, with little or no change in characteristics over time.

- *Seborrheic keratosis (SK)*: Tan-brown-black color, sharply circumscribed, round/oval shape. Can be flat or minimally raised and are often scaly. A key characteristic is their "stuck-on" appearance. They most commonly appear on the face, trunk, and upper extremities and are more common with increasing age. SK has no malignant potential (**Fig. 72.1**).

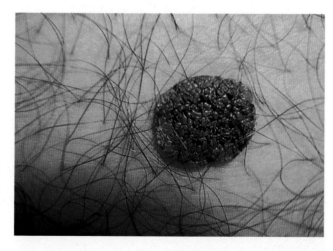

Fig. 72.1 Seborrheic keratosis. Brown, oval sessile plaque with characteristic "stuck on" appearance. (Courtesy of DermAtlas, Johns Hopkins University, www.dermatlas.org.)

- *Actinic keratosis (AK)*: Yellow-brown scaly patches found most often on sun-exposed skin. A key characteristic is their rough "sandpaper" like texture, often appreciated on light palpation rather than clinical examination. AKs occur on exposed surfaces, most commonly the face, ears, dorsum of the hands, and legs. More commonly seen in middle-aged and elderly with a greater predominance in males and fair-skinned individuals with a history of sun exposure. Most importantly, AKs have a documented malignant potential and 10 to 20% of AKs will progress to squamous cell carcinoma (**Fig. 72.2**).
- *Lentigo*: Tan, brown to black, small, well circumscribed, evenly pigmented macules that do not darken with sun exposure, thus differentiating them from ephelides (freckles). The two most common are lentigo simplex and solar lentigo.

  - *Lentigo simplex*: The most common form; may arise anywhere on the body. They most commonly arise in childhood and are unassociated with sun exposure. They have no malignant potential.
  - *Solar lentigo*: Present in sun-exposed skin. Most common in middle-aged individuals and those with a history of sun exposure. They have no malignant potential, but are considered markers for individuals who have had previous sunburns and are therefore at increased risk for developing skin cancer (**Fig. 72.3**).
  - *Lentigo maligna*: Subtype of melanoma in situ that develops in sun-damaged skin in the middle-aged and elderly. Typically a large, brown-black patch with indefinite borders. It has an estimated 5% lifetime risk of progression to lentigo maligna melanoma (**Fig. 72.4**).

- *Nevi*: Can be congenital or acquired

  - *Congenital nevus*: Sharply demarcated pigmented areas that can vary greatly in size, configuration, and color. By definition, these lesions are present at birth. Most common locations include the trunk, extremity, or

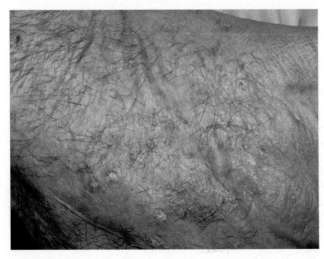

Fig. 72.2 Actinic keratosis. Multiple diffusely scattered stellate papules with scaly centers found on sun-exposed areas such as the dorsum of the hand as seen in this image. Palpation would reveal sandpaper-like texture characteristic of these lesions. (Courtesy of DermAtlas, Johns Hopkins University, www.dermatlas.org.)

Fig. 72.3 Solar lentigo. Multiple, variable-sized, hyperpigmented macules on the back of a young, fair-skinned man with a history of multiple sunburns. (Courtesy of DermAtlas, Johns Hopkins University, www. dermatlas.org.)

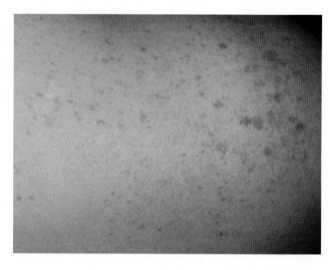

face. They can appear with or without hair. **Small** congenital nevi (< 1.5 cm in diameter) have an extremely low incidence of malignant degeneration. Although **medium-sized** congenital nevi (1.5 to 20.0 cm) have a slightly greater risk of malignancy, lifelong medical observation is recommended over immediate prophylactic excision. **Large** congenital nevi (> 20 cm) have a reported incidence of malignant transformation from 5 to 40%, and removal is recommended by many. It is also important to rule out leptomeninges involvement when these are encountered in the head and neck.

- *Acquired*: Extremely common. Each individual has an average of 18 to 40 acquired nevi. They vary in size (but are usually less than 6 mm in diameter), shape, color, and surface characteristics, as do malignant melanomas. A key distinguishing characteristic is that each individual nevus, unlike melanoma, tends to have a uniformly distributed color and

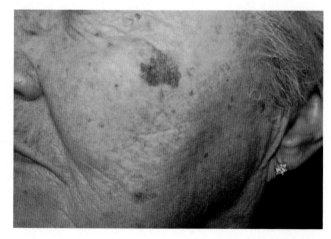

Fig. 72.4 Lentigo maligna. A 72-year-old woman with a 5-year history of a slowly expanding, irregular, dark brown, 2.5 cm patch with scalloped borders on her cheek. Biopsy revealed lentigo maligna, a type of melanoma in situ. (Courtesy of DermAtlas, Johns Hopkins University, www.dermatlas. org.)

symmetry both in its initial presentation and over time. Any **changing** skin lesion should raise suspicion for melanoma. Acquired nevi appear between early childhood to age 40 and often begin to involute at age 60. Any **new** pigmented skin lesion in an individual greater than 40 years of age should be critically examined.

- *Dysplastic or atypical mole*: Have variable color (pink, brown, tan, or black) and the variation is present within each lesion, which helps to distinguish them from benign acquired nevi. They have irregular borders and can be flat or have a raised center ("fried-egg" lesion). Unlike benign acquired nevi, they are usually irregular in shape and color, and often the patient notices its appearance changing over time (**Fig. 72.5**). In the instance where melanoma occurs in multiple family members (atypical mole-melanoma syndrome), atypical moles are thought to be precursors to melanoma with a 100% and 60% association with familial and sporadic melanoma, respectively.

◆ Malignant Skin Lesions

- *Nonmelanoma skin cancer (NMSC)*: Typically found in anatomical areas of sun exposure. Fair skin, blue eyes, red hair, a tendency to sunburn, and immunosuppression are all increased risk factors for developing NMSC.

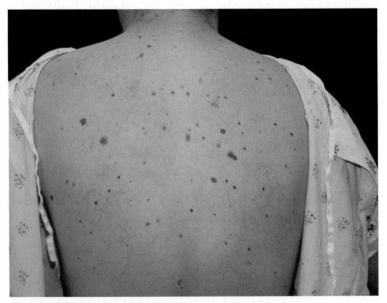

Fig. 72.5 Dysplastic mole. Multiple 2.0- to 1.5-cm hyperpigmented macules, papules, and plaques with variable pigmentation and irregular borders. Note that the color variation occurs within each nevus, helping to distinguish it from a benign nevus. Several family members also have a large number of atypical nevi. (Courtesy of DermAtlas, Johns Hopkins University, www.dermatlas.org.)

- ○ *Basal cell carcinoma (BCC)*: There are many types of clinical variants; however, the most common one is a pearly nodule that typically develops central ulceration, rolled borders, and telangiectasias. BCC is the most common malignant cutaneous neoplasm. The majority of BCC tumors appear in the head and neck, the nose being the most common site. However, one third of BCC cases occur in sun-protected sites, including the inner canthus and behind the ear. They occur more frequently in the elderly but they are not limited to that age group; 20% occur in patients younger than age 50. Patients frequently present with recurring bleeding or scabbing at the site. Metastatic potential is described but exceedingly rare. BCC tumors have great potential for local invasion and destruction (**Fig. 72.6**).
- ○ *Squamous cell carcinoma (SCC)*: Erythematous, hyperkeratotic, scaling plaque that generally occurs in the elderly. Left untreated, SCC is locally destructive and capable of regional or distant metastasis (**Fig. 72.7**).

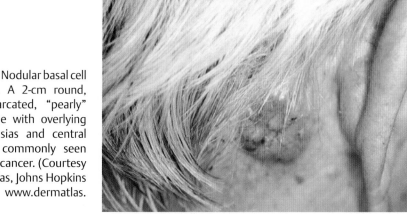

Fig. 72.6 Nodular basal cell carcinoma. A 2-cm round, well demarcated, "pearly" pink plaque with overlying telangiectasias and central ulceration commonly seen in this skin cancer. (Courtesy of DermAtlas, Johns Hopkins University, www.dermatlas.org.)

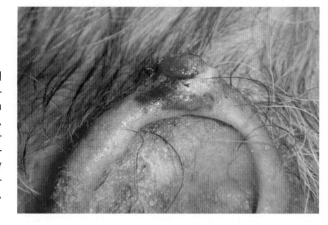

Fig. 72.7 Squamous cell carcinoma. A 1.5-cm erythematous oval nodule with eroded gelatinous surface, characteristic of its locally destructive nature, in this sun-exposed area of an elderly man. (Courtesy of DermAtlas, Johns Hopkins University, www.dermatlas.org.)

○ *Merkel cell carcinoma (MCC)*: MCC is often clinically misdiagnosed as a cyst because its clinical appearance typically mimics a cyst: red, pink, or bluish, painless, shiny dermal or subcutaneous nodules. The distinguishing feature from a cyst is that typically MCC exhibits rapid growth. These occur mostly in sun-exposed areas with 60% appearing in the head and neck. They most commonly occur in whites more than 60 years of age. Locally aggressive behavior and regional and distant metastases are common (**Fig. 72.8**).

● *Malignant melanoma (MM)*: The classic ABCDE criteria are *a*symmetry, *b*order irregularity, *c*olor variegation, *d*iameter > 6 mm, and *e*volving. These criteria aid in distinguishing melanoma from a benign nevus. Melanoma is primarily a diagnosis in white individuals with the mean age of diagnosis being 53. The incidence, however, is increasing in younger individuals. Dysplastic nevi, fair-complexioned individuals, a history of excessive sun exposure, particularly blistering sun burns, a family history of melanoma, a personal history of any prior skin cancer, and the presence of xeroderma pigmentosum all confer greater risk of developing melanoma. Its tendency to metastasize and high lethality make it the leading cause of skin cancer–related deaths. There are four subtypes to be aware of:

○ *Superficial spreading*: Aged 30 to 50, trunk in men, legs in women
○ *Nodular melanoma*: Legs and trunk, thick, nodular appearance, can ulcerate, has a very rapid growth phase (**Fig. 72.9**).
○ *Lentigo maligna melanoma*: Head, neck, and arms, > 65 years of age
○ *Acral lentiginous*: Palms, soles, or subungual, least common of all the subtypes but accounts for 60% of melanoma in dark-skinned individuals.

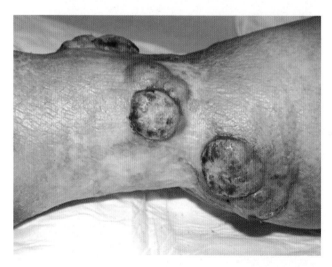

Fig. 72.8 Merkel cell carcinoma. Capable of distant metastases, this is an example of Merkel cell carcinoma appearing in the leg of a 70-year-old woman 2 years after initial resection. They appear as multiple, pink, cystic nodules overlying hemorrhagic erosions and crusts. (Courtesy of DermAtlas, Johns Hopkins University, www.dermatlas.org.)

Fig. 72.9 Nodular melanoma. An 87-year-old man with a pigmented, ulcerated, nodular lesion of his right frontal skin and right submandibular lymphadenopathy, consistent with nodular melanoma's high metastatic rate. (Courtesy of DermAtlas, Johns Hopkins University, www.dermatlas. org.)

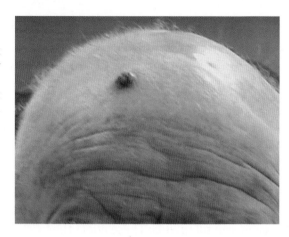

Suggested Reading

Fuchs A, Marmur E. The kinetics of skin cancer: progression of actinic keratosis to squamous cell carcinoma. Dermatol Surg 2007;33:1099–1101

Habif TP. Clinical Dermatology. 4th ed. St. Louis: Mosby; 2004:Chapter 22

Hussein MR. Melanocytic dysplastic naevi occupy the middle ground between benign melanocytic naevi and cutaneous malignant melanomas: emerging clues. J Clin Pathol 2005;58:453–456

Hutcheson AC, McGowan JW IV, Maize JC Jr, Cook J. Multiple primary acral melanomas in African-Americans: a case series and review of the literature. Dermatol Surg 2007;33:1–10

McKenna JK, Florell SR, Goldman GD, Bowen GM. Lentigo maligna/lentigo maligna melanoma: current state of diagnosis and treatment. Dermatol Surg 2006;32:493–504

Menzies SW. Cutaneous melanoma: making a clinical diagnosis, present and future. Dermatol Ther 2006;19:32–39

Tannous ZS, Mihm MC Jr, Sober AJ, Duncan LM. Congenital melanocytic nevi: clinical and histopathologic features, risk of melanoma, and clinical management. J Am Acad Dermatol 2005;52:197–203

Veness MJ, Palme CE, Morgan GJ. Merkel cell carcinoma: a review of management. Curr Opin Otolaryngol Head Neck Surg 2008;16:170–174

73 Brow Deformity or Dysfunction

Noah E. Meltzer

The upper face is bounded by the hairline superiorly and the glabella inferiorly. The orbits span the border between the upper and midface. The aesthetic subunits in the upper face are the forehead and upper eyes. Abnormalities of the upper face can be due to various conditions, such as aging, neurological, autoimmune, or other disorders. Upper face abnormalities can impair appearance or eye protection or be signs of systemic disease (eg, myasthenia gravis).

Rhytids and aging changes can be caused by the following:

- *Horizontal rhytids*: These affect the forehead and are due to frontalis muscle activity.
- *Horizontal, oblique, and vertical rhytids of the glabella*: These are due to corrugator supercilii and procerus muscle activity.
- *Crow's feet*: These are found in the lateral canthal region and are due to orbicularis oculi activity.
- *Sun exposure*

Brow ptosis is the inferior displacement of the brow at or below the superior orbital rim, usually affecting the temporal portion more significantly. This inferolateral displacement may cause temporal hooding, obstructing the superolateral visual fields. Brow ptosis can be caused by the following:

- *Aging*
- *Facial paralysis* may cause unilateral brow ptosis.
- *Congenital facial asymmetry*

Lid ptosis is a reduced vertical palpebral fissure due to an inferiorly placed upper lid margin. The normal vertical distance between lids should be 10 mm, and the margin of the upper eyelid should cover 1 to 2 mm of the superior limbus. Lid ptosis can be unilateral (such as in Horner syndrome) or bilateral (usually due to aging). Lid ptosis must be evaluated in relationship to brow position because of the intimate relationship between these two elements. The differential includes the following:

- Aging (*senile ptosis*)
- *Horner syndrome*
- *Myasthenia gravis*, especially when presence is intermittent.
- *Levator disinsertion*, due to surgery or trauma.
- Prior remote minor lid trauma

Lagophthalmos refers to incomplete eye closure. This may be due to the following:

- *Facial weakness or paralysis*
- *Overresection of tissue* in blepharoplasty

Orbital dystopias are either overly wide-spaced or close-set eyes. By convention, the distance between the medial canthi should be approximately equal to the width of one eye measured from lateral to medial canthus, or about half the interpupillary distance. Typical interpupillary distance is 60 to 70 mm, making the normal intercanthal distance ~30 to 35 mm. **Hypertelorism** refers to eyes set overly far apart. **Hypotelorism** refers to eyes set too closely. True hypertelorism means the globes and/or orbits are displaced; displacement of the medial canthus (such as in a naso-orbital-ethmoid fracture) results in **telecanthus** (or **pseudohypertelorism**—the appearance of hypertelorism). Vertical orbital dystopia describes when one orbit is out of horizontal alignment with the other.

- Orbital dystopias are typically caused by *congenital craniofacial abnormalities.*

Puffy eyelids may be caused by the following:

- *Fat pseudoherniation* of inferior orbital fat pads; this is a hereditary predisposition to laxity and relative protrusion of the orbital fat pads.
- *Lacrimal gland ptosis* must be recognized in the evaluation of the upper eyelid and is found in the lateral aspect of the superior orbit.
- *Orbicularis oculi hypertrophy* may occur due to hyperactivity.
- *Orbicularis oculi redundancy* occurs as part of the aging process.
- *Blepharochalasis* is a rare disease thought to be autoimmune that presents with recurrent bilateral (rarely unilateral) periorbital edema and gradual atrophy of the periorbital skin.

Suggested Reading

Friedman O, Wang TD, Cook TA. Management of the aging periorbital area. In: Cummings CW, Haughey BH, Thomas JR, et al, eds. Otolaryngology–Head and Neck Surgery. Philadelphia: Elsevier Mosby; 2005

Pastorek NJ. Blepharoplasty. In: Bailey Head and Neck Surgery–Otolaryngology. Philadelphia: Lippincott Williams & Wilkins; 2001

74 Midface Deformity

Noah E. Meltzer

The midface is bounded by the glabella superiorly and the subnasale inferiorly. Aesthetic subunits in the midface are the lower eyes, cheeks, and nose. Midface abnormalities can dramatically impair appearance, they can produce pooling of tears (in ectropion), or be a sign of systemic illness such as human immunodeficiency virus (HIV).

Rhytids and **aging changes** can be seen in the midface.

- *Prominence of the nasolabial (also called melolabial) folds*: Due to descent of the malar fat pad inferomedially. This descent produces a deepened nasolabial crease with a more prominent nasolabial fold.
- *Sun exposure*

Malar ptosis is the inferomedial displacement of the malar fat pad. Causes include the following:

- *Aging*
- *Trauma* and failure to resuspend the malar periosteum may result in unilateral malar ptosis.

Malar hypoplasia produces a short and retruded midface, often with bite malocclusion. This can occur in isolation or be associated with a *congenital craniofacial syndrome*.

Submalar wasting is the progressive atrophy of the submalar fat pads. This is often seen in conjunction with progressive fat atrophy throughout the face and body. Causes include the following:

- *Aging*
- *Facial wasting syndrome* can be due to highly active antiretroviral therapy (HAART) for HIV; this can also include insulin resistance, central adiposity, and hyperlipidemia.
- *HIV-associated lipodystrophy* is the atrophy of fat in the face, as well as the rest of the body, seen in untreated patients with HIV.

Ectropion is the sagging of the lower eyelid away from the globe (**Fig. 74.1**). Causes of this include the following:

- *Aging*
- *Facial paralysis*, which allows the lower lid to fall away from the globe as gravity overcomes facial muscle tone.
- *Trauma*, which can produce scarring that retracts the lower lid skin.
- *Excessive resection* of skin/muscle during blepharoplasty

Entropion refers to a lower eyelid margin that is rolled in toward the globe. This may be caused by the following:

Fig. 74.1 Lower eyelid ectropion due to an age-related increase in horizontal lid length and laxity. Note increased scleral show, mild bulbar conjunctival injection, and visible palpebral conjunctiva. Pooling of tears and epiphora are often associated with this condition.

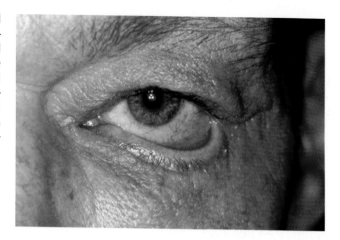

- *Trauma to the bulbar conjunctiva* can produce scarring and contracture that draws the lid margin inward.
- *Transconjunctival approaches* to the orbital floor can also produce scarring and contracture.

Proptosis is abnormal anterior displacement of the globe. Proptosis may be due to the following:

- *Thyroid eye disease*, which produces proptosis secondary to conal hypertrophy.
- *Vascular orbital lesions*
  - *Lymphangioma*
  - *Hemangioma*
  - *Cavernous hemangioma*
- *Wegener granulomatosis*
- *Lymphoma or leukemia*
- *Neuroblastoma*
- *Orbital pseudotumor*
- *Infectious processes*
  - *Orbital cellulitis*
  - *Orbital abscess*
  - *Subperiosteal abscess*
  - *Cavernous sinus thrombosis*

Scleral show refers to inferior displacement of the lower eyelid margin below the lower limbus margin; the lower lid normally covers ~1 mm of the lower limbus. Causes of scleral show include the following:

- *Aging*
- *Facial paralysis*

- *Prior trauma*
- *Overresection of skin/muscle* during blepharoplasty

Trichiasis means inverted eyelashes, which may be due to the following:

- *Eyelid trauma*
- *Transconjunctival approach* for orbital fracture or blepharoplasty
- *Blepharoplasty*
- *Burns* (chemical or thermal)
- *Ocular cicatricial pemphigoid*
- *Stevens-Johnson syndrome*
- *Vernal keratoconjunctivitis*
- *Trachoma*
- *Herpes zoster*

Suggested Reading

Friedman O, Wang TD, Cook TA. Management of the aging periorbital area. In: Cummings CW, Haughey BH, Thomas JR, et al, eds. Otolaryngology–Head and Neck Surgery. Philadelphia: Elsevier Mosby; 2005

Pastorek NJ. Blepharoplasty. In: Bailey Head & Neck Surgery–Otolaryngology. Philadelphia: Lippincott Williams & Wilkins; 2001

75 Lip Lesion or Deformity

Bruce K. Tan

Lips form the anatomical boundary at which mucosalized epithelium transitions to become keratinized squamous epithelium. As a result, diseases affecting both mucosa as well as skin can manifest on the lips. Because lips play a prominent role in facial aesthetics, enunciation, and maintaining oral competence, lip lesions or defects are readily noticeable and can be devastating for social interaction. Lip abnormalities include congenital errors of embryological development, acquired lesions resulting from trauma and aging, manifestations of systemic disease or infection, and both benign and malignant neoplasms. This section focuses on those conditions that may involve treatment by the facial plastic surgeon.

◆ Congenital Lip Abnormalities

Congenital lip abnormalities are among the most common craniofacial developmental abnormalities. Of these cleft lip is the most common, and is associated with a cleft palate in 68 to 86% of patients.

- *Cleft lip*: Can be either unilateral or bilateral and occurs only on the upper lip (**Fig. 75.1**). Cleft abnormalities result from the nasal and maxillary prominences failing to fuse in midline during the fifth and sixth week of intrauterine development. The severity of clefting can also vary:
  - *Microform cleft lip* is a dehiscence of the orbicularis muscle with associated vermilion notching but intact overlying skin.
  - *Incomplete cleft lip* spares some of the superior upper lip.
  - *Complete cleft lip* involves all three layers with none of the upper lip crossing midline.

- *Labial frenulum*: May involve the upper or lower lips. In infants, the labial frenulum typically extends over the alveolar ridge and should regress after the eruption of teeth. An aberrant frenulum can lead to periodontal disease and bone loss.
- *Congenital double lip*: May present in isolation or as a component of *Ascher syndrome*. Patients with a double lip have a fold of excess or redundant tissue that appears on the mucosal side of the lip when the lip is tensed during smiling.
- *Congenital lip pit*: A depressed sinus lined with stratified squamous epithelium that communicates with the minor salivary glands. Saliva can be expressed from these pits when pressure is applied. This may occur at the oral commissure, the midline upper lip, or the lower lip. Children with the

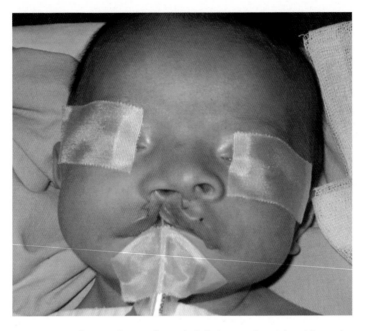

Fig. 75.1 Infant with a unilateral cleft lip on the right side and a cleft-associated nasal deformity characterized by an inferior and lateral displacement of the nasal alar.

autosomal dominant *Van der Woude syndrome* have bilateral lip pits on the vermilion of the lower lip and cleft lip or palate.

- *Microstomia*: Commonly associated with *holoprosencephaly* as well as other congenital syndromes such as the *Freeman-Sheldon syndrome*.
- *Macrostomia*: Extremely rare but can result from abnormalities of branchial arch development.

◆ Lip Trauma

Lip trauma can result from a variety of mechanisms ranging from blunt force trauma to avulsion or electrical injury. In repairing traumatic injury to the lip, attention must be paid to restoring both cosmesis and functionality.

- *Lip contusion*: Results from blunt force injury of the perioral soft tissue. Substantial soft tissue swelling can occur in this area.
- *Lip laceration*: If the vermilion border is lacerated, special attention must be paid to reapproximation during closure.
- *Lip avulsion*: These injuries result in the loss of soft tissue.
- *Lip burn*: Burn injuries can result from thermal, electrical, or caustic exposure. Electrical injuries to the oral commissure are relatively common

in young children and can result in significant functional and aesthetic debilitation.

- *Traumatic keratosis*: Granular hyperkeratotic surface alterations that result from chronic friction trauma such as habitual lip biting.
- *Lip mucocele*: Presents as a painless, smooth, freely movable, soft, and fluctuant mass, usually on the lower lip. These are caused by trauma resulting in a shear injury to a minor or accessory salivary gland duct.
- *Fibroma*: A sessile, pedunculated, firm mass that forms in response to chronic irritation.
- *Pyogenic granuloma*: A smooth, dome-shaped, or pedunculated papule or nodule with a glistening surface. The papules have a soft texture and range from bright red, to dusky red, to violaceous, to brown-black. Predisposing factors can include trauma but also include hormonal influences, growth factors, infections, and microscopic arteriovenous anastomoses.

◆ Cosmetic due to Aging

Aging results in progressive loss of lip volume and definition. Addressing cosmetic concerns surrounding the aging lip requires attention toward reversing the following:

- *Volume loss*
- *Loss of lip definition*
- *Vertical rhytids*

◆ Neoplasms: Benign

- *Neurofibroma*: Presents as a soft, painless, slowly growing mass. The oral cavity and lips are common areas of involvement in von Recklinghausen neurofibromatosis.
- *Keratoacanthoma*: A benign neoplasm that has an initial rapid growth phase after which it stabilizes and spontaneously regresses after several weeks to months. It appears as an ulcerated, circumscribed lesion with an indurated base.
- *Hemangioma* of the lip: Relatively common and usually presents at birth. These undergo a rapid proliferative phase and tend to spontaneously regress with aging.
- *Papilloma*: Soft, pedunculated mass with numerous tiny fingerlike surface projections. Human papilloma virus (HPV)-6 and HPV-11 are the most commonly associated viral subtypes.
- *Granular cell tumor*: Presents as a small, firm, painless, sessile and nodular-appearing lesion. Synchronous lesions can often be found in 15% of patients. Malignant degeneration can occur in ~1% of all cases.
- *Minor salivary gland tumors*: Twenty to forty percent of minor salivary gland neoplasms are benign.

- ○ *Pleomorphic adenoma*
- ○ *Monomorphic adenoma*
- ○ *Oncocytoma*
- ○ *Other rare benign tumors*
- ● *Melanotic macules/nevi*

◆ Neoplasms: Premalignant

- ● *Actinic cheilitis*: Presents as rough, scaly lips with fissures and ulcerations. The lower lip is more commonly affected because it receives more ultraviolet-ray exposure.
- ● *Leukoplakia*: A heterogeneous clinical entity that can vary in appearance ranging from a thin grayish surface alteration with ill-defined margins to sharply demarcated, thick, opaque plaques. It is generally associated with use of tobacco products. Several distinct histopathological subtypes of leukoplakia deserve special mention.
  - ○ *Proliferative verrucous leukoplakia*: A multifocal and persistent lesion that evolves from a thin, flat, white patch that slowly evolves into a papillary and verrucous lesion. Unlike most leukoplakia, patients with proliferative verrucous leukoplakia are not usually tobacco users, but malignant transformation occurs in over 70% of cases.
  - ○ *Hairy leukoplakia*: The lesion does not always appear "hairy"; it is usually white plaque(s) that may be contiguous or separate and can appear corrugated or "hairy." Typically, occurs on the lateral border of the tongue.
- ● *Erythroplakia*: A red mucosal plaque with a high risk of progression to carcinoma

◆ Neoplasms: Malignant

- ● *Squamous cell carcinoma*: The most common malignancy of the lip. It typically presents as an area of crusting within an area of leukoplakia on the lower lip. As it progresses, it enlarges into a large bleeding, ulcerated mass. Smoking, chronic sun exposure, poor dental hygiene, and chronic alcoholism have been shown to be contributing factors.
- ● *Basal cell carcinoma*: The second most common malignancy after squamous cell carcinoma and tends to occur on the upper lip. These tumors appear as pearly white nodules with central dimpling.
- ● *Melanoma* of the lip: Usually manifests as flat, heterogeneously pigmented lesions with irregular borders, although nodular varieties are not uncommon. Desmoplastic neurotropic melanoma is a nonpigmented type of melanoma that presents on the lower lip as an ulceration.

- *Microcystic adnexal carcinoma*: A rare, low-grade sweat gland carcinoma with a predilection for the upper lip. It is locally aggressive but it is rarely metastatic.
- *Merkel cell tumor*: An aggressive malignancy that manifests as red or violaceous dome-shaped nodules. Regional metastases are common. Recent studies have linked the tumor to the Merkel cell polyomavirus.
- *Kaposi's sarcoma (KS)*: Can present as a lip nodule or macule and is usually associated with immunosuppression. The HHV-8 virus agent is responsible for KS.
- *Minor salivary gland tumors*: Sixty to eighty percent of minor salivary gland neoplasms are malignant.
  - *Mucoepidermoid carcinoma*
  - *Adenoid cystic carcinoma*
  - *Acinic cell carcinoma*
  - *Carcinoma ex-pleomorphic adenoma*
  - *Other rare malignant tumors*

- *Tumors of mesenchymal origin (ie, sarcoma)*: Very rare

Suggested Reading

Arosarena OA. Cleft lip and palate. Otolaryngol Clin North Am 2007;40:27–60, vi

Bentley JM, Barankin B, Guenther LC. A review of common pediatric lip lesions: herpes simplex/recurrent herpes labialis, impetigo, mucoceles, and hemangiomas. Clin Pediatr (Phila) 2003;42:475–482

Esclamado RM, Krause CJ. Lip cancer. In: Bailey BJ, eds. Head and Neck Surgery Otolaryngology. Philadelphia: JB Lippincott; 1993

Lian TS. Benign tumors and tumor-like lesions of the oral cavity. In: Cummings CW, Haughey BH, Rhomas JR, eds. Otolaryngology–Head and Neck Surgery. Philadelphia: Elsevier Mosby; 2005

Mueller DT, Callanan VP. Congenital malformations of the oral cavity. Otolaryngol Clin North Am 2007;40:141–160, vii

Perkins SW, Sandel HD IV. Anatomic considerations, analysis, and the aging process of the perioral region. Facial Plast Surg Clin North Am 2007;15:403–407, v

Sciubba JJ. Oral mucosal lesions. In: Cummings CW, Haughey BH, Rhomas JR, eds. Otolaryngology–Head and Neck Surgery. Philadelphia: Elsevier Mosby; 2005

Ship JA, Ghezzi EM. Oral manifestations of systemic disease. Cummings CW, Haughey BH, Rhomas JR, eds. Otolaryngology–Head and Neck Surgery. Philadelphia: Elsevier Mosby; 2005

Wein RO, Weber RS. Malignant neoplasms of the oral cavity. Cummings CW, Haughey BH, Thomas JR, eds. Otolaryngology–Head and Neck Surgery. Philadelphia: Elsevier Mosby; 2005

76 Neck Aging

Babar Sultan

The aging neck can be a great cause of preoccupation for a patient, and any intervention lies in a thorough understanding of the interplay of heredity and aging with anatomy. The anatomical components of concern can be divided into skin, fat, muscle, and bone. As one examines the neck, it is helpful to define what is ideal. The neck should have a clear delineation from the inferior border of the mandible with a cervicomental angle of ~90 degrees. There should be a slight depression inferior to the hyoid bone followed by a prominence of the thyroid cartilage.

◆ Horizontal Cervical Rhytids

- *Skin degeneration* of collagen and elastin fibers leads to redundant and sagging skin.
- *Dynamic lines* are created perpendicular to the vectors of muscle (eg, platysma) contraction.

◆ Effacement of Cervicomental Angle

- *Unequal or excess fat deposition*: Either acquired or hereditary
- *Supraplatysmal fat deposition*
- *Subplatysmal, submental fat deposition*
- *Overdevelopment of suprahyoid bone musculature*
- *Low hyoid bone position*: Below the fourth cervical vertebra
- *Congenital microgenia or senile absorption of alveolar bone*: Weakens chin contour, not to be confused with retrognathia.

◆ Jowling

- *Facial fat deposition*: Classically associated with the jowl appearance. *Jowl* comes from the Middle English word *cholle*, meaning prominence and laxity of the flesh of the lower cheek and jaw.
- *Ptotic malar fat pad*: Contributes to the fullness of the jowl.
- *Laxity of superficial musculoaponeurotic system flap*
- *Submandibular gland ptosis*: Causes unsightly appearance of bilateral neck masses, which can be seen as jowls.

◆ Platysmal Banding

Seventy percent of the population has no platysmal decussation at midline, and with aging comes atrophy causing the muscle to fall in the midline. With further loss of tone, an anterior banding appearance can occur.

Suggested Reading

Adamson PA, Litner JA. Surgical management of the aging neck. Facial Plast Surg 2005;21:11–20

Kamer FM, Pieper PG. Surgical treatment of the aging neck. Facial Plast Surg 2001;17:123–128

Mendelson BC, Freeman ME, Wu W, Huggins RJ. Surgical anatomy of the lower face: the premasseter space, the jowl, and the labiomandibular fold. Aesthetic Plast Surg 2008;32:185–195

Williams EF, Pontius AT. The aging neck. In: Bailey BJ, Johnson JT, eds. Head and Neck Surgery—Otolaryngology. 4th ed. Philadelphia: Lippincott Williams & Wilkins; 2006:2651–2662

77 Bony Deformity

Eugene A. Chu

There is a wide range of craniomaxillofacial deformities. Appropriate management is based on obtaining the proper diagnosis. This may be facilitated by organizing the broad differential into three categories: congenital, traumatic, and neoplastic. Despite advances in imaging, the history and the physical remain critical aspects to arriving at the correct diagnosis.

◆ Congenital

Craniofacial anomalies are a group of deformities of the bones of the face and skull. They may occur in isolation, such as cleft lip, or as part of a recognized syndrome. The etiology of most craniofacial abnormalities is multifactorial involving both environmental and genetic factors. **Table 77.1** lists some common craniofacial syndromes.

Table 77.1 Common Craniofacial Syndromes

Syndrome	Clinical Findings
Waardenburg syndrome	Sensorineural hearing loss, partial albinism (white forelock usually), heterochromic iris, laterally displaced medial canthi
Pierre Robin syndrome	Micrognathia with glossoptosis, mandibular hypoplasia, cleft palate
Treacher Collins syndrome	Malformed external ear, mandibular and malar hypoplasia, antimongoloid slant of the palpebral fissures, coloboma of the lower eyelid, conductive hearing loss
Goldenhar syndrome	Facial asymmetry, unilateral malformed external ear with preauricular tags and sinuses, conductive hearing loss, microphthalmia, epibulbar lipodermoid, macrostomia with mandibular hypoplasia, vertebral abnormalities
Velocardiofacial syndrome	Cleft palate, hypernasal speech, cardiac abnormalities, characteristic facies

Other congenital bony deformities include the following:

- *Cleft lip*: Usually soft tissue only, but a complete cleft can include the entire lip and the underlying premaxilla.
- *Cleft palate*: Occurs during fetal development when there is incomplete fusion of the palate. The degree of clefting can vary from a submucous cleft where the musculature of the palate is deficient to a complete cleft palate with involvement of the hard palate, soft palate, and uvula.
- *Craniosynostosis*: Premature fusion of the cranial sutures resulting in an abnormal head shape. Simple craniosynostosis involves a single suture, whereas compound craniosynostosis involves two or more sutures.
- *Deformational plagiocephaly*: From the Greek words *plagio* for oblique and *cephale* for head. Refers to asymmetry of the cranium from external molding such as a tight intrauterine environment. Noncongenital forms of deformational plagiocephaly may be related to sleeping position (on the back) or muscular torticollis.
- *Hemifacial microsomia*: One side of the face is underdeveloped, most notably affecting the ears, midface, and mandible. Ear malformations can result in hearing loss, whereas retrognathia and malformation of the mandible can lead to feeding difficulties and respiratory distress.

◆ Trauma

Maxillofacial fractures may result from blunt or penetrating trauma. Blunt trauma predominates and includes motor vehicle accidents, sports-related trauma, occupational injuries, and falls. Penetrating trauma involves gunshot wounds, stabbings, and explosive injuries. Diagnosis involves careful history and physical examination and select radiographic imaging.

- *Temporal bone fracture*: May present with cranial nerve abnormalities (ie, facial paralysis), hearing loss, or nystagmus with involvement of the labyrinthine system. Mastoid (Battle sign) or periorbital (raccoon eyes) ecchymosis is commonly associated with skull base injuries. Fractures may be classified as longitudinal or transverse based on the orientation of the fracture to the long axis of the petrous pyramid. Hemotympanum or otorrhagia may be present and is more commonly associated with longitudinal fractures and injury of the external auditory canal.
- *Frontal sinus fracture*: There may be a history or signs of trauma to the forehead. An obvious deformity or bony step-off may be present. Categorized according to involvement of anterior table only or posterior table as well. Clear rhinorrhea suggests a posterior table fracture with *cerebrospinal fluid (CSF) rhinorrhea* secondary to dural injury.
- *Nasal fracture*: Most commonly fractured bone of the face. Signs and symptoms include cosmetic deformity, epistaxis, nasal congestion or airway obstruction, external swelling, periorbital ecchymosis, crepitus, and tenderness to palpation. Rarely emergent but often associated with other injuries. Must rule out septal hematoma and open nasal fracture with exposed bone

or cartilage. The presence of cerebrospinal fluid (CSF) rhinorrhea indicates more severe injury and warrants further radiological evaluation.

- *Orbital fracture*: Presents with history of periocular or facial trauma. The patient may complain of diplopia, pain, or visual disturbance, and there is usually significant swelling in this area. Clinical examination must assess for proptosis, enophthalmos, retrobulbar hemorrhage, palpable bony step-off, orbital emphysema, extraocular movements, visual acuity, and sensation of the periorbital region. With many orbital floor blow-out fractures, the only clinical finding will be enophthalmos, which will not be apparent at presentation because of soft-tissue swelling. Radiological evaluation is key in this scenario.
- *Nasal-orbital-ethmoid fracture*: Telecanthus indicates probable involvement of the naso-orbital-ethmoid complex.
- *Maxilla/mandible fracture*: Presents with a history of trauma to the head and neck region. Patients often complain that bite is "off" or that the teeth do not come together properly. Paresthesias of the lip or chin indicate involvement of the inferior alveolar or mental nerve, whereas cheek numbness comes from injury to the infraorbital nerve. Trismus may be due to pain, muscle injury, or the fracture. Examination must assess occlusion, the status of the dentition, and the presence or absence of bony step-off or mobile segment as well as any mucosal injuries. Maxillary and mandibular fractures are classified according to the location of the fracture, whether it is displaced or nondisplaced, whether it is compound, simple, or comminuted, and whether its orientation is considered favorable or unfavorable.

◆ Neoplasm

Bony tumors of the maxillofacial region are categorized as either primary bone tumors or secondary bone tumors.

Primary Bone Tumors

The most common symptom of bone tumors is pain; however, many patients will not experience any symptoms, except for the mass. Some bone tumors may weaken the structure of the bone causing pathological fractures.

- *Benign tumors: Osteoma, osteochondroma, aneurysmal bone cyst, enchondroma, giant cell tumor*
- *Fibroosseous lesions: Fibrous dysplasia, ossifying fibroma, cherubism*
- *Malignant tumors: osteosarcoma, chondrosarcoma, Ewing sarcoma, other sarcomas, multiple myeloma, chordoma, hemangiopericytoma, malignant fibrous histiocytoma*

Secondary Bone Tumors

Can be subdivided into metastatic tumors, tumors resulting from contiguous spread of adjacent soft tissue neoplasms, and tumors resulting from malignant transformation of preexisting benign lesions. Metastatic cancers are more frequently seen than primary malignancies of bone. For adults most originate from carcinomas of the *prostate, breast, kidney, lung, thyroid,* and *colon.* For children most are related to *neuroblastoma, rhabdomyosarcoma,* or *retinoblastoma.*

◆ Inflammatory and Metabolic

Inflammatory lesions usually present with other findings, such as fever, overlying cellulitis, and signs of systemic disease.

- *Osteomyelitis*: Can be due to bacteria or tuberculosis
- *Langerhans cell histiocytosis*: Lesions can be unifocal or multifocal; in multifocal disease there is often solid organ involvement as well.
- *"Brown tumor" of hyperparathyroidism*: Reactive lytic lesion caused by excess osteoclast activity.
- *Paget disease*: hyperostosis

Suggested Reading

Ellis EI III. Treatment methods for fractures of the mandibular angle. J Craniomaxillofac Trauma 1996;2:28–36

Kawamoto HK, Heller JB, Heller MM, et al. Craniofrontonasal dysplasia: a surgical treatment algorithm. Plast Reconstr Surg 2007;120:1943–1956

Kellman R. Maxillofacial trauma. In: Cummings CW, CH, BH; Thomas JR, Harker LA, Flint PW, eds. Cummings Otolaryngology–Head and Neck Surgery. Vol 1. 4th ed. St. Louis: Mosby; 2004:602–638

Manson PN, Clark N, Robertson B, et al. Subunit principles in midface fractures: the importance of sagittal buttresses, soft-tissue reductions, and sequencing treatment of segmental fractures. Plast Reconstr Surg 1999;103:1287–1306, quiz 1307

78 Alopecia

Lisa E. Ishii

Alopecia, or hair loss where there was formerly hair growth, is a common problem that affects more than half of the male population, and up to 40% of females over the age of 70. Scalp alopecia is of particular concern because the length and fullness of hair on the scalp are associated with youthfulness and physical attractiveness, and this hair frames the face to draw attention to the eyes. Gray, thinning hair is associated with increasing age and maturity and areas of balding draw attention away from the eyes to the forehead and scalp. Although alopecia can be the result of many different processes, the most common cause is androgenetic alopecia (AGA). When evaluating a patient with alopecia, a detailed history and physical are necessary to properly diagnose and treat the underlying condition. Alopecia can be distinguished as diffuse or focal, and nonscarring or scarring (also known as cicatricial).

Diffuse nonscarring alopecia can be caused by the following:

- *Androgenetic (or androgenic) alopecia (AGA)*: AGA is the most common cause of alopecia in men and women. AGA may begin in puberty for men and typically increases in incidence per decade, with 30% of men noticing some baldness in their thirties, 40% in their forties, and so forth, until ultimately 60 to 80% of all men eventually experience AGA. The onset is typically later for women and ultimately less common. The incidence varies by ethnic group, with Chinese, Japanese, and black men less frequently affected than whites, but for all groups the incidence increases with age.
- *Alopecia areata*: This is an autoimmune disease that affects ~1 to 2% of the population and occurs in males and females. Although it can occur in people of all ages, it most commonly presents in the late teenage or early adult years. It typically presents with small, round patches of hair loss, which range in severity from small areas that spontaneously regrow to extensive, persistent patches.
- *Anagen effluvium*: This hair loss occurs after insults or injury to the follicle that cause impaired mitotic activity. Usually the result of chemotherapeutic agents, the arrest of cell division can lead to a narrow, weakened hair shaft segment that is easily fractured, or the complete failure to produce a hair shaft. It is more common and severe with combination chemotherapy than single drug chemotherapy.
- *Telogen effluvium*: This typically occurs when an insult or trauma causes multiple hair follicles to enter the telogen phase at once. Telogen effluvium can occur at any age and is typically self-correcting.

Focal nonscarring alopecia can be caused by the following:

- *Androgenetic alopecia*: See above.
- *Alopecia areata*: See above.

- *Trichotillomania*: Patients with trichotillomania have an impulse control disorder that manifests as pulling out scalp, eyelash, eyebrow, or pubic hairs. They may have scalp bald patches or patches of missing hair in other areas. The vast majority of patients are women, and onset is typically in the pre- or early-adolescent years.
- *Traction alopecia*: This is a common cause of hair loss resulting from traction forces on the scalp, typically from various hairstyling practices such as braids, weaves, or cornrows.
- *Tinea capitis*: This disease, also known as "ringworm of the scalp" is caused by superficial fungal infections of the skin that typically affect the hair shafts of the scalp, eyebrows, or eyelashes.
- *Syphilis*: Secondary syphilis may present with patchy alopecia of the scalp or other parts of the body. It should be suspected as a cause in patients with other symptoms of secondary syphilis such as lymphadenopathy, fatigue, myalgia, weight loss, and sores.

Scarring or cicatricial alopecia is caused by the following:

- *Traumatic injury*: Patients who have a history of injuries such as *burn, laceration*, or *radiation* may have alopecia in the affected area.
- *Primary cicatricial alopecia*: This group of hair disorders is linked by the potential to develop permanent loss of scalp hair follicles in affected areas. Examples of causes include *discoid lupus erythematosis, sarcoidosis, dermatomyositis*, and *lichen planopilaris*.

Suggested Reading

Ali A. Dermatology: A Pictorial Review. McGraw-Hill; 2002

DeBerker DAR, Messenger AG, Sinclair RD. Disorders of Hair: Rooks Textbook of Dermatology. Boston: Blackwell; 2004

Loos BM, Kabaker SS. Hair restoration: medical and surgical techniques. In: Cummings CW, Haughey BH, Thomas JR, et al, eds. Otolaryngology–Head and Neck Surgery. Philadelphia: Elsevier Mosby; 2005

79 Internal or External Nasal Deformity

Murugappan Ramanathan Jr.

◆ Internal

Nasal obstruction is one of the most common complaints encountered by an oto-laryngologist/facial plastic surgeon. Nasal obstruction is a symptom, not a diagnosis, and is therefore caused by numerous medical and structural conditions. Airflow within the nasal cavity is both laminar and turbulent. Laminar airflow causes air to reach from the nose to the lower respiratory tract during inspiration. Turbulent airflow facilitates exchange of heat and moisture. The most common medical cause of nasal obstruction is chronic mucosal inflammation/chronic sinusitis, whereas common structural causes include deformities of the external and/or internal nasal valve. When evaluating a patient with nasal obstruction, a detailed history and physical including examination of the nasal septum, inferior turbinate, and internal/external nasal valves is necessary to properly diagnose and treat the underlying condition.

Mucosal and Soft Tissue Etiologies

Mucosal inflammation can decrease the cross-sectional area of the nasal valve, therefore causing nasal obstruction. This is typically intermittent or fluctuating but can be fixed (see Chapters 27 and 28). Common causes include the following:

- *Inflammatory rhinosinusitis*
- *Allergic rhinitis*
- *Nonallergic rhinitis*
- *Rhinitis medicamentosa*
- *Nasal polyposis*: Usually fixed, but size and symptoms can fluctuate.
- *Sinonasal neoplasm* (see Chapter 30)

Structural Etiologies

Structural causes usually cause fixed obstruction. However, patients can have both structural and mucosal causes of obstruction, causing some level of fluctuation even when there is a fixed structural problem. A common area of structural nasal obstruction is the nasal valve. Anatomically, the nasal valve is defined by the septum medially, the nasal floor and inferior turbinate head inferiorly, and the internal nasal valve superiorly. Structural nasal obstruction can be divided into **static** and **dynamic** dysfunction. **Static** dysfunction includes decreased nasal airflow at rest and is usually caused by a deviated septum, inferior turbinate hypertrophy, or narrowed internal nasal valve. **Dynamic** dysfunction is obstruction that varies with respiratory effort and is related to weakened structural support of the lateral nasal wall. Common structural causes include static dysfunction, dynamic dysfunction, and external factors.

Static Dysfunction

- *Deviated septum*: The nasal septum is composed of the quadrangular cartilage anteriorly, the bony vomer inferiorly, and the perpendicular plate of the ethmoid posteriorly. The floor of the septum is composed of the bony maxillary crest. Deviation of either the cartilaginous or the bony septum can contribute to nasal obstruction.
- *Inferior turbinate hypertrophy*: An enlarged anterior portion of the inferior turbinate can narrow the nasal valve and cause symptomatic obstruction.
- *Internal nasal valve*: The internal nasal valve is the narrowest portion of airflow and functions as the primary regulator of flow and resistance. Nasal airflow is proportional to the radius of the narrowest portion of the nasal passage to the fourth power (Poiseuille's law); therefore small differences can affect airflow greatly. The internal nasal valve can also cause dynamic obstruction. Etiologies of internal valve obstruction include the following:
  - *Congenitally weak lower lateral cartilages*
  - *Cephalic malposition of the lower lateral cartilages* (**Fig. 79.1**)
  - *Overresection* of the dorsal septum and upper lateral cartilages in rhinoplasty
  - *Overresection* of the lateral crura from cephalic trims in rhinoplasty
  - *Disarticulation* of the upper lateral cartilages from trauma or previous surgery

Dynamic Dysfunction

- *External nasal valve*: External nasal valve collapse (alar collapse) occurs during maximal inspiration and results from poor cartilaginous support of the alar sidewalls.
  - *Weak lower lateral cartilages*
  - *Vestibular stenosis*: Cicatricial scarring after trauma or previous surgery

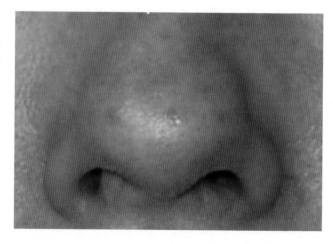

Fig. 79.1 Depiction of cephalic malpositioning of the lower lateral cartilages, which is a normal anatomical variant. Classically, this has been referred to as a "parenthesis tip deformity" where the supra-alar crease is moved medially and cephalically oriented, thereby resembling a pair of parentheses that frames the nasal tip.

- Postsurgery dysfunction
  - *Dome division*
  - *Overresection of cephalic trims*

◆ External

Deformities of the nose can arise from congenital, acquired, or traumatic etiologies. Correction of these deformities presents the otolaryngologist/facial plastic surgeon with numerous challenges. It is critical not to compromise the structural support of the nose while achieving facial harmony. Ironically, rhinoplasty itself can often be the primary cause of newly acquired nasal deformity. Nonetheless, a thorough physical examination including a nasal analysis is crucial to identify and address the various deformities. Some commonly encountered deformities include the following:

- *Crooked nose*: Encompasses deviations that can arise from the caudal septum, bony and cartilaginous dorsum, or nasal tip creating asymmetry. Most cases involve the lower two thirds of the nose. It is important to describe the deviation in each area of the nose—upper, middle, and lower thirds.
  - *Congenital*
  - *Posttraumatic*
- *Saddle nose deformity*: A significant loss of the bony and cartilaginous septum usually caused by *aggressive dorsal reduction* or *septal hematoma/trauma*. Resembles the shape of a saddle. It can also be caused by destructive or inflammatory processes such as *cocaine abuse* or *Wegener granulomatosis*.
- *Midvault collapse*: Seen *after resection of a dorsal hump* and is caused by destabilized upper lateral cartilages falling medially toward the anterior septal angle.
- *Dorsal hump*: A prominence of the nasal dorsum that may involve the bony and/or cartilaginous vaults of the nose. Most of the hump is typically cartilaginous.
- *Cephalic malposition of the lower lateral cartilages*: Alar cartilages normally lie at a 30- to 40-degree angle from the alar rim. Cephalic malposition is a condition in which alar cartilages are positioned along the dorsal septum causing an abnormal fullness over the anterior septal angle, tip bulbosity, or a pollybeak deformity. It may be associated with alar retraction. This condition is a commonly overlooked cause of supratip fullness and can cause dynamic or static nasal valve collapse.
- *Pollybeak deformity*: A dorsal nasal convexity resembling a parrot's beak. Usually a *complication of rhinoplasty* with a disproportionate tip/supratip relationship.
- *Tip bulbosity*: Fullness and bulblike appearance of the nasal tip often caused by *prominence of the domes of the lateral crura* of the lower lateral cartilage.

- *Tip ptosis*: Caused by excessive tip rotation, often due to a contracted naso-labial angle. Can be secondary to *abnormally weakened nasal cartilage* that is acquired or through the aging process. Relative shortness of the medial crura can also cause this.
- *Alar retraction*: Often caused by malposition or weakness of the lateral crura (**Fig. 79.2**). It may be congenital or secondary to previous rhinoplasty.
- *Excessive width of nostrils*: Alar base width may manifest as excessive width of the alar attachments to the face, as excessive "flaring," or both (**Fig. 79.3**).

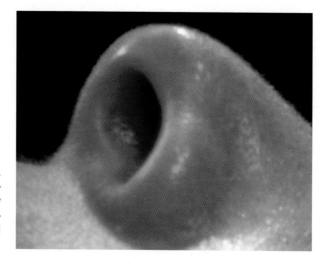

Fig. 79.2 Alar retraction, which is one of the most common complications of primary rhinoplasty secondary to arching, malpositioning, or surgical weakening of the lateral crura.

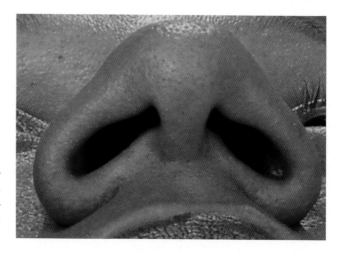

Fig. 79.3 Excessive alar base width associated with "flaring." This can be corrected most commonly using a "wedge" or "sill" excision.

Suggested Reading

Kim DW, Rodriguez-Bruno K. Functional rhinoplasty. Facial Plast Surg Clin North Am 2009;17:115–131, vii

Toriumi DM, Checcone MA. New concepts in nasal tip contouring. Facial Plast Surg Clin North Am 2009;17:55–90, vi

XI Using New and Forthcoming Technologies for Differential Diagnosis

Section Editor: *Thomas A. Tami*

80 Advances in Audiologic and Vestibular Testing

Jill M. Anderson, Fawen Zhang, and Ravi N. Samy

Although the mainstays of the diagnosis of patients with audiologic or vestibular disorders are history and physical examination, the differential diagnosis may be narrowed with a battery of tests. Unfortunately, the varying pathologies often cause similar symptomatology. Advances in these tests have improved the understanding of the disease processes as well as improved the determination of the site-of-lesion. Newer testing modalities have allowed greater objectivity with less subjective variability. As the field of audiology continues to expand, it is prudent for the practicing otolaryngologist to dialogue with the audiologist to improve and further the understanding of otologic diseases and to stay at the forefront of diagnosis and management. Before proceeding to the newest advances in audiologic and vestibular testing, it is prudent to review the basic testing.

◆ Vestibular Testing

The sense of balance requires the integrity of the visual, somatosensory, and vestibular system. Balance disturbance can be present in the form of dizziness, vertigo, or disequilibrium. Clinical assessment of balance disorders includes observation of spontaneous eye movement, Romberg and Fukuda testing, gait and tandem gait testing, and head shake and thrust tests. During clinical testing, the observation of nystagmus is enhanced through the use of special glasses called Frenzel lenses to avoid central suppression caused by fixation. In addition to physical examination and clinical assessment, multiple established vestibular tests exist.

Vestibular tests include identification of gaze-evoked nystagmus, evaluation of dynamic positionally induced vertigo and nystagmus using the Dix-Hallpike and other positioning maneuvers, evaluation of static positionally induced nystagmus, and evaluation of the vestibular ocular reflex (VOR). Testing for the VOR includes saccade and smooth pursuit testing. Finally, horizontal semicircular canal function is measured by caloric stimulation using warm and cool air or water.

Electronystagmography

Electronystagmography (ENG) is a technique that objectively records nystagmus by measuring the corneoretinal potential resulting from the VOR when the balance system is stimulated. The resulting nystagmus is measured using the slow phase velocity (SPV, the angle of the slow phase of the nystagmus in degrees per second) to identify the existence of vestibular pathology.

ENG includes a series of test categories such as spontaneous nystagmus, ocular-motor tests, the Dix-Hallpike maneuver, positional tests, and caloric tests. The spontaneous nystagmus test is performed to identify pathological unprovoked nystagmus and to rule out the influence of spontaneous nystagmus on the response in other vestibular tests.

The ocular-motor test battery evaluates the function of VOR pathway with the saccade test, the gaze fixation test, the sinusoidal tracking test/smooth pursuit test, and the optokinetic test. Abnormalities of these tests are more suggestive of central disorders of the vestibular nuclei or cerebellum.

The Dix-Hallpike maneuver evaluates the function of the posterior semicircular canal by observing evoked nystagmus directly or via video-recording equipment. Usually, this test is used to provoke nystagmus and vertigo commonly associated with benign paroxysmal positional vertigo (BPPV).

The positional test assesses eye movements as the head is slowly positioned in different directions. Abnormalities may reflect peripheral or central abnormalities depending on the results of the test.

The caloric test evaluates the eye movements as warm (44°C) or cold (30°C) water (or air) is circulated in the ear canal. The function of the left and right horizontal semicircular canal can be evaluated separately and compared in the caloric test. Abnormalities of this test correlate with inner ear vestibular pathology.

Sinusoidal Harmonic Acceleration/Rotational Chair Tests

The sinusoidal harmonic acceleration (SHA) test battery assesses the eye movement induced by back-and-forth sinusoidal movement on a motorized chair rotated at several different speeds. SHA tests can be performed in addition to ENG testing to confirm a diagnosis. The SHA test battery includes a saccadic eye movement test, smooth pursuit, optokinetic nystagmus, gaze nystagmus, spontaneous nystagmus, and fixation of nystagmus during rotational testing. This motion stimulates the horizontal semicircular canals in both ears simultaneously and so cannot separate out unilateral vestibular pathology. The measurements of the results include gain (response amplitude divided by stimulus amplitude), phase (timing of the response relative to the stimulus), bias (average value of slow phase eye velocity over a complete cycle), and gain asymmetry (comparison of gain during rotation to the right versus rotation to the left).

Dynamic Platform Posturography/Computerized Dynamic Posturography

Dynamic platform posturography (DPP) and computerized dynamic posturography (CDP) constitute a test battery that assesses the ability to use sensory (eg, visual, vestibular, or somatosensory) input to coordinate the motor responses for balance maintenance. Changes in the sensory information (somatosensory or visual) such as tilting the platform or providing inaccurate visual reference result in the change of the patient's center of gravity (COG). Sensors located under the feet measure voltage changes caused by the change of COG. The patients utilize the sensory input and adjust their position to avoid falling. In the case of vestibular disorders, the cues from other sensory systems become more important. Information gleaned from this test can identify malingering patients or may be used to craft treatment plans for vestibular rehabilitation.

The motor control test (MCT) assesses the patient's responses to sudden movements of the platform. The adaptation test (ADT) evaluates a patient's ability to minimize sway when exposed to a series of platform rotations in the toes-up or toes-down direction. In the posture-evoked response (PER) test, surface electrodes are placed on the medial gastrocnemius and tibialis anterior muscles to record compound muscle contraction activity of each muscle group when rapid rotations of the platform are used.

◆ Innovations in Vestibular Testing

Newer vestibular tests should have advantages over established testing. They should be more convenient to perform, and they should be able to assess the function of more components of the vestibular system because arguably the most important objective vestibular examination, caloric testing, measures only the function of the lateral semicircular canal. New vestibular tests should yield objective and quantitative data and are discussed following here.

Videonystagmography (VNG) is quite similar to ENG, but there are some important differences. For this test the subject wears goggles while video cameras are used to record eye movements in the horizontal and vertical axes. The greatest advantage of the video-oculographic system is its ability to record and analyze eye movement from each individual eye when the vestibular tests are executed. Video systems are typically more accurate than the standard ENG method because they are less sensitive to lid artifact and are not affected by electrical noise. Moreover, the calculation of measurements such as precision (gain or accuracy), latency, or peak velocity based on eye movements is more accurate. Computer-driven systems are used to better control variables and provide greater accuracy of stimulus presentation, data collection, and data analysis. These systems may use light-emitting diodes (LEDs) on a light bar anchored to the wall or in a self-contained oculomotor stimulator, promising a high level of control over stimulus presentation. More sophisticated measurements such as the short and long time constants of the SPV versus time function have been used to characterize the dynamic changes of the vestibular system response during stimulation. Results can be compared with normative data. The contemporary analysis techniques may integrate algorithms that can be used to separate the contributions of the peripheral and central vestibular system and the visual-oculomotor system.

More naturally occurring stimulating situations may be better models for physiological function. For example, the Vestibular Autorotation Test (VAT, Western Systems Research, Inc., Pasadena, CA) is a fast test lasting 18 seconds that evaluates the VOR function under more natural conditions. The patient is instructed to look at the visual target and perform horizontal and vertical head movement. The VAT may be more sensitive than other vestibular tests. It records responses of both the horizontal and two vertical canals, the superior and posterior canals. Due to these advantages, the VAT can be used as the first screening test for patients with balance problems as well as to monitor the effectiveness of vestibular rehabilitation.

Portability of a testing system is an important feature. For example, the IntelliNetx VNG I Video ENG System (Eye Dynamics, Inc., Torrance, CA) allows ENG tests to be performed anywhere. ICS Chartr 200 system (GN Otometrics, Taastrup, Denmark) combines VOG and ENG in a single convenient device and comes with features such as a remote control and built-in fixation light as well as software for automatic calculation and interpretation analysis.

Tests evaluating not only horizontal but also other semicircular canals and otolith organs have been developed. For example, VNG can evaluate the function of the vertical semicircular canal. Further, to test the function of semicircular canals other than the posterior semicircular canal, a series of modified Dix-Hallpike maneuvers have been developed with head positioning in the plane of the vertical semicircular canals.

A high torque rotary chair test provides the ability to perform unilateral utricular assessment. The chair is fitted with a translation sled that can move the subject along an interaurally oriented axis, during which one utricle becomes aligned with the axis of rotation. Thus the utricle on the stimulated side is assessed. This stimulus induces ocular counterrolling (OCR) that can be measured with three-dimensional video-oculography (3D VOG). The OCR output is a measure of the utricular function of the stimulated side.

Off-vertical axis test evaluates the function of the otolith organ by assessing the eye movement during rotation about an axis that is tilted away from earth vertical.

The subjective visual vertical (SVV) test is a method to evaluate the perception of the head position relative to gravity. The subject is instructed to adjust a visible luminus line in complete darkness to what they consider to be gravitational vertical. This test is used to evaluate utricular function.

The galvanic vestibular test might be a test of otolith function. It consists of using a direct current of 1 to 5 mA on the mastoid process in an attempt to stimulate the vestibular while eye movement and postural sway are recorded.

Vestibular evoked myogenic potentials (VEMPs) are used to assess the function of the saccule. The saccule is virtually unresponsive to auditory stimulation but is sensitive to vibratory information resulting from high-intensity sound. This neural information reaches the vestibular nucleus in the brainstem, from which nerve impulses are sent to the sternocleidomastoid (SCM) muscles via the medial vestibulospinal tract (MVST). In the VEMP test, electrodes are placed over the upper half of each SCM muscle, and a reference electrode is placed on the lateral end of the upper sternum. The electromyographic activity is recorded as the patients rotate their head toward the contralateral shoulder to tense the SCM muscle. At the same time the patient is stimulated with intense (eg, 95 dB HL) air-conduction stimuli or bone-conduction stimuli.

Vestibular evoked potentials (VEPs) are scalp-recorded compound action potentials of the vestibular nerve and/or central system that are elicited by vestibular stimuli (ie, head motion) that activate the vestibular neural pathway. VEPs can test the function of different vestibular organs depending on the stimulus characteristics. Due to the lack of test standards, VEPs are not used for human clinical vestibular assessment.

Tests that evaluate the response of the vestibular system to higher frequencies have been developed. In the Active Head Rotational Test (AHR), the patient is instructed to rotate the head from side to side horizontally or vertically at frequencies ranging from 2 to 6 Hz while eye movement is recorded with ENG/VNG. These frequencies of head motion occur in normal locomotion. This examination evaluates active head movements at higher frequencies than conventional vestibular tests.

In summary, evaluation of balance disorders is complex due to the contributions from the vestibular, somatosensory, and visual system. With the use of vestibular testing battery, it is possible to assess the function of components separately or simultaneously. With the knowledge of the testing procedures and their updated development, otolaryngologists and audiologists can work together for efficient evaluation and optimal management of their patients.

◆ Auditory Testing

The essentials of the complete audiometric evaluation are well established and may include the pure tone audiogram, speech audiometry, tympanometry, and acoustic reflex assessment. Newer forms of auditory testing are in clinical use but may not be familiar to all clinicians, including otoacoustic emissions and electrocochleography. A brief review of these examinations follows. Finally, this chapter will conclude with brief presentations of highly innovative audiologic testing that may ultimately become as familiar to the clinician as the tympanogram.

Otoacoustic Emissions

Otoacoustic emissions (OAEs) occur spontaneously, but the greatest information from these emissions can be obtained in response to stimuli. The most commonly used evoked tests include transient evoked (TEOAE) and distortion product (DPOAE) otoacoustic emissions (**Fig. 80.1A,B**). These two types of OAEs are reflected wave energies generated by active properties of normally functioning cochlear outer hair cells (OHCs) in response to the sound-induced,

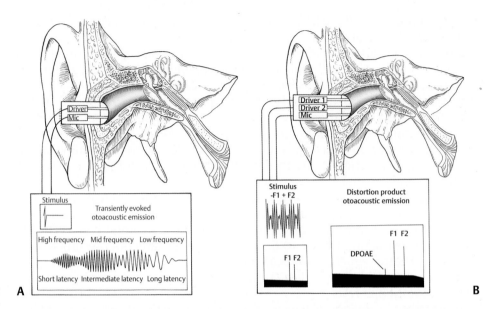

Fig. 80.1 **(A)** An example of how the transient evoked otoacoustic emission (TEOAE) is recorded (top) and the waveform generated (bottom). **(B)** An example of how distortion product otoacoustic emission (DPOAE) is recorded (top) and the waveform and spectrum of primary stimuli (bottom left) as well as the spectrum of DPOAE (bottom right).

forward-propagated traveling intracochlear wave. These emissions travel backward through the middle ear system and are measured in the ear canal as minute sounds. OAEs can be elicited by either a broad spectrum click (TEOAE) or by a dual-tone stimulus DPOAE. Responses from both tests may detect frequency specific OHC impairment, as may result from noise exposure, congenital loss, hypoxic injury, aging, or ototoxicity. TEOAEs are absent to click stimuli when OHC damage causes hearing loss greater than 20 to 30 dB HL. Because OAEs have such high specificity for OHC pathology, they can be essential in differentiating cochlear pathology from retrocochlear pathology. They are especially useful in cases of suspected auditory neuropathy. However, because OAEs are dependent on a normal middle ear mechanism for accurate detection in the ear canal, middle ear pathology can diminish or eliminate these responses.

Perhaps the most widely used application of OAEs is as a hearing screening device in neonatal hearing screening programs because the majority of permanent hearing impairment in neonates originates from OHC pathology. OAEs are an ideal screening method due to their ease of administration and rapid test responses. OAEs do not require placement of scalp electrodes and are easily obtained by simply placing a small probe tip containing both a transducer and a receiver into the ear canal. Accurate bilateral responses can be measured in a cooperative infant in seconds to minutes. However, common occurrences of transient middle ear effusion and ear canal occlusion in neonates may obscure accurate cochlear assessment and contribute to the need for a repeat OAE screening or a follow-up auditory brainstem response (ABR) evaluation.

It must be emphasized that OAE assessments are not hearing tests but rather tests of the mechanical functioning of the cochlear OHC. Normal OAEs are highly correlated with but do not insure normal hearing sensitivity.

Electrocochleography

Electrocochleography (ECoG) is the objective electrophysiological measure used for the detection of endolymphatic hydrops, which is believed to be the pathophysiological correlate to Meniere disease. This test provides information on the cochlear receptor potentials and auditory nerve. The cochlear potentials consist of the cochlear microphonic (CM), which is generated by the alternating current (AC) arising from OHC activity, and the summating potential (SP), which is generated by the direct current (DC) arising from both the outer and inner hair cell activity in response to an acoustic stimulus. The compound action potential (AP) is the postsynaptic response, which reflects the synchronous firing of the sum of the auditory nerve fibers; it is labeled as N1 in the ECoG recording. This N1 waveform peak is equivalent to wave I in an ABR.

Acceptable placement sites for a near-field ECoG recording electrode are either on the wall of the ear canal, directly on the tympanic membrane, or transtympanic, to rest on the cochlear promontory. The acoustic stimuli used to elicit the cochlear potentials may consist of a click stimulus or tone burst stimulus delivered through an insert earphone, a headphone, or in free field. The reference electrode is typically placed on the ipsilateral mastoid.

Results of the ECoG are reported as the ratio of the amplitude of the SP to the AP. An increased ratio is associated with increased endolymphatic pressure. An increase in fluid pressure causes an increase in the stiffness of the cochlear transmission system, which produces a greater activation of the hair cells, which is reflected by a larger SP. An SP:AP ratio of 0.5 or larger is considered abnormal. However, the ratios obtained are usually compared between the patient's pathological ear to the unaffected ear, or alternatively to results obtained from the beginning of the disease to later stages. Because Meniere disease is dynamic and variable, repeated SP amplitudes may progressively increase over time as the disease progresses.

There are disadvantages to the use of ECoG as a diagnostic tool. One potential procedural problem is the difficulty in recording a reliable response clearly detectable from background electrical noise. The placement of transtympanic electrodes can usually provide an enhanced signal-to-noise ratio for better recordings, but patients may find the procedure uncomfortable. In addition, variability of responses obtained from test to test and the lack of standardization in the methodology make it difficult to compare results to normative data. Examiner bias is also a potential problem in the interpretation of results. In addition, the overall sensitivity of ECoG to Meniere disease may only approximate 60 to 70%, and the presence of permanent high frequency hearing loss in patients who are symptomatic may obscure or eliminate reliable responses.

Innovations in Auditory Testing

Innovative auditory testing to be discussed in the last section includes the stacked auditory brainstem response examination, the auditory steady-state response, wide band reflectance, and laser-Doppler vibrometry.

Stacked Auditory Brain Stem Response

To best understand the stacked ABR, a review of the fundamentals of ABR will be presented. The ABR test currently remains the gold standard of auditory electrophysiological tests. It has multiple uses in the clinical setting. The scalp-recorded electrophysiological response provides essential temporal information of the neural conductivity of a large portion of the auditory brainstem pathways beginning from the distal portion of the acoustic nerve to the level of the lateral lemniscus. The first five prominent peaks (waves I through V) in a normal ABR waveform correspond to the major nerve tracts and auditory nuclei along the auditory pathway (**Fig. 80.2**). Calculations of the absolute and inter-peak latencies are made for the identification of anomalies that may impede normal neural conduction. Middle ear pathology contributes to an overall delay in the absolute latencies of all the peaks in the waveform. Retrocochlear pathol-

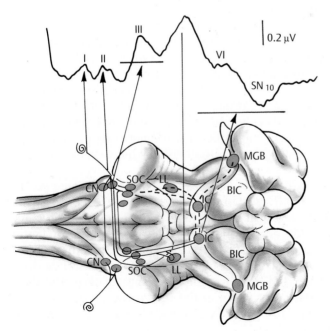

Fig. 80.2 The auditory brainstem response (ABR) recorded from a normal auditory pathway. The neural generators (bottom) correspond to the respective wave peaks (top) in ABR.

ogy typically affects absolute delays at and beyond the site of the pathology with subsequent effects on the interwave latencies as well.

The ABR is an essential tool to diagnose the presence of retrocochlear pathology. The hallmark of auditory neuropathy is an abnormal ABR in the presence of normal OAEs. The presence of internal auditory canal/cerebellopontine angle pathology (eg, acoustic neuromas, meningiomas, etc.) may also be determined with ABR evaluation. These lesions affect neural conduction by their compressive effects on the acoustic nerve fibers or internal auditory artery. However, because the spectrum of the click stimulus used to elicit an ABR waveform primarily activates the high frequency region of the basilar membrane, a standard ABR evaluation with a click stimulus may not show anomalies if a tumor is not near enough or large enough to impinge on the high frequency neural fibers. As a result, small tumors (≤ 1 cm) often go undetected with conventional ABR tests. Therefore, when an acoustic neuroma is suspected but standard ABR tests reveal normal responses, the current trend is to conduct follow-up testing with a stacked ABR.

In addition to providing the status of the neural conduction of the auditory pathways, the ABR is also a fundamental objective tool for estimating behavioral thresholds in infants and other difficult to test populations. Estimates of hearing sensitivity are made by first establishing the presence of an ABR waveform at suprathreshold levels and then incrementally decreasing the intensity levels of the acoustic stimulus until no observable wave V response is recorded. The acoustic stimuli for behavioral threshold estimation may include a broad spectrum click stimulus or frequency-specific tonal stimuli delivered by air conduction or bone conduction. This behavioral estimation method is a time-intensive procedure and requires patient immobility to reduce muscle artifact that may be introduced into the responses. Therefore, infants and young children may require sedation for this procedure.

The stacked ABR procedure is a modification of conventional ABR to be used in the diagnosis of suspected acoustic neuromas. Because the conventional ABR procedure utilizes an unmasked broad spectrum click stimulus, it is primarily sensitive to larger tumors or those that impinge on the high-frequency acoustic nerve fibers. Smaller (≤ 1 cm) tumors or those that are located on low frequency acoustic nerve fibers may go undetected with the conventional ABR. Therefore, follow-up assessment with the stacked ABR procedure is recommended by some because it has been reported to yield 95% specificity.

The stacked ABR method differs from the conventional method in both the auditory stimuli used to elicit the response and the recording procedures used to calculate the response. The stimulus that is used in the stacked ABR method is a broad spectrum band masked click that is divided into five equal and distinct frequency bands. Recordings are made as this modified click stimulates one unmasked frequency band of the cochlea while filtering out the other four frequency bands through masking. ABR responses to each frequency band region of the cochlea are sequentially obtained, and then all five band responses are added together, aligning the large wave Vs, to obtain a summed neural response.

The stacked ABR also differs from conventional ABR in that with conventional ABR the wave V latency is measured, whereas with the stacked ABR, the wave V amplitude is measured (**Fig. 80.3**).

Auditory Steady State Response

The auditory steady state response (ASSR) is one of the newer clinical tools in the audiologic test battery. The ASSR technique was developed to provide a faster and more objective frequency-specific estimation of hearing thresholds in infants and young children than is available with ABR. This electrophysiological test differs from the ABR in several ways. First, this procedure utilizes amplitude-modulated pure tones that provide better frequency selectivity due to a narrower spectrum of energy than found with transient acoustic stimuli (tone bursts) typically used in the ABR evaluation. In addition, the ASSR technique is designed to employ multiple binaural simultaneous frequency stimulation to obtain accurate behavioral threshold estimations in a reduced time period. With this technique, up to four separate frequency threshold estimations can be calculated in each ear simultaneously (**Fig. 80.4**). This can be accomplished because the ASSR displays dominant energy at a frequency corresponding to the modulation frequency of the stimuli; it is possible to provide different modula-

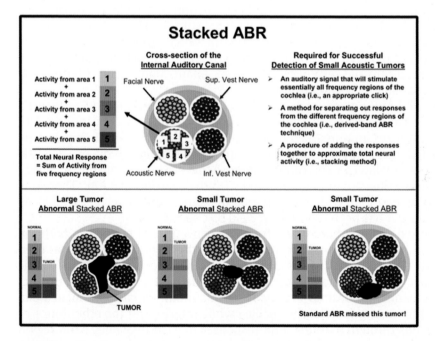

Fig. 80.3 Illustrations of the location of various tumors and their effects on the stacked ABR response. (Courtesy of the House Ear Institute, Los Angeles, CA.)

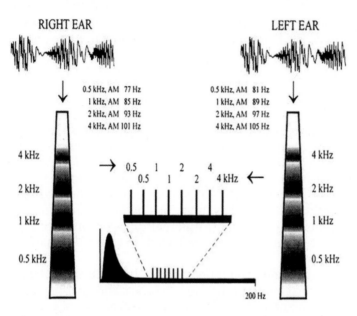

RIGHT EAR   LEFT EAR

0.5 kHz, AM 77 Hz   0.5 kHz, AM 81 Hz
1 kHz, AM 85 Hz   1 kHz, AM 89 Hz
2 kHz, AM 93 Hz   2 kHz, AM 97 Hz
4 kHz, AM 101 Hz   4 kHz, AM 105 Hz

4 kHz   4 kHz

0.5 1   2   4
0.5   1   2   4 kHz

2 kHz   2 kHz

1 kHz   1 kHz

0.5 kHz   0.5 kHz

200 Hz

Fig. 80.4 A demonstration of the acoustic stimuli used to elicit binaural simultaneous responses to four different frequencies and the frequency specificity of the stimulation of the basilar membrane.

(Adapted from Lins OG, Picton TW, Boucher BL, et al. Frequency-specific audiometry using steady-state responses. Ear Hear 1996;17(2):81–96. Used with permission.)

tion frequencies for four carrier frequencies to each ear at the same time without compromising the response. Another benefit is that the presence or absence of a response to the ASSR stimulus is determined by an automated statistical analysis on the response spectrum. Therefore, subjective decisions on the part of the examiner are eliminated and can help reduce analysis time.

A possible additional benefit of the ASSR technique is that audiometric threshold estimations can be made beyond the typical diagnostic range of the ABR in patients with severe to profound hearing losses. Patients who have hearing sensitivity levels in the range of 80 to 100 dB nHL may be more effectively identified as potential candidates for cochlear implantation. However, some reports in the literature suggest that the high intensity stimuli used for this purpose may produce artifactual responses, which could potentially be mistaken for true threshold responses.

Despite the potential for this electrophysiological technique to provide rapid binaural multiple simultaneous threshold estimations in infants, it is not currently the electrophysiological test of choice in newborn hearing screening programs. One disadvantage of this method in the neonatal population is that it can be difficult to maintain the head position required to accurately collect simultaneous binaural responses. In addition, the ASSR technique may be more suitable for a diagnostic follow-up measure than as an initial screening tool because some researchers report obtaining more accurate and reliable threshold measures in infants older than 1 month of age as opposed to those obtained in the neonatal period.

Wide Band Reflectance

Acoustic reflex test measures using a wideband signal (click or chirp) with multiple frequencies ranging from 250 to 8000 Hz may provide a more accurate and sensitive assessment of the middle ear muscle reflex (MEMR) arc, than conventional methods using a 226 Hz probe tone. The simultaneous multiple frequency stimulation of the wide band reflectance provides the most favorable frequencies needed to elicit MEMRs in various patient populations. This method also holds promise to differentiate different types of conductive hearing loss based upon the frequencies that are reflected back from the middle ear system.

Another advantage of the wide band reflectance is that it does not require a hermetically sealed ear canal for pressurization. Pressurization has been found to obscure the MEMR in infants. The infant ear canal is capable of expanding during conventional tympanometric measures with pressurization, which may in turn indicate normal tympanograms even when abnormal middle ear conditions are present. Middle ear problems such as transient effusion or ear canal obstruction are responsible for a large portion of the neonates who fail infant hearing screening. This tool holds promise as a valuable tool for the assessment of middle ear status in those infants who fail screening with OAE.

Laser-Doppler Vibrometry

An additional technological advance in middle ear analysis is the use of laser-Doppler vibrometry (LDV). LDV provides a spatial analysis of the impedance of the middle ear ossicles not available through conventional impedance measures. These measures are achieved by the calculation of the velocity of a reflected laser beam from the umbo of a vibrating tympanic membrane (**Fig. 80.5**). LDV velocity measures have the potential to aid in the differential diagnosis of conductive hearing loss related to ossicular disorders. LDV may also aid in presurgical planning, potentially increasing the rate of successful surgical outcomes.

Fig. 80.5 Drawing of a laser-Doppler vibrometry middle ear analyzer attached to a standard operating microscope.

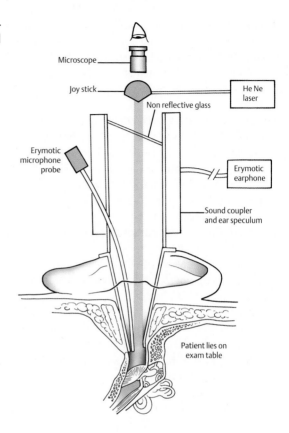

Suggested Reading

Burkard RF, Don M, Eggermont JJ. Auditory Evoked Potentials: Basic Principles and Clinical Application. Baltimore: Lippincott Williams & Wilkins; 2007

Don M, Kwong B, Tanaka C. The stacked ABR: a successful small acoustic tumor screening method. House Ear Institute; 2003. Available at: http://www.hei.org/research/electro/stkabrinfo.htm

Don M, Kwong B, Tanaka C, Brackmann D, Nelson R. The stacked ABR: a sensitive and specific screening tool for detecting small acoustic tumors. Audiol Neurootol 2005;10:274–290

Don M, Masuda A, Nelson R, Brackmann D. Successful detection of small acoustic tumors using the stacked derived-band auditory brain stem response amplitude. Am J Otol 1997;18:608–621, discussion 682–685

Feeney MP, Keefe DH. Acoustic reflex detection using wide-band acoustic reflectance, admittance, and power measurements. J Speech Lang Hear Res 1999;42:1029–1041

Ferraro JA. Clinical electrocochleography: overview of theories, techniques and applications. 2003. Available at: http://www.audiologyonline.com/articles/article_detail.asp?article_id=452

Jacobson GP, Shepard NT, eds. Balance Function Assessment and Management. San Diego, CA: Plural Publishing Inc. 2008

Joint Committee on Infant Hearing (JCIH). Available at: http://www.jcih.org/posstatemts.htm

Kemp DT. Otoacoustic emissions, their origin in cochlear function, and use. Br Med Bull 2002;63:223–241

Laboratory Evaluation of Dizziness Recommended by iVertigo by Troost. Available at: http://ivertigo.net/vertigo/verevaluation.html

Lins OG, Picton TW. Auditory steady-state responses to multiple simultaneous stimuli. Electroencephalogr Clin Neurophysiol 1995;96:420–432

Lins OG, Picton TW, Boucher BL, et al. Frequency-specific audiometry using steady-state responses. Ear Hear 1996;17:81–96

Manuel D, Kwong B, Tanaka, C. The Stacked ABR: A Successful Small Acoustic Tumor Screening Method. 2003

Picton TW, Dimitrijevic A, Perez-Abalo MC, Van Roon P. Estimating audiometric thresholds using auditory steady-state responses. J Am Acad Audiol 2005;16:140–156

Rosowski JJ, Mehta RP, Merchant SN. Diagnostic utility of laser-Doppler vibrometry in conductive hearing loss with normal tympanic membrane. Otol Neurotol 2003;24:165–175

Setting the Standard in Balance and Mobility Recommended by NeuroCom. Available at: http://www.onbalance.com/neurocom/protocols/sensoryImpairment/SOT.aspx

Hain TC. Vestibular testing. Available at: http://www.tchain.com/otoneurology/testing/engrot.html

Utah State University. National Center for Hearing Assessment and Management (NCHAM). Available at: http://www.infanthearing.org/index.html

Whittemore KR Jr, Merchant SN, Poon BB, Rosowski JJ. A normative study of tympanic membrane motion in humans using a laser Doppler vibrometer (LDV). Hear Res 2004; 187:85–104

Calculating Slow Phase Velocity of Nystagmus Recommended by AudiologyOnline. Available at: http://www.audiologyonline.com/askexpert/display_question.asp?question_id=244

81 The Genetic Revolution

John H. Greinwald Jr.

Genetic analysis of human disease has moved from the laboratory to the outpatient clinic, yet it can be confounding to the clinician unfamiliar with this field. This chapter presents a genetic review, followed by the current state of genetic analysis of pediatric sensorineural hearing loss—one of the prime examples of clinical genetics in otolaryngology.

◆ Genetic Overview

Human genes are molecular codes for inherited factors. Genes are arranged linearly on 23 pairs (ie, 46) of chromosomes. These chromosomes consist of 22 pairs of autosomes and one pair of sex chromosomes. Males have an X and a Y pair of sex chromosomes, whereas females have two X chromosomes. The location of a gene on a chromosome is termed a *locus*. Each chromosome pair carries a distinctive set of gene **loci**, and on any given gene, the genetic codes may differ (**alleles**). The genetic code for a specific trait (**genotype**) consists of either two identical alleles (**homozygous**) or two disparate alleles (**heterozygous**). The physical manifestation of a trait, referred to as the **phenotype**, is determined by which alleles are present and how they interact. An allele is considered **dominant** if its presence results in a specific phenotype. It is considered **autosomal recessive** if both alleles are required for the expression of its phenotype. An X-linked recessive gene is present in only one allele (**hemizygous**) in males because the Y chromosome generally does not carry an allele complementary to the X chromosome. There may be several different types of base pair changes. A truncating mutation causes premature cessation of protein formation and may be either a *nonsense* or a splice site mutation. A *missense* mutation allows the protein to be produced, though an altered amino acid code is present.

Dominant traits are transmitted from one generation to another. There is a 50% chance that an affected heterozygous individual will transmit an abnormal gene to offspring. **Penetrance** is the ability of a gene to manifest any of the phenotypic characteristics related to that gene. In a family with a dominant condition, not all persons carrying the affected gene display the disease phenotype. This occurrence is called **incomplete penetrance**. Dominant disorders can also have variable **expressivity**, whereby family members present with different manifestations of the affected gene. It is thus presumed that environmental influences or interaction with other genes can modify phenotypic expression.

In the absence of consanguinity, an **autosomal recessive trait** is usually seen in offspring in small nuclear families. The offspring of heterozygous (ie, carrier) parents have a 25% risk of being affected. Being heterozygous for two different genes (**double heterozygous**) may cause hearing loss. An X-linked recessive trait can lack phenotypic expression if it is carried by a heterozygous female, but male offspring of this female would have a 50% chance of inheriting the gene.

Also, heritable disorders that are caused by abnormalities at the chromosomal level and involve extra or absent chromosomal material are characterized by developmental delays and various congenital anomalies.

Disparate genotypes can produce a similar phenotype. This phenomenon, referred to as **genetic heterogeneity**, often makes it difficult to identify causative genes. In patients with nonsyndromic hearing loss, gene identification is difficult because there is a high degree of heterogeneity and an absence of obvious phenotypic traits. By contrast, patients with syndromic hearing loss have definable traits that assist in gene identification.

Gene Structure

Each gene generally consists of (1) **exons**, which are DNA that codes for the actual protein; (2) **introns**, which are areas interspersed between exons; (3) **splice sites**, which are DNA at the exon–intron junction; and (4) untranslated regulatory regions, which are DNA that is **upstream** and **downstream** of the first and last exons, respectively.

◆ Sensorineural Hearing Loss

Approximately one in 1000 children has a bilateral severe to profound sensorineural hearing loss (SNHL) at birth or in early childhood. In more than 50% of these children, the etiology of SNHL is genetic. In ~70% of cases attributed to genetic mutations, an isolated (nonsyndromic) hearing impairment is the only phenotypic manifestation. In the remaining 30%, hearing impairment exists along with other abnormalities (syndromic hearing impairment). The majority (80%) of patients with SNHL display an autosomal recessive mode of transmission. Another 15% are estimated to have an autosomal dominant mode of inheritance. A small percentage (~5%) are X-linked or mitochondrial (**Fig. 81.1**).

As previously stated, nonsyndromic hearing loss is associated with a high degree of genetic heterogeneity; over 50 loci have been identified as causing this condition. In a small number of genes, allelic variants can cause both syndromic and nonsyndromic SNHL as well as both dominant and recessive inheritance patterns. Additionally, some syndromes involving SNHL do not manifest their full phenotype in young children. This may lead to a misdiagnosis of nonsyndromic hearing loss until later in childhood or adulthood.

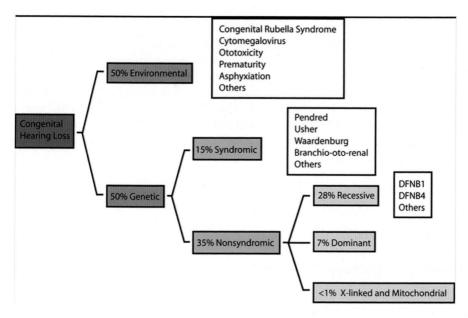

Fig. 81.1   Differential diagnosis of pediatric sensorineural hearing loss.

Genetic Testing for Sensorineural Hearing Loss

Approximately 40% of children with SNHL are diagnosed by either genetic testing (20%) or temporal bone imaging (20%). Because of cost and time restrictions, it is impossible to screen for mutations in all genes related to SNHL. A more targeted approach to genetic testing is thus warranted.

GJB2 Mutations

The most common gene involved in SNHL is *GJB2* (gap junction β-2 protein), also known as connexin 26 (CX 26). Studies have identified over 100 different mutations in *GJB2* as a cause for hearing loss. The most common mutation is 35delG, which accounts for about one third of all *GJB2* mutations. In patients with severe to profound SNHL, ~30% have biallelic mutations in *GJB2*. In patients with less severe hearing impairment, the prevalence of biallelic *GJB2* mutations is ~10%. Genotypes with biallelic truncating mutations have a high risk (~90%) of severe to profound hearing impairment. Hearing loss in patients with *GJB2* mutations is generally bilateral, symmetric, and nonprogressive, with patients displaying flat audiograms. Occasionally, however, patients display asymmetric hearing loss, sloping audiometric patterns, or borderline hearing loss. These findings are generally associated with at least one missense mutation.

Other Gene Mutations

Mutations in several other genes are also thought to be causative for a significant proportion of cases of SNHL. Research has shown that molecular genetic testing of *OTOF, MYO7A, CDH23,* and *SLC26A4* together can identify a genetic etiology in 14% of patients with non-*GJB2*-related hearing loss, and possible genetic etiology in an additional 11%. Testing that includes *MYO7A, CDH23,* and *SLC26A4* identifies Usher syndrome and Pendred syndrome at younger ages, allowing for early diagnosis and intervention. Mutations in the *12SrRNA* gene are found in ~1% of the population in the United States. Mutations in *tRNA*[ser] are uncommon.

◆ New Horizons

Microarray Technology

Recent advances have made it possible to rapidly screen DNA samples for thousands of possible genetic mutations. This can be done through a technique called *microarray technology.* Arrays can be used to analyze DNA for sequence changes or to analyze RNA for detecting gene expression. To detect DNA sequence changes, the array simultaneously analyzes multiple DNA fragments, determining if sequence variants are present in a specific DNA sequence. This technology offers several advantages over the standard method of detecting sequence changes (referred to as **dideoxy sequencing**), including accuracy, simplicity, efficiency, and cost effectiveness.

The concept of how an array works is relatively straightforward. Target array DNA is placed in tiny wells (ie, 8 μm) on a glass slide. DNA from a patient is then placed in each well. Through a process called **hybridization**, array DNA and patient DNA chemically bond. This bonding process is linked to another reaction, which causes fluorescence. The specific base pair at each location on the DNA can then be determined. This entire process is called **resequencing**.

Alternatively, some arrays seek to detect only single nucleotide polymorphisms (SNPs; specific abnormal base pair changes) linked to disease. This process is known as *genotyping.* Most mutations that cause disease are relatively common; hence, if a finite number of known mutations are selectively screened, a more efficient and less costly management algorithm can be developed. There are, nevertheless, several important drawbacks of this technology. It can yield false-negative results, leading to an underdiagnosis of the genetic cause of hearing loss. Also, novel mutations cannot be detected. As well, any abnormal results would require confirmation by some type of sequencing technology, though this would focus on specific mutations of interest.

Our research team is currently analyzing several SNP chip arrays to use as a clinical screening tool. We are also analyzing newer hybrid arrays that offer the benefits of both resequencing and genotyping on a single chip.

Resequencing Microarray for Sensorineural Hearing Loss

The identification of more than 40 genes causative for SNHL makes it practical to organize these genes on a single hearing loss gene chip that allows for a more comprehensive diagnostic evaluation. Application of this technology makes array-based screening an exciting tool because it can more than double the yield of genetic screening of children with SNHL. A better understanding of the genotype–phenotype correlations that exist for each of the genes would allow for a more accurate prognosis and disease-specific interventions. Our research team (Affymetrix, Santa Clara, CA) has therefore developed a resequencing array containing seven genes implicated in nonsyndromic SNHL, including *CDH23, MYO7A, OTOF, SLC26A4, GJB6, KCNQ1*, and *KCNE1* (deafness GeneChip). We have compared the results of our array to those with dideoxy sequencing in a cohort of 37 children with non-*GJB2*-related SNHL. We have also developed an integrative analysis plan using genetic epidemiology, sequence conservation, and bioinformatic predictions to assess the putative pathogenicity of each sequence variant. In our cohort, we found disease-causing mutations in *CDH23, MYO7A, OTOF*, and *SLC26A4*. Overall, a genetic cause of hearing loss was identified in five of 37 (13.5%) patients. A possible genetic cause of hearing loss was found in four of 37 (10.8%) patients who are double heterozygotes. No genetic cause of hearing loss was found in 28 of 37 (75.7%) patients. Statistical analysis of audiometric data revealed no phenotypic differences among the three genotypic categories. Over 98% of all hybridized DNA yielded results. There was a strong correlation between the results of the deafness GeneChip and dideoxy sequencing, with false-negative and false-positive rates of less than 2%. The results of this study indicate that comprehensive genetic testing (ie, testing for *GJB2* and deafness GeneChip) can identify a genetic etiology of SNHL in greater than 40% of patients. Our deafness GeneChip represents the first resequencing array for molecular testing of pediatric SNHL, providing a rapid, cost-effective diagnostic tool.

Suggested Reading

Cutler DJ, Zwick ME, Carrasquillo MM, et al. High-throughput variation detection and genotyping using microarrays. Genome Res 2001;11:1913–1925

Kothiyal P, Cox S, Ebert J, et al. High-throughput detection of mutations responsible for childhood hearing loss using resequencing microarrays. BMC Biotechnol 2010;10:10

Preciado DA, Lawson L, Madden C, et al. Improved diagnostic effectiveness with a sequential diagnostic paradigm in idiopathic pediatric sensorineural hearing loss. Otol Neurotol 2005;26:610–615

Putcha GV, Bejjani BA, Bleoo S, et al. A multicenter study of the frequency and distribution of GJB2 and GJB6 mutations in a large North American cohort. Genet Med 2007;9:413–426

Snoeckx RL, Huygen PL, Feldmann D, et al. GJB2 mutations and degree of hearing loss: a multicenter study. Am J Hum Genet 2005;77:945–957

Van Camp G, Smith RJH. Hereditary Hearing Loss Homepage. Available at: http://webho1.ua.ac.be/hhh/

82 New Diagnostic Techniques for Otolaryngologists

Thomas A. Tami

Technological advances in otolaryngology–head and neck surgery continue to change the way we approach diagnosis and treatment. Although this serves as a primer for current diagnostic methods in otolaryngology, diagnostic approaches will undoubtedly continue to evolve. The evolution in genetically based diagnosis, innovations in audiology, and imaging breakthroughs for head and neck surgery have been touched upon previously in this section. Computer-aided differential diagnosis utilizing artificial intelligence, and electronic olfaction are but two of the many other areas of contemporary technology that may soon be impacting our specialty. This chapter offers a very brief overview of these cutting edge technologies.

◆ Artificial Intelligence in Medicine

Starting with the initial description of artificial intelligence (AI) by Isaac Asimov in his classic 1950 novel *I, Robot*, the attempts to achieve this elusive goal have been met with only limited success and acceptance. From a diagnostic standpoint AI in medicine (AIM) could be a tremendous tool for both medical training as well as clinical practice. Already, from financial systems, billing and coding programs, diagnostic laboratory reporting, to electronic medical records, computers have been playing an increasing role in the medical arena. The combination of decision models, flow charts, clinical histories, clinical laboratory, and procedural data with the mathematics of decision theory can result in systems to augment the decision-making activities of practitioners. This knowledge can be expressed in the form of simple rules, or as a decision tree. A classic example of this type of system is KARDIO, which was a system developed to interpret electrocardiograms (ECGs).

AIM can be extended to explore poorly understood areas of medicine. Investigators are now discussing "data mining" processes and "knowledge discovery" systems. It is now possible, using patient data, to automatically construct pathophysiological models that describe the functional relationships among clinical datasets. For example, in 1993, Hau and Coiera described a learning system that used patient data obtained during cardiac bypass surgery to create models of normal and abnormal cardiac physiology. These models could be used to detect real-time changes in a patient's clinical status. Alternatively, in a research setting, these models could help establish initial hypotheses to drive further experimentation.

AIM also has a potential role in the development of clinical guidelines. In situations where there are several alternate treatments for a condition, analysis of databases of clinical outcomes from competing treatments can be used to facilitate the selection of ideal treatment regimens. DXplain is one of these clinical decision support systems that was developed and implemented at the Massachusetts General Hospital in the mid-1980s. This system assists in the diagnostic process by analyzing clinical data such as signs, symptoms, and laboratory data. It then produces a ranked list of possible diagnoses based on probability while also suggesting further diagnostic testing.

Not surprisingly, direct-to-consumer applications of AI diagnostic software are now available. One on-line program is EasyDiagnosis. The parent company, MathMedics, develops and markets Web-based interactive medical decision support software for both consumers and health care providers. This online program begins by investigating the chief complaint or symptom and then allowing the patient to navigate the diagnostic process, ultimately establishing a group of possible diagnoses listed in order of probability. For example, say a patient has vertigo. By answering a series of pointed clinical questions, users are ultimately guided to a probability-based differential diagnosis of their condition. The parent company also produces AI-based managed care intelligent process software for physician organizations to help with various issues such as eligibility, authorization/certification, and outcomes analysis.

The entire field of medical informatics and computer-based data analysis is in its infancy. However, with the widespread use and expansion of the electronic medical record and the inherent data sharing that will result, computers will have an increasing role, not only in diagnosis, but in outcomes analysis and ultimately public reporting of quality data. The field of medicine, and in particular otolaryngology, is in the midst of a computer-driven (r)evolution that will ultimately change the paradigm of medical diagnosis, patient management, clinical outcomes, and quality initiatives.

◆ The Electronic Nose for Ear, Nose, and Throat Diagnosis

The concept of an electronic nose was first introduced in 1982 to try to mimic mammalian olfaction. By using metal oxide gas sensors, this device could correctly identify several different substances, but it never really came close to fulfilling the original goal of identifying multiple odors. Over time, other technologic approaches have been applied in addition to gas sensors. Optical sensor systems, mass spectrometry, ion mobility spectrometry, gas chromatography, and infrared spectroscopy have all been applied to this problem, but even after 25 years, the ability to recognize and describe actual odors is still not possible.

Although the potential applications for an electronic nose device are multiple (food quality and spoilage, air quality, emission toxicity, and environmental safety monitoring), its most exciting role may lie in medical diagnostic applications. Smell has traditionally been an important component of diagnosis, beginning with Hippocrates who stated that much could be learned about patients using the sense of smell as a diagnostic tool. By analyzing for substances in the exhaled gases of patients, the electronic nose can assist in several diagnostic areas: ethanol and acetone can be detected and used as markers to screen for diabetes mellitus; nitric oxide, a gas produced in the breath of asthmatic patients, can now be quantified to determine disease severity; or uremia can be detected and quantified in patients with chronic renal dysfunction. One of the most interesting studies of the electronic nose was for the detection of lung cancer. In one study, the predictive value of this technology to detect volatile organic compounds in exhaled gases was comparable to computed tomography used to screen for lung cancer.

Probably the most useful medical application for otolaryngology, however, lies in the ability to detect and identify the odorants produced by various organisms causing infections. The Cyranose 320 was used to evaluate in vitro bacterial samples from patients with upper respiratory infections and was able to detect and discriminate among *Staphylococcus aureus, Streptococcus pneumoniae, Haemophilus influenzae,* and *Pseudomonas aeruginosa.* As this technology improves, the goal might be to use this technology in the setting of acute infection so that organism-specific antibiotic therapy can be instituted before culture results are available. Currently it is unknown whether this technology will ever fulfill its potential as a diagnostic tool in otolaryngology. However, it certainly offers exciting possibilities for the clinical practice of the specialty.

Suggested Reading

Coiera E. Guide to Health Informatics. 2nd ed. New York: Oxford University Press; 2003. Available at corporate site for EasyDiagnosis: http://mathemedics.com/index.html

Röck F, Barsan N, Weimar U. Electronic nose: current status and future trends. Chem Rev 2008;108:705–725

Thaler ER. Candidate's thesis: the diagnostic utility of an electronic nose: rhinologic applications. Laryngoscope 2002;112:1533–1542

Index

Note: Page numbers followed by *f* and *t* indicate figures and tables, respectively.

SCC. *See* Squamous cell carcinoma
Schizophrenia, and olfactory disturbance, 165
Schwannoma
  consistency, 332
  facial nerve, 99, 314
    and facial paralysis, 100
  intranasal, 152
  jugular foramen, middle ear or mastoid
    involvement in, 57
  of middle ear or skull base, 57
  nasal obstruction caused by, in children, 176
  vestibular. *See* Vestibular schwannoma
Scleral show, 403–404
Scleroderma
  dysphagia caused by, 273
  hearing loss in, 53
  odynophagia in, 267
  telangiectasias in, 309
  and throat clearing, 280
  xerostomia in, 182, 214
Scleroderma esophagus, and regurgitation, 287
Scleroma, laryngitis in, 221
Scorbutic gingivitis, 186
Scrofula, 379
  and fistula formation, 355–356
Scurvy. *See also* Vitamin C deficiency
  epistaxis in, 146
SDS. *See* Speech discrimination score (SDS)
Sebaceous cyst, 354
Sebaceous gland carcinoma, of external auditory
  canal, and facial nerve dysfunction, 99
Sebaceous hyperplasia, 306
Seborrheic dermatitis, 292t, 293–294, 294f, 303
  in children, 362
  of external auditory canal, 68, 81
  neonatal, 377
Seborrheic keratosis, 305, 322, 393, 393f
Seizure(s). *See also* Temporal lobe seizures
  and aspiration, 277
  complex partial, vertigo and disequilibrium
    caused by, 90
Selective antibody immune deficiencies, in
  children, 175
Sellar tumor, 348
Semicircular canal(s). *See also* Superior
    semicircular canal
  and dizziness, 5
  lateral, fistula, cholesteatoma with, and vertigo,
    89
  posterior, dehiscence, vertigo and disequilibrium
    caused by, in children, 110
Senile sebaceous hyperplasia, 320
Sensorineural hearing loss. *See* Hearing loss,
  sensorineural
Serology, 22
Seromucous glands, of nasal mucosa and
  submucosa, 131
Serous glands, of nasal mucosa and submucosa,
  131
Serpigio, 377
SHA. *See* Sinusoidal harmonic acceleration (SHA)
  tests
Shingles, 296t, 297, 299
Shprintzen syndrome, 385

Sialadenitis, 326
  acute
    fistulas caused by, 354
    suppurative, 212
  bacterial, 354
  chronic, 212
  parotid, 354
  and taste disorders, 205
  viral, 354
Sialadenosis, 211, 214
Sialolithiasis, 198, 212
Sialometaplasia, necrotizing, 201
Sialorrhea, 215
  definition, 211
Sialosis, benign, of parotid, 329
Single nucleotide polymorphisms (SNP), 442
Sinonasal undifferentiated carcinoma, 152
  and epistaxis, 144
  and nasal obstruction, 123
Sinus
  branchial cleft, 79, 382, 383f
    first, 381
    second, 382, 383f
  paranasal. *See* Paranasal sinus(es)
  preauricular, 374, 381
    draining, 78
    otalgia caused by, in children, 106
Sinusitis, 239t, 245
  acute, in children, 173
  allergic fungal, and nasal polyposis, 121
  bacterial, nasal obstruction in, 126
  in children, 5 A's, 177t
  chronic
    and globus, 281
    and throat clearing, 279
  fungal. *See also* Allergic fungal sinusitis
    and halitosis, 216
  nasal/perinasal swelling caused by, 318
  periorbital swelling caused by, 316
  viral, rhinorrhea in, 134
Sinus mass. *See* Mass(es), sinonasal
Sinusoidal harmonic acceleration (SHA) tests, 426
Sinus tract(s). *See also* Sinus
  in children, 381–384
Sjögren syndrome
  epidemiology, 214
  periorbital swelling in, 316
  and regurgitation, 286
  signs and symptoms, 214–215
  and taste disturbance, 207
  xerostomia in, 182, 214
SK. *See* Seborrheic keratosis
Skin cancer, 393
  nonmelanoma, 396–398
Skin disorders
  drug-induced, odynophagia in, 267
  infectious, in children, 377–380
Skin lesion(s)
  benign, 393–396
  cosmetic, 393–399
  infectious, in children, 377–380
  malignant, 396–398
  of syphilis, 299
  of tuberculosis, 299